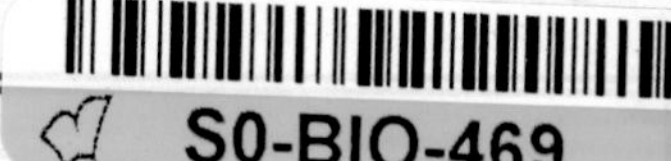


# ESSENTIALS OF CARDIOVASCULAR MEDICINE

*Abridged Pocket Guide*

**Mark Freed, M.D.**
**Cindy Grines, M.D.**

Division of Cardiovascular Diseases
William Beaumont Hospital
Royal Oak, Michigan

*First Edition*

**Physicians' Press**
Birmingham, Michigan

**Notice**. The explosive growth of new pharmacologic and non-pharmacologic therapies has resulted in the rapid evolution and acceptance of practice patterns often based on retrospective nonrandomized data and personal experience. Their ultimate role will require close inspection of prospective randomized trials. The clinical recommendations set forth in this book are those of the authors; they are offered as *general guidelines only and are not to be construed as absolute indications*. In addition, not all medications have been accepted by the U.S. Food and Drug Administration (USFDA) for usages described in this manual. The use of any drug should be preceded by a careful review of the package insert, which provides indications and dosages as approved by the USFDA. The reader is advised to consult the package insert before using any therapeutic agent. The authors and publisher disclaim responsibility for adverse effects resulting from omissions or undetected errors.

Expanded reviews of the topics contained in this manual—including principles of diagnosis, recent clinical trials and controversies—and chapters on Cardiac Surgery and ECG Interpretation may be found in the *Unabridged Edition* of Essentials of Cardiovascular Medicine (see page 268).



Comments and suggestions should be referred to:

**Physicians' Press**
555 South Woodward Ave., Suite 908
Birmingham, Michigan 48009
Tel/Fax: (810) 642-4949

Printed in the United States of America ISBN 0-9633886-3-0

# TABLE OF CONTENTS

# CONTRIBUTORS

**Rose Anton, M.D.**
Department of Pathology, Baylor University Medical Center, Dallas, Texas. *Angina Pectoris.*

**Jeffrey D. Band, M.D.**
Clinical Associate Professor of Medicine, Wayne State University. Director, Division of Infectious Disease and Clinical Epidemiology, William Beaumont Hospital, Royal Oak, Michigan. *Infectious and Inflammatory Cardiac Diseases, Pericardial Disease.*

**James Boatman, M.D.**
Cardiologist, William Beaumont Hospital, Royal Oak, Michigan
*Adult Congenital Heart Disease.*

**Louis R. Caplan, M.D.**
Professor and Chairman, Department of Neurology, Tufts University School of Medicine. Neurologist-in-Chief, New England Medical Center, Boston, Massachusetts. *Cerebrovascular Disease.*

**Kanu Chatterjee, M.B., F.R.C.P.**
Professor of Medicine, Lucie Stern Professor of Cardiology, Director, Cardiac Care Unit, Moffitt Hospital, San Francisco, California. *Heart Failure.*

**John P. DiMarco, M.D., Ph.D.**
Professor of Medicine, Director, Clinical Electrophysiology Laboratory, University of Virginia Health Sciences Center, Charlottesville, Virginia. *Cardiac Arrhythmias and Conduction Disturbances.*

**Pamela S. Douglas, M.D.**
Associate Professor, Harvard Medical School. Director, Noninvasive Cardiology, Beth Israel Hospital, Boston, Massachusetts. *Cardiac Disease and Pregnancy.*

**Mark Freed, M.D.**
Cardiologist, William Beaumont Hospital, Royal Oak, Michigan
*Shock, Pericardial Disease.*

**James A. Goldstein, M.D.**
Assistant Professor of Medicine, Washington University School of Medicine. Medical Director, Cardiac Transplantation, Barnes Hospital, St. Louis, Missouri. *Valvular Heart Disease.*

**Antonio M. Gotto, Jr., M.D., D.Phil.** Distinguished Professor and Chairman, Department of Medicine, Baylor College of Medicine. Chief, Internal Medicine, The Methodist Hospital, Houston, Texas. *Dyslipidemia.*

**Cindy L. Grines, M.D.**
Director, Cardiac Catheterization Laboratories, William Beaumont Hospital, Royal Oak, Michigan. *Myocardial Infarction.*

**Matthew H. Johnson, Pharm.D.**
Adjunct Assistant Professor of Pharmacy Practice, Wayne State Univ. College of Pharmacy, Detroit, Michigan. Assistant Director of Pharmaceutical Services, William Beaumont Hospital, Royal Oak, Michigan. *Cardiac Drugs.*

**Norman M. Kaplan, M.D.**
Professor of Internal Medicine, Chief, Hypertension Division, University of Texas Southwestern Medical Center, Dallas, Texas. *Hypertension.*

**Thomas H. Lee, M.D.**
Associate Professor, Harvard Medical School. Director, Clinical Initiatives Development Program, Chief, Section for Clinical Epidemiology, Brigham and Womens Hospital, Boston, Massachusetts. *Non-Cardiac Surgery for the Cardiac Patient.*

**Richard L. Lucarotti, Pharm.D.**
Adjunct Associate Professor, Wayne State University College of Pharmacy and Allied Health Professions, Detroit, Michigan. Director of Pharmacy, William Beaumont Hospital, Royal Oak, Michigan. *Cardiac Drugs.*

**William A. Murray, M.D.**
Senior Fellow, Division of Cardiology, University of Washington, Seattle, Washington. *Cardiac Arrest and Life-Threatening Arrhythmias.*

**Carl J. Pepine, M.D.**
Professor of Medicine, Co-Director, Division of Cardiology, University of Florida College of Medicine, Gainesville, Florida.
*Angina Pectoris.*

**Heidi A. Pillen, Pharm.D.**
Clinical Pharmacist, William Beaumont Hospital, Royal Oak, Michigan. *Cardiac Drugs.*

**Jun Anthony V. Quion, M.D.**
Research Fellow, Section of Atherosclerosis, Baylor College of Medicine, Dallas, Texas. *Dyslipidemia.*

**Stuart Rich, M.D.**
Professor of Medicine, Chief, Section of Cardiology, University of Illinois at Chicago, Chicago, Illinois. *Pulmonary Vascular Disease.*

**Mary Beth Sancimino, Pharm.D.**
Clinical Pharmacist, William Beaumont Hospital, Royal Oak, Michigan. *Cardiac Drugs.*

**Maureen A. Smythe, Pharm.D.**
Assistant Professor of Pharmacy Practice, Wayne State University College of Pharmacy and Allied Health Professions, Detroit, Michigan. Clinical Education Coordinator, William Beaumont Hospital, Royal Oak, Michigan. *Cardiac Drugs.*

**John A. Spittell, Jr., M.D.**
Professor of Medicine, Mayo Medical School. Emeritus Consultant, Mayo Clinic, Rochester, Minnesota. *Peripheral Vascular Disease.*

**Peter C. Spittell, M.D.**
Senior Associate Consultant, Division of Cardiovascular Diseases, Mayo Clinic, Assistant Professor of Medicine, Mayo Clinic, Rochester, Minnesota. *Peripheral Vascular Disease.*

**W. Douglas Weaver, M.D.**
Professor of Medicine, Director, Cardiovascular Critical Care, Division of Cardiology, University of Washington, Seattle, Washington. *Cardiac Arrest and Life-Threatening Arrhythmias.*

# DEDICATION

Some climb mountains to look down from atop
Others, to view the next highest peak

— *To those who strive toward the next highest peak*

Mark Freed, M.D.

I thank my past and present mentors Charlie Wooley, Bob Vogel, Eric Topol, Steve Nissen, Tony DeMaria and Bill O'Neill for their advice, encouragement, and for motivating me to higher achievements; my family for all their love and support; and my children, Derek and Jessica, for making paper airplanes out of only 80% of the edited pages.

Cindy Grines, M.D.

# ABBREVIATIONS & DEFINITIONS

ABC (airway, breathing, circulation)
ACE (angiotensin converting enzyme)
ACLS (advanced cardiac life support)
ACT (activated coagulation time)
AFIB (atrial fibrillation)
APSAC (anisoylated plasminogen streptokinase activator complex)
ARDS (adult respiratory distress syndrome)
AS (aortic stenosis)
ASD (atrial septal defect)
AV (atrioventricular, as in AV block)
AVR (aortic valve replacement)
BID (twice daily)
BP (blood pressure)
CABG (coronary artery bypass grafting)
CAD (coronary artery disease)
CCB (calcium channel blocker)
CCU (cardiac care unit)
CEN (carotid endarterectomy)
CHD (coronary heart disease)
CHF (congestive heart failure)
CNS (central nervous system)
COPD (chronic obstructive pulmonary disease)
CPR (cardiopulmonary resuscitation)
CrCl (creatinine clearance; estimated by [(140-age) x (ideal body wt, kg)] *divided by* [72 x serum creatinine (mg/dL)]. For females, multiply by 0.85.
CT (computerized tomography)
CV (cardiovascular)

D (day)
DIC (disseminated intravascular coagulation)
DL (deciliter)
DVT (deep venous thrombosis)
DX (diagnosis)
ECG (electrocardiogram)
ECHO (echocardiogram, echocardiography)
EP (electrophysiology)
ET (endotracheal tube)
G, GM (gram)
GI (gastrointestinal)
GFR (glomerular filtration rate)
GU (genitourinary)
HDL-C (high-density lipoprotein cholesterol)
HOCM (hypertrophic obstructive cardiomyopathy)
HR (heart rate)
HRS (hours)
IABP (intra-aortic balloon pump counterpulsation)
ICD (internal cardioverter-defibrillator)
IVCD (intraventricular conduction delay)
IM (intramuscular)
INR (international normalized ratio)
IPC (intermittent pneumatic compression)
ISA (intrinsic sympathomimetic activity)
IV (intravenous)
IVC (inferior vena cava)
IVPB (intravenous piggy back)
J (joules)
JPC (junctional premature contraction)

JVD (jugular venous distension)
JVP (jugular venous pressure)
K+ (potassium)
L (liter)
LAFB (left anterior fascicular block)
LBBB (left bundle branch block)
LDL-C (low-density lipoprotein cholesterol)
LP (lumbar puncture)
LPFB (left posterior fascicular block)
LV (left ventricle; left ventricular)
LVEF (left ventricular ejection fraction)
LVH (left ventricular hypertrophy)
MBC (minimum bacteriocidal concentration)
MCG (microgram)
MCL (microliter)
MG (milligram)
MI (myocardial infarction)
MIC (minimum inhibitory concentration)
MIN (minute)
ML (millimeter)
MR (mitral regurgitation)
MRI (magnetic resonance imaging)
MS (mitral stenosis)
MVP (mitral valve prolapse)
Na++ (sodium)
NPO (nothing by mouth)
NSAID (nonsteroidal anti-inflammatory drug)
NSVT (nonsustained ventricular tachycardia)
PCWP (pulmonary capillary wedge pressure)
PDA (patent ductus arteriosus)
PE (pulmonary embolism)
PHTN (pulmonary hypertension)
PO (per os - by mouth; oral)
PR (portion of ECG corresponding to atrial depolarization and repolarization)
PRN (as needed)
PT (prothrombin time)
PTCA (percutaneous transluminal coronary angioplasty)
PTT (partial thromboplastin time)
PVC (premature ventricular contraction)
PVR (pulmonary vascular resistance)
Q (every)
QD (every day)
QID (four times daily)
QOD (every other day)
RBBB (right bundle branch block)
RBC (red blood cell)
RCA (right coronary artery)
RVH (right ventricular hypertrophy)
RX (treatment, therapy)
SAH (subarachnoid hemorrhage)
SBP (systolic blood pressure)
SC (subcutaneous)
SIADH (syndrome of inappropriate antidiuretic hormone)
SK (streptokinase)
SL (sublingual)
SQ (subcutaneous)
SVR (systemic vascular resistance)
SVT (supraventricular tachycardia)
TID (three times daily)
TPA (tissue plasminogen activator)
TR (tricuspid valve regurgitation)
VF (ventricular fibrillation)
VSD (ventricular septal defect)
VT (ventricular tachycardia)
WPW (Wolff-Parkinson-White syndrome)

# 1. HYPERTENSION

Norman M. Kaplan, M.D.

## I. OVERVIEW

50 million Americans (25% of adult population) have hypertension, defined by a systolic blood pressure (BP) >140 mmHg ± diastolic BP >90 mmHg. Untreated, hypertension is associated with an increased incidence of nonfatal and fatal coronary artery disease, stroke, renal disease, and all-cause mortality. More than 90% of hypertension is idiopathic (primary or essential), while 5-10% can be ascribed to an identifiable cause (secondary hypertension). Among patients with hypertension, 1-2% will develop a hypertensive emergency at some point in their clinical course. Proper treatment results in decreased morbidity and mortality from stroke and coronary heart disease; yet, only 35% of those with hypertension are aware of their diagnosis, 49% are receiving medications, and 21% of treated patients have BP's < 140/90 mmHg (Arch Int Med 1993; 153:149).

## II. PRINCIPLES OF THERAPY

- Blood pressures ≥ 140/90 mmHg are usually treated. However, if BP is 140-150/90-94 mmHg with no evidence of target organ damage or other cardiovascular risk factors, some clinicians readdress the need for active intervention after 3-6 mos. of observation. Goal of therapy: BP < 140/90 mmHg; in diabetic hypertensives, more aggressive control is recommended (BP ≤ 130/80 mmHg).
- **Lifestyle modifications** (Step 1, p. 3) **should be initiated *prior to* drug therapy for mild-moderate hypertension and *simultaneous with* drug therapy for severe hypertension** (BP > 180/110 mmHg). Lifestyle modifications lower blood pressure, improve lipid profile, and reduce overall cardiovascular risk.
- **Optimize patient compliance:** Education about dietary, hygienic, and pharmacologic measures is essential. A drug(s) should be should be chosen that is affordable, treats coexistent disease when present, has convenient dosing and a favorable side-effect profile. If a diuretic is not initially chosen and the first line agent proves inadequate as monotherapy, a diuretic should probably be added next. Diuretics enhance the effects of most antihypertensive medications. It may take several months to achieve BP lowering goals.
- **Stepdown therapy:** Monotherapy ultimately provides adequate BP control for > 50% of patients. If BP has been well-controlled on 2 drugs for ≥ 6 months, gradual withdrawal of the first drug may be attempted. Close monitoring is advised; hypertension may return after months to years. Attempts to completely discontinue antihypertensive therapy are generally not recommended.

## FIGURE 1. TREATMENT OF HYPERTENSION: *STEPPED-CARE APPROACH*

***Step 1*** **Lifestyle modifications:**

- Lose weight if overweight
- Limit alcohol intake to ≤1 oz/d of ethanol (24 oz. of beer, 8 oz. of wine, or 2 oz. of 100-proof whiskey)
- Exercise (aerobic) regularly
- Reduce sodium intake to <100 mmol/d (<2-3 g of sodium or <6 g of NaCl)
- Maintain adequate dietary potassium, calcium, and magnesium intake
- Stop smoking and reduce dietary saturated fat and cholesterol intake for overall cardiovascular health

→ ***Step 2*** **If BP remains >140/90 mmHg:**

- Continue lifestyle modifications
- Initiate drug therapy based on presence of associated patient conditions (see pp. 4-7). If none are present, a diuretic or β-blocker is preferred since they— unlike other agents— have been tested and shown to reduce mortality.

→ ***Step 3*** **If BP remains >140/90 mmHg:**

- Increase drug dose *or*
- Substitute another drug *or*
- Add 3rd agent from different class

→ ***Step 4*** **If BP remains >140/90 mmHg:**

- Add 2nd or 3rd agent and/or diuretic if not already prescribed.

→ ***Step 5*** **If BP remains >140/90 mmHg:**

- See Resistant Hypertension, p. 11

## III. TREATMENT OF ESSENTIAL HYPERTENSION (NON-EMERGENT)

| Associated Condition | Drug Therapy | Comments |
|---|---|---|
| Angina | CCB, **β**-blocker, or nitrates; reduce BP gradually to prevent hypotension and myocardial ischemia. | Avoid monotherapy with hydralazine or nifedipine (↑ heart rate and myocardial oxygen consumption). Thiazide diuretics should be used sparingly (unfavorable effects on insulin resistance, lipids, electrolytes). |
| Arrhythmia<br>*Sinus bradycardia, Sick Sinus Syndrome* | Diuretic, ACE inhibitor, or **α**-blocker. | Avoid antihypertensives that depress sinus node function such as **β**-blockers, clonidine, aldomet, diltiazem, and verapamil. |
| *AFIB/flutter or SVT (without pre-excitation)* | **β**-blocker, diltiazem, verapamil, or clonidine. | Avoid monotherapy with hydralazine or nifedipine (may accelerate AV conduction). |
| AV block | ACE inhibitor, diuretic, or **α**-blocker. | Avoid **β**-blockers, verapamil, and diltiazem (may ↑ block). |
| Benign prostatic hypertrophy | **α**-blocker. | Provides relief of obstructive symptoms. |
| Blacks | Diuretic, CCB, or **α**-blocker. | **β**-blockers & ACE inhibitors are less effective as monotherapy. |
| COPD with bronchospasm/asthma | CCB or ACE inhibitor. | **β**-blockers may provoke bronchospasm. ACE inhibitor-induced cough may complicate bronchospastic disease. CCBs may worsen gas exchange in severe COPD. |
| Diabetes | ACE inhibitor, CCB, or **α**-blocker. | Control BP to ≤ 130/85 mmHg. **ACE inhibitors slow progression of diabetic nephropathy** (NEJM 1993;329:1456). **β**-blockers may prolong insulin-induced hypoglycemia and mask hypoglycemic symptoms. |

*CCB = calcium channel blocker, ACE = angiotensin converting enzyme.* *See p. 1 for abbreviations and p. 199 for drug information.*

## III. TREATMENT OF ESSENTIAL HYPERTENSION (NON-EMERGENT)

| Associated Condition | Drug Therapy | Comments |
|---|---|---|
| Elderly (age > 65) | Diuretic, CCB, ACE inhibitor, or *α*-blocker; start at low dose to avoid postural hypotension. | *β*-blockers effective but more likely to cause side effects. Avoid drugs associated with postural hypotension (e.g., labetalol, guanethidine). **Sudden onset of hypertension suggests atherosclerotic renovascular disease.** |
| Gout | All drug classes except diuretics. | Diuretics may be used in asymptomatic hyperuricemia. |
| Heart failure, systolic | ACE inhibitor, diuretic, or *α*-blocker. | Newer CCBs (amlodipine, felodipine) appear promising. *β*-blockers are generally not recommended, although they may be of value in selected CHF patients and in acute MI. |
| Hypertrophic obstructive cardiomyopathy | *β*-blocker or verapamil if systolic function preserved. | Avoid nitrates and vasodilators (may ↑ LV outflow obstruction). |
| Hyperlipoproteinemia | *α*-blocker, ACE inhibitor, or CCB. | Aggressive attempt at lifestyle modification (p. 3) may lower BP, improve lipid profile, and decrease cardiovascular risk. Thiazides ↑ total cholesterol and triglycerides.<br>*β*-blockers ↑ triglycerides, ↓ HDL (*β*-blocker-ISA may ↑ HDL). |
| Liver disease | All agents except methyldopa and labetalol. | Many antihypertensives are hepatically-metabolized and require dosage adjustment. |
| Left ventricular hypertrophy (LVH) | ACE inhibitor, CCB, *β*-blocker, or *α*-blocker. | Weight loss, low sodium diet, and all drugs except direct vasodilators have been shown to cause regression of LVH. It is unknown whether reversal of LVH improves outcome. If severe diastolic dysfunction is present, avoid nitrates and diuretics (may ↓↓ BP). |

*CCB = calcium channel blocker, ACE = angiotensin converting enzyme.* *See p. 1 for abbreviations and p. 199 for drug information.*

## III. TREATMENT OF ESSENTIAL HYPERTENSION (NON-EMERGENT)

| Associated Condition | Drug Therapy | Comments |
|---|---|---|
| Post-MI | ACE inhibitor and/or **β**-blocker. | Diltiazem may reduce cardiac event rate in patients with non-Q MI and preserved LV function (Ch. 4). |
| Osteoporosis | Thiazide diuretic. | Thiazides may prevent hip fracture in osteopenic post-menopausal females (JAMA 1991;265:370). |
| Peripheral vascular disease | Vasodilator, ACE inhibitor, CCB, or **α**-blocker. | Claudication may worsen as BP is lowered and if non-selective **β**-blockers are used. |
| Pregnancy | See p. 160. | |
| Pulmonary hypertension | See pp. 184-185. | |
| Pre-op | See p. 138. | |
| Renal insufficiency (creatinine > 2 mg/dL) | Loop diuretics (may require high doses), ACE inhibitor, CCB, **α**-blocker, and/or labetalol. Diabetic nephropathy: ACE inhibitor (NEJM 1993;329:1456). | Combination therapy is often required. May need to add minoxidil in refractory cases. End-stage renal disease may require dialysis or renal transplantation for BP control. Avoid $K^+$-sparing diuretics and $K^+$ supplements. Many BP drugs are excreted by the kidneys and require dosage adjustment. |
| Smoker who won't quit | **α**-blocker, ACE inhibitor, or CCB. | Hepatically-metabolized **β**-blockers (propranolol, timolol, metoprolol, labetalol) are often less effective in smokers. |
| Systolic hypertension (isolated) in the elderly | Diuretic, CCB, ACE inhibitor, or **α**-blocker: start at low dose and adjust in small increments to ↓ risk of cerebral ischemia. | Goal of therapy is to reduce systolic BP ≤ 160 mmHg. Lifestyle modifications (p. 3) may be sufficient to control hypertension. **β**-blockers are effective but associated with more side effects. |

*CCB = calcium channel blocker, ACE = angiotensin converting enzyme.* *See p. 1 for abbreviations and p. 199 for drug information.*

## III. TREATMENT OF ESSENTIAL HYPERTENSION (NON-EMERGENT)

| Associated Condition | Drug Therapy | Comments |
|---|---|---|
| Valvular heart disease<br>*Aortic stenosis, severe* | Valvuloplasty or surgery (Ch. 9). | Avoid nitrates, ACE inhibitors, vasodilators, **α**-blockers **β**-blockers and CCBs. |
| *Mitral stenosis* | **β**-blocker or CCB. | |
| *Aortic/mitral regurgitation, chronic* | ACE inhibitor, vasodilator, or nitrates. | Diuretics for pulmonary congestion. |
| *Mitral valve prolapse* | **β**-blocker. | **β**-blockers also for arrhythmias and psychogenic symptoms. |
| Young patient | ACE inhibitor or **α**-blocker. | These agents cause little sexual dysfunction or exercise intolerance. |

*CCB = calcium channel blocker, ACE = angiotensin converting enzyme.* *See p. 1 for abbreviations and p. 199 for drug information.*

## IV. INDICATIONS AND EFFECTS OF OUTPATIENT ANTIHYPERTENSIVES

| Drug Class | 1° Indications | Chol | TG | HDL | $K^+$ | $Mg^+$ | Uric acid | Insulin resistance | LVH regression | Secondary Cardioprotection |
|---|---|---|---|---|---|---|---|---|---|---|
| ACE inhibitors | Diabetes with nephropathy; Post-MI; CHF | 0 | 0 | 0 | ↑ | 0 | 0 | ↓ | ↓↓ | + |
| *β*-blockers without ISA | Post-MI, migraine, tremor, tachycardia | 0/↑ | ↑↑ | ↓ | ↑ | 0 | 0 | ↑↑ | ↓ | + |
| *β*-blockers with ISA | Same as above | 0 | ↑ | 0 | 0 | 0 | 0 | ↑ | ↓ | + |
| Calcium channel blockers | Elderly, black, CAD, renal insufficiency | 0 | 0 | 0 | 0 | 0 | 0 | 0 | ↓ | Perhaps with verapamil or diltiazem |
| Diuretics | Elderly, blacks, renal failure, CHF | ↑ | 0 | 0 | ↓ | ↓ | ↑ | ↑ | 0 | 0 |
| Central *α*-blockers | Sedative effect desired | 0 | 0 | 0 | 0 | 0 | 0 | ? | ↓ | ? |
| Peripheral *α*-blockers | Diabetes, dyslipidemia, BPH | ↓ | ↓ | ↑ | 0 | 0 | 0 | ↓ | ↓ | ? |
| Vasodilators | Peripheral vascular disease, vasculitis | ↓ | 0 | 0 | 0 | ? | 0 | ? | 0 | 0 |

0 = no significant effect; ↑ (↓) = increased (decreased) effect; ? = unknown or no consistent group effect; ACE = angiotensin converting enzyme; Chol = cholesterol; TG = triglycerides; HDL = high density lipoprotein cholesterol; LVH = left ventricular hypertrophy; CAD = coronary artery disease; CHF = congestive heart failure; ISA = intrinsic sympathomimetic activity; BPH = benign prostatic hypertrophy.

## V. TREATMENT OF HYPERTENSIVE URGENCIES
### (Requires Oral or Parental Therapy to Reduce BP Within Hours)

| Presentation | First Line Therapy | Comments |
|---|---|---|
| Diastolic BP > 130 mmHg with retinal hemorrhage or papilledema | Nitroprusside (IV) or labetalol (IV). | 30% of non-blacks will have renovascular hypertension as the etiology. |
| Cerebral infarction with severe hypertension | Nitroprusside (IV). | Marked falls in BP may provoke cerebral hypoperfusion; **drug therapy should be withheld unless diastolic BP > 120 mmHg.** |
| Severe rebound (overshoot) hypertension post-drug withdrawal | Labetalol (IV) or $\alpha$-blocker; restart drug that lead to rebound. | Clonidine rebound is associated with high circulating catecholamines. Avoid $\beta$-blockers during clonidine-induced hypertension (may further increase BP due to unopposed $\alpha$-receptor stimulation). |
| Severe hypertension pre-urgent surgery or post-op hypertension | Labetalol (IV), CCB (IV), or $\beta$-blocker (IV). | Avoid direct vasodilators (e.g., hydralazine), which may increase shear forces and the risk of bleeding from vascular suture lines. |

## VI. TREATMENT OF HYPERTENSIVE EMERGENCIES
### (Requires Parental Therapy to Reduce BP Within Minutes)

| Presentation | First Line Therapy | Comments |
|---|---|---|
| Cardiac<br>*Aortic dissection* | See p. 172. | Monotherapy with direct vasodilators (e.g., hydralazine) may ↑ vascular shear forces and extend the dissection. |
| *Acute heart failure* | See Ch. 8. | |

*CCB = calcium channel blocker, ACE = angiotensin converting enzyme. See p. 1 for abbreviations and p. 199 for drug information.*

## VI. TREATMENT OF HYPERTENSIVE EMERGENCIES
**(Requires Parental Therapy to Reduce BP Within Minutes)**

| Presentation | First Line Therapy | Comments |
|---|---|---|
| *Acute myocardial infarction (MI)* | Bed rest, analgesia, and sedation. Drug therapy: IV **β**-blocker, IV nitroglycerin and/or ACE inhibitor (Ch. 4). | Nitrates should be avoided in the presence of low filling pressures or RV infarction. Nifedipine and diltiazem should be used with caution, if at all. |
| *Post-CABG* | Nitroprusside ± CCB/**β**-blocker. Resume oral BP meds post-op day #2. | Avoid hydralazine/diazoxide (↑ cardiac work) and labetalol/**β**-blockers if moderate-severe systolic dysfunction is present. |
| Cerebrovascular<br>*Hypertensive encephalopathy* | Nitroprusside or labetalol (IV). | Goal of therapy: Decrease diastolic to BP 110 mmHg within the first hour. Maintain BP at an even higher level if neurologic status deteriorates during therapy. Avoid methyldopa & reserpine (sedation), and diazoxide (↓ cerebral blood flow). |
| *Intracerebral hemorrhage (hem)* | Same as for cerebral infarction (p. 9). | |
| *Subarachnoid hem* | Nimodipine (p. 194). | Nimodipine shown to ↓ vasospasm & recurrent stroke. |
| Eclampsia | See p. 161. | |
| Epistaxis, severe | Oral antihypertensive of choice. Labetalol (IV) may rarely be needed. | Cocaine-saturated nasal pledgets, posterior pack, cauterization, arterial ligation, and blood transfusions as needed. |
| Food/drug interactions with MAO inhibitors | Phentolamine (IV **α**-blocker). Avoid **β**-blockers (may further elevate BP due to unopposed **α**-receptor stimulation). | Drugs that may interact with MAO inhibitors: levodopa, methyldopa, sympathomimetic amines (including over-the-counter decongestants), guanadrel, and meperidine (fatal cardiovascular collapse). Foods that may precipitate this reaction: avocados, bananas, bean curd (including soy sauce), |

*CCB = calcium channel blocker, ACE = angiotensin converting enzyme. See p. 1 for abbreviations and p. 199 for drug information.*

## VI. TREATMENT OF HYPERTENSIVE EMERGENCIES
**(Requires Parental Therapy to Reduce BP Within Minutes)**

| Presentation | First Line Therapy | Comments |
|---|---|---|
| Interactions with MAO inhibitors (cont.) | See previous page. | beer and ale, certain cheeses, processed meats, canned figs, sausage, shrimp paste, red wines, yeast extracts, caffeine, chocolate, broad beans. |
| Head injury | Labetalol (IV); gradually ↓ BP to avoid cerebral hypoperfusion. | Avoid methyldopa & reserpine (sedation), and diazoxide (↓ cerebral blood flow). |
| Pheochromocytoma crisis | Phentolamine (IV ***α***-blocker). | Avoid ***β***-blockers (unopposed ***α***-receptor stimulation by ↑↑ circulating catecholamines may further elevate BP). |
| Post-op bleeding from suture lines | Labetalol (IV), CCB, or ***β***-blocker. | Avoid hydralazine (may increase vascular shear forces and the risk of bleeding). |

## VII. RESISTANT HYPERTENSION

Inability to achieve adequate BP control despite 3-drug therapy occurs in 3-11% of patients with hypertension. Treatment consists of identifying and correcting the cause:

1) **Non-adherence to therapy**: Use once or twice-a-day dosing and patient education.
2) **Overdiagnosis:** "White coat" hypertension (hypertension which occurs only in response to stress of office visits), pseudohypertension (artificial elevation of BP due to failure of BP cuff to completely compress rigid brachial arteries).
3) **Drug related:** Dosage too low, inappropriate combinations (e.g., two drugs from same class), rapid inactivation (e.g. hydralazine), co-administration of drugs that ↑ BP (diet pills, nasal decongestants, antidepressants, adrenal steroids, nonsteroidal anti-inflammatory drugs, cocaine, oral contraceptives, exogenous thyroid hormone replacement, cholestyramine binding of antihypertensives, caffeine or tobacco within one hour of BP reading).
4) **Volume overload:** Inadequate diuretic therapy, excess sodium intake, fluid retention from ↓ BP and progressive renal damage.
5) **Associated conditions:** Obesity, ethanol > than 1 ounce/day, cigarette smoking, renal insufficiency, renovascular hypertension and other causes of secondary hypertension as described below.

## VIII. SECONDARY HYPERTENSION

| | |
|---|---|
| Definition | Hypertension that can be ascribed to an identifiable cause. |
| Prevalence | 5-10% of the total hypertensive population. |
| Indications for work-up | History, physical exam, and labs suggest a secondary cause; resistance to triple drug therapy; BP worsening after a period of good control; accelerated or malignant hypertension; negative family history and diastolic BP > 110 mmHg. |
| Therapy | See specific disorders, below. |

### A. RENAL PARENCHYMAL DISEASE

| | |
|---|---|
| Diagnosis | Renal ultrasound (bilateral small scarred kidneys), renal biopsy. |
| Treatment | • **Drug therapy: Loop diuretics** (may require high dose). Nonresponders: One approach is to use an ACE inhibitor and/or CCB, followed by *α*-blocker and/or labetalol; add minoxidil when further therapy is required. Avoid NSAIDs (inhibit production of vasodilatory renal prostaglandins), $K^+$ sparing diuretics and $K^+$ supplements.<br>• **Hemodialysis or renal transplantation** may be required for hypertensive control in end-stage renal disease. |

### B. RENOVASCULAR HYPERTENSION

| | |
|---|---|
| Presentation | Suspect diagnosis in those with onset of hypertension < 30 years of age or rapid onset after 50 years; resistance to 3-drug therapy; deterioration in renal function after administration of ACE inhibitors; uncontrolled hypertension after period of good control; malignant hypertension; recurrent acute pulmonary edema; sudden worsening of renal function in hypertensive patient; epigastric, subcostal or flank bruit; extensive atherosclerosis elsewhere. |

*CCB = calcium channel blocker, ACE = angiotensin converting enzyme.* *See p. 1 for abbreviations and p. 199 for drug information.*

## B. RENOVASCULAR HYPERTENSION

| | |
|---|---|
| Screen | **Captopril renography**: Test requirements: Normal sodium intake, no diuretic or ACE inhibitor, no antihypertensives x 3 wks (if possible). Have patient sit for ≥ 30 min, then draw venous blood for plasma renin activity (PRA) at baseline and 60 min. after 50 mg of oral captopril (diluted in 10 ml of water). Positive test: Stimulated PRA of ≥ 12 ng/ml/hr, an absolute increase in PRA ≥ 10 ng/ml/hr, and a ≥ 150% increase in PRA above baseline (≥ 400% if baseline below 3 ng/ml/hr). Isotopic renography demonstrates a decrease in renal blood flow or GFR by ≥ 20%. |
| Diagnosis | Renal arteriography with renal vein renins vs. "therapeutic trial" of balloon angioplasty. |
| Treatment | • Renal artery revascularization relieves hypertension in 85% of cases.<br>- **Atherosclerotic disease: Surgery is the most reliable form of therapy**. If the lesion is short, segmental, and unilateral, balloon angioplasty results compare favorably with surgical correction; restenosis, which may occur in up to 25% of cases, usually responds to repeat dilatation. When plaque extends from the abdominal aorta to involve the renal artery orifice, balloon angioplasty success and longterm patency rates are reduced. Most agree that revascularization is indicated for (1) poorly-controlled hypertension; (2) deterioration in renal function on medical therapy; (3) those intolerant/noncompliant with medical therapy; and (4) young patients.<br>- **Fibromuscular dysplasia: Balloon angioplasty** is treatment of choice (high success, low restenosis).<br>• **Medical therapy: CCB, β-blockers, or diuretics**. Longterm medical therapy is generally reserved for poor revascularization candidates and when hypertension persists after revascularization. *Even when BP is adequately controlled on medical therapy, renal dysfunction and loss of renal mass may develop.* Renal function and size should be followed q 3-6 mos. |

*CCB = calcium channel blocker, ACE = angiotensin converting enzyme.* *See p. 1 for abbreviations and p. 199 for drug information.*

| C. PRIMARY ALDOSTERONISM | |
|---|---|
| Presentation | **Hypertension with hypokalemia** (may first become evident during treatment with diuretics); muscle pain, cramping or weakness; polyuria/polydipsia; metabolic alkalosis; impaired carbohydrate tolerance; and development of multiple renal cysts. |
| Screen | • **Plasma renin activity (PRA):** Levels < 1 ng/ml/hr and plasma aldosterone-to-renin ratio > 20 suggest the diagnosis.<br>• **24 hour $K^+$ urine potassium** performed while patient is hypokalemic, ingesting a normal $Na^+$ intake (urinary $Na^+$ excretion > 100 meq/day), and not receiving supplemental $K^+$ or diuretics. If the urinary $K^+$ is < 30 meq/day, primary aldosteronism is essentially excluded; if > 30 meq/day, continue workup as described below. |
| Diagnosis | • **24 hour urine for aldosterone, sodium, and cortisol with upright PRA and serum potassium**. Discontinue diuretics and replenish normal body stores and serum levels of $K^+$ (may take weeks-months). Administer either a high sodium diet for 5 days or IV normal saline (2 liters over 4 hours). Primary aldosteronism is diagnosed if Cushing's disease is excluded and sodium loading does not suppress aldosterone (i.e., either urinary aldosterone is significantly elevated if high sodium diet is prescribed or recumbent serum aldosterone > 10-20 ng/dL following IV saline load).<br>• To distinguish **bilateral adrenal hyperplasia from adrenal adenoma**, a **CT scan** should be obtained. If nondiagnostic, an MRI or adrenal scintillation scan with iodinated cholesterol derivative is often of value. If these tests continue to be nondiagnostic, consider bilateral adrenal vein catheterization (less than 2-fold difference in aldosterone suggests hyperplasia). |
| Treatment | • **Bilateral adrenal hyperplasia: $K^+$-sparing diuretic (spironolactone**, amiloride or triamterene) ± nifedipine.<br>• **Adrenal adenoma:** Preoperative spironolactone followed by **surgical resection.** 75% of patients are cured; 25% remain hypertensive and require drug therapy. |

*CCB = calcium channel blocker, ACE = angiotensin converting enzyme.* *See p. 1 for abbreviations and p. 199 for drug information.*

| D. CUSHING'S SYNDROME | |
|---|---|
| Presentation | Truncal obesity, moon facies, ecchymosis, muscle atrophy, edema, striae, acne, hirsutism, osteoporosis, glucose intolerance and/or hypokalemia. |
| Screen | • **24 hour urinary free cortisol**: Levels > 100 mcg suggest the diagnosis.<br>• **Overnight dexamethasone suppression test:** 1 mg of dexamethasone at midnight followed by plasma cortisol at 8:00 a.m. If level > 7 mcg/dL, proceed with *prolonged* dexamethasone suppression test (see below). |
| Diagnosis | Measure **basal plasma ACTH levels** and perform a **prolonged dexamethasone suppression test**: Administer 0.5 mg dexamethasone every 6 hrs x 2 days followed by 2 mg every 6 hrs x 2 days. Measure urinary free cortisol and plasma cortisol on the second day of each dose:<br>- *Adrenal tumor*: Failure to suppress cortisol with low or high dose dexamethasone; basal ACTH undetectable.<br>- *Ectopic ACTH syndrome*: Failure to suppress on low or high dose; ACTH elevated.<br>- *Cushing's disease* (excess pituitary ACTH → bilateral adrenal hyperplasia): Failure to suppress on low dose but suppressed to < 50% of control value by high dose; ACTH normal to elevated.<br>Note: 10% of patients with Cushing's disease do not suppress adequately while 5% with ectopic ACTH do suppress. |
| Treatment | • **Pituitary adenoma: Transphenoidal microsurgery** improves signs and symptoms in ~80%. Bilateral adrenalectomy reserved for disabling symptoms unresponsive to other forms of therapy. Ketoconazole and mitotane inhibit adrenal cortisol secretion and may be of adjunctive value.<br>• **Ectopic ACTH syndrome: Remove tumor when feasible.** Adjunctive ketoconazole, metapyrone, aminoglutethimide, alone or in combination, may be of value.<br>• **Adrenal adenoma or carcinoma: Surgical resection.** Mitotane for residual or nonresectable tumor.<br>• Antihypertensive medications are not considered primary therapy, although they may be of adjunctive value (diuretic plus spironolactone). |

| E. PHEOCHROMOCYTOMA | |
|---|---|
| Presentation | Hypertension (persistent in 50%, paroxysmal in 50%; normotensive in a few), episodic palpitations, headache, sweating, orthostatic hypotension, weight loss and glucose intolerance. |
| Screen | • **24 hour urinary total metanephrines**: Levels > 1.3 mg suggest the diagnosis. False positive tests are much more likely if the patient is taking sympathomimetic drugs, MAO inhibitors (e.g., phenelzine, tranylcypromine), or labetalol. False negative results have been seen after x-ray contrast media containing methylglucamine (Renografin, Hypaque).<br>• **Plasma catecholamines:** Levels > 2000 pg/mL suggests the diagnosis. If 500-2000 pg/mL, the clonidine suppression test is used to make the diagnosis (see below). When drawing samples for plasma catecholamines, the patient must be resting at least 30 minutes prior to venipuncture (note: some patients have normal levels during asymptomatic normotensive periods). Contact lab for details of sample collection, handling, storage, and drugs that may affect interpretation of results. Many acute illnesses (e.g., MI, diabetic ketoacidosis, shock, stroke) and chronic disorders (e.g., hypothyroidism, peptic ulcer, depression, COPD, CHF) can cause elevations in plasma catecholamines and false positive test results. |
| Diagnosis | • **Clonidine suppression test:** Failure to suppress plasma catecholamine levels by ≥ 50% 3 hours after oral administration of 0.3 mg of clonidine is indicative of pheochromocytoma (note: may cause marked hypotension).<br>• **Tumor localization: CT scan** able to localize tumor in 90% of cases (i.e., when tumor is > 1 cm in diameter). Others: $^{131}$I-MIBG scan or selective arteriography with regional catecholamine levels. |
| Treatment | • **Immediate treatment** of severe hypertension: **Phentolamine** (IV). **Long-term therapy: Surgical resection** is the treatment of choice. **Pre-operative α-receptor blockade** (phenoxybenzamine or doxazosin until normotensive x 5-10 days) is often recommended to avoid extreme hypertension during tumor manipulation and allow re-expansion of intravascular volume depletion, which is typical of pheochromocytoma. May develop post-op hypoglycemia (treat with IV dextrose) ± hypotension (treat with volume expanders and phenylephrine). Longterm clinical follow-up is important to identify late recurrences.<br>• **If surgical resection is not possible,** chronic medical therapy with **phenoxybenzamine** (oral α-blocker) or **alpha-methyl-tyrosine** (oral inhibitor of catechol synthesis) is recommended. |

*CCB = calcium channel blocker, ACE = angiotensin converting enzyme.* *See p. 1 for abbreviations and p. 199 for drug information.*

## F. COARCTATION OF THE AORTA

| | |
|---|---|
| Presentation | May complain of **cold feet and leg claudication**. Findings on physical exam include arm BP > leg BP, thrill in suprasternal notch, systolic flow murmur best heard in left posterior thorax, and absent femoral pulses in most. Chest x-ray may demonstrate rib notching (increased collateral flow through intercostal arteries) and indentation of the aortic knob ("figure 3 sign"). **One-third of patients have bicuspid aortic valves.** Complications include congestive heart failure, endocarditis, and stroke. Without corrective surgery, 80% ultimately die prematurely from complications of hypertension. |
| Diagnosis | Aortography. |
| Treatment | **Surgical repair or angioplasty** is the treatment of choice. Transient post-op worsening of hypertension can usually be prevented by prophylactic $\beta$-blockade. Drug therapy: ACE inhibitor or CCB. |

## G. PRIMARY HYPERPARATHYROIDISM

| | |
|---|---|
| Presentation | Patients are frequently asymptomatic: 10-20% of cases are first diagnosed after routine chemical screening. The first manifestation may be **hypercalcemia after initiating therapy with thiazide diuretics**. Other manifestations variably include fatigue, weakness, renal symptoms in 50% (polyuria, nocturia, renal stones, nephrocalcinosis), proximal muscle weakness, and nonspecific joint and back symptoms. |
| Diagnosis | Elevated levels of serum calcium and parathyroid hormone. |
| Treatment | **Surgical parathyroidectomy** is the treatment of choice. Although hypertension may persist, surgery generally halts the formation of renal stones and allows skeletal remineralization in those with bone disease. **Post-op hypocalcemia** is not uncommon; acute treatment with IV calcium and longterm therapy with vitamin D and oral calcium may be needed. For elderly patients and patients with mild elevations of serum calcium only, optimal therapy is controversial (i.e., surgery vs. conservative medical follow-up). Thiazide diuretics should be avoided (may further ↑ serum $Ca^{++}$). |

*CCB = calcium channel blocker, ACE = angiotensin converting enzyme.* *See p. 1 for abbreviations and p. 199 for drug information.*

## H. DRUG-INDUCED HYPERTENSION

| | |
|---|---|
| Glucocorticoids | Treat with diuretics ± spironolactone. |
| Licorice | Present in some chewing tobaccos. Treat with diuretics ± spironolactone. |
| Sympathomimetics | Present in diet pills and street drugs. Treat with labetalol. |
| Nonsteroidal anti-inflammatory drugs | Substitute acetaminophen or increase the dose of BP drug. |
| Alcohol | Etiology in up to 10% of young males with hypertension. |
| Oral contraceptives | All patients receiving oral contraceptives should have their BP checked after 3-6 months of use. If BP is elevated, other forms of contraception should be considered. When medical therapy is required, a diuretic-spironolactone combination is often effective. |
| Cocaine | Phentolamine for hypertension and $\beta$-blockers for arrhythmias. |
| Cyclosporine | Treat hypertension with labetalol or a central $\alpha$-agonist. Avoid diltiazem, nicardipine, verapamil and other drugs that increase cyclosporine levels. |

*CCB = calcium channel blocker, ACE = angiotensin converting enzyme.* *See p. 1 for abbreviations and p. 199 for drug information.*

# 2. DYSLIPIDEMIA

Jun Anthony V. Quion, M.D.
Antonio M. Gotto, Jr., M.D., D.Phil.

## I. OVERVIEW

It is estimated that 20% of U.S. adults have high total cholesterol ($\geq$ 240 mg/dL) and that another 31% have borderline-high total cholesterol (200–239 mg/dL). Several large-scale randomized placebo-controlled trials have shown reductions in cardiovascular morbidity and mortality with lipid-lowering therapy, both in primary and secondary prevention. Intensive LDL cholesterol lowering, to below ~ 100 mg/dL, slows the progression of atherosclerotic plaques and may induce their regression. However, the response of coronary lesions to lipid-lowering therapy is small and appears to depend on the stage of lesion development. The effect of regression on clinical outcome awaits definition.

## II. STEPPED CARE MANAGEMENT OF HYPERCHOLESTEROLEMIA

### Step 1: Initial Classification and Follow-up

Total serum cholesterol and HDL-cholesterol should be measured in all persons over age 20 and classified according to Figure 1.

### STEP 2: Once a Dyslipidemia is Identified

1) Screen for the presence of secondary dyslipidemia, including alcohol abuse, diabetes mellitus, thyroid disorders, nephrotic syndrome, obstructive jaundice, and medications (thiazide diuretics, $\beta$-blockers, estrogen, progestin, androgen, glucocorticoids).
2) Carefully review family history for genetic causes. If severe hypercholesterolemia is present, screen family members.
3) Assess possible contribution of lipid abnormalities to history (e.g., angina, claudication, pancreatitis) and physical examination findings (e.g., xanthomas, xanthelasma, hepatosplenomegaly).
4) Estimate risk for coronary heart disease and other atherosclerotic disease to guide intensity of further management (see below).

## STEP 3: Initiate Therapy with Dietary and Hygienic Measures

**Dietary modification and hygienic measures (exercise, weight control, smoking cessation, etc.) are considered first-line therapy** for all patients with hypercholesterolemia (Figure 4). Drug therapy should be initiated only after an adequate trial of dietary therapy has failed to lower LDL cholesterol levels to within desired range after 6 months. Exceptions include (1) Patients with established CHD; drug therapy is usually started after a shorter period of--or concurrently with--dietary therapy, and (2) Patients with very high LDL levels (above 220 mg/dL); drug therapy may be initiated concurrently with Step II diet.

## STEP 4: Drug Therapy (Figure 5, Tables 2-3)

| Special groups | |
|---|---|
| *Young adults ♂, premenopausal ♀* | Most young adults males (age < 35 years) and premenopausal females with LDL cholesterol levels between 160-220 mg/dL are at low risk of CHD in the short-term. **In general, drug therapy can be withheld** in these groups unless extreme elevations in LDL cholesterol (>220 mg/dL) or multiple risk factors are present--especially diabetes mellitus and patients with a family history of premature coronary heart disease. |
| *Post-menopausal females* | In the absence of contraindications such as breast cancer, postmenopausal women should benefit from **estrogen replacement therapy**, which has been shown to reduce the incidence of CHD and beneficially affect LDL and HDL cholesterol levels. Although oral preparations are generally preferable, they tend to exacerbate hypertriglyceridemia; topical forms are therefore preferred in such instances. |
| *Elderly patients* | Age by itself should not preclude diet and drug therapy when hypercholesterolemia is present. |
| *Diabetics* | There appears to be a synergistic effect between diabetes mellitus and hypercholesterolemia in the development of CHD. Therefore, **initiation levels and therapeutic goals, *even in the absence of coronary heart disease*, should be similar to recommendations for those with established CHD** (initiation level, LDL > 100 mg/dL; therapeutic goal, LDL < 100 mg/dL). |

| STEP 5: When Diet and Drugs Fail | |
|---|---|
| LDL-apheresis | May be considered for all patients with homozygous familial hypercholesterolemia (FH), for patients with heterozygous FH and established CHD, and for any patient with established CHD if LDL cholesterol remains above 190 mg/dL despite maximal dietary and pharmacological intervention. Plasmapheresis (plasma exchange) may be used for the acute management of severe hypertriglyceridemia to reduce the risk for pancreatitis. |
| Others | • Gene therapy: Experimental option for treating homozygous FH and other rare dyslipidemias caused by gene defects.<br>• Antioxidants, fish oil: Routine use has not yet been established as beneficial by clinical trials. |
| Referral to a lipid specialist | Made on an individual basis, usually after a primary-care physician finds combination drug therapy ineffective, or before such therapy is initiated when he or she is uncomfortable monitoring the metabolic impact of combination drug therapy. In general, patients with severe refractory lipid disorders and those who require complex management, such as LDL-apheresis therapy, should receive the attention of a lipid specialist. |

## Figure 1. Primary Prevention in Adults Without Coronary Heart Disease (CHD): *Initial Classification Based on Total and HDL-Cholesterol*

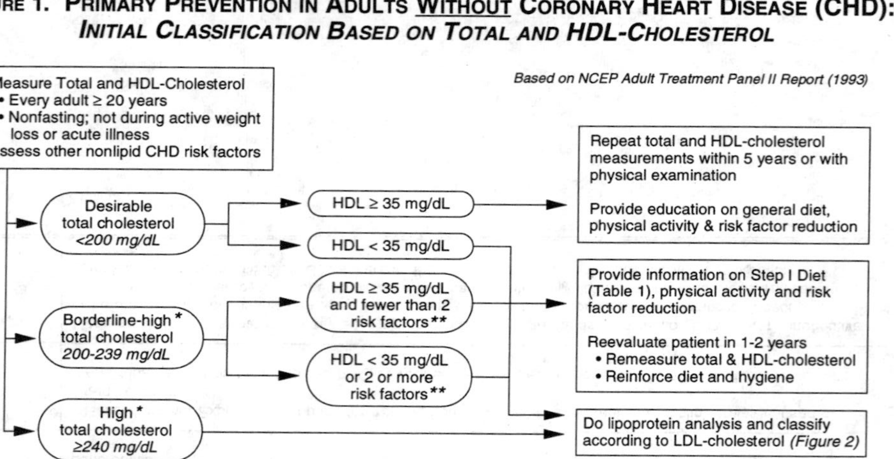


****CHD Risk Factors:**
Age *(male ≥ 45, female ≥ 55 or premature menopause without estrogen replacement).*
Family history *(MI or sudden death in father [mother] or other male [female] first - degree relative before age 55 [65]).*
Current cigarette smoking
Hypertension *(BP ≥ 140/90 mmHg or taking antihypertensive medication)*
Low HDL-cholesterol *(< 35 mg/dL).*
Diabetes mellitus
**NOTE:** *If HDL > 60 mg/dL, subtract 1 from risk factor total.*

* *Must be confirmed by repeat measurement 1-8 weeks apart; If values vary by > 30 mg/dL, obtain 3rd test 1-8 weeks later and use average of 3 values.*

## Figure 2. Primary Prevention in Adults Without Coronary Heart Disease (CHD): *Subsequent Classification Based on LDL-Cholesterol*

*Based on NCEP Adult Treatment Panel II Report (1993)*

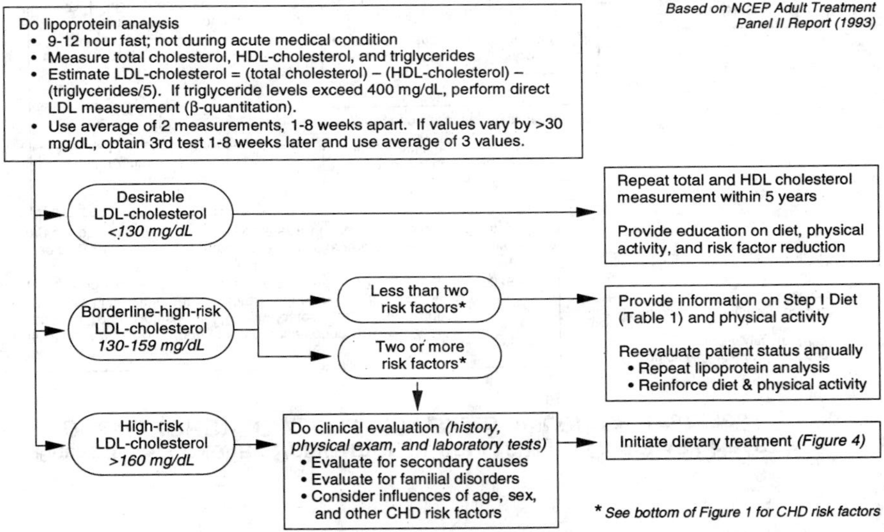

Do lipoprotein analysis
- 9-12 hour fast; not during acute medical condition
- Measure total cholesterol, HDL-cholesterol, and triglycerides
- Estimate LDL-cholesterol = (total cholesterol) – (HDL-cholesterol) – (triglycerides/5). If triglyceride levels exceed 400 mg/dL, perform direct LDL measurement (β-quantitation).
- Use average of 2 measurements, 1-8 weeks apart. If values vary by >30 mg/dL, obtain 3rd test 1-8 weeks later and use average of 3 values.

Desirable LDL-cholesterol *<130 mg/dL* → Repeat total and HDL cholesterol measurement within 5 years

Provide education on diet, physical activity, and risk factor reduction

Borderline-high-risk LDL-cholesterol *130-159 mg/dL*
- Less than two risk factors* → Provide information on Step I Diet (Table 1) and physical activity

  Reevaluate patient status annually
  - Repeat lipoprotein analysis
  - Reinforce diet & physical activity
- Two or more risk factors* → Do clinical evaluation

High-risk LDL-cholesterol *>160 mg/dL* → Do clinical evaluation *(history, physical exam, and laboratory tests)*
- Evaluate for secondary causes
- Evaluate for familial disorders
- Consider influences of age, sex, and other CHD risk factors

→ Initiate dietary treatment *(Figure 4)*

* *See bottom of Figure 1 for CHD risk factors*

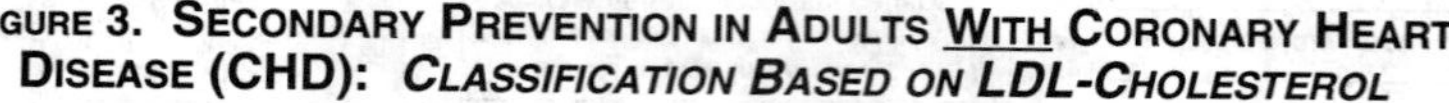

# FIGURE 3. SECONDARY PREVENTION IN ADULTS WITH CORONARY HEART DISEASE (CHD): *CLASSIFICATION BASED ON LDL-CHOLESTEROL*

*Based on NCEP Adult Treatment Panel II Report (1993)*

** See bottom of Figure 1 for CHD risk factors*

Do lipoprotein analysis

- 9-12 hour fast; not during acute medical condition
- Measure total cholesterol, HDL-cholesterol, and triglycerides
- Estimate LDL-cholesterol = (total cholesterol) – (HDL-cholesterol) – (triglycerides/5). If triglyceride levels exceed 400 mg/dL, perform direct LDL measurement (β-quantitation).
- Use average of 2 measurements, 1-8 weeks apart. If values vary by >30 mg/dL, obtain 3rd test 1-8 weeks later and use average of 3 values.

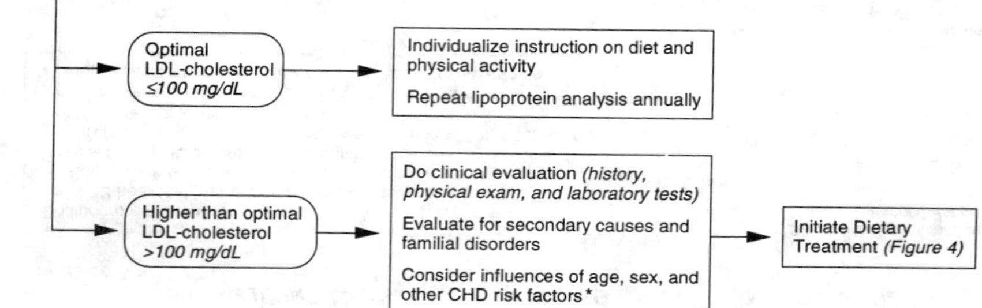

# FIGURE 4. DIETARY TREATMENT OF HYPERCHOLESTEROLEMIA

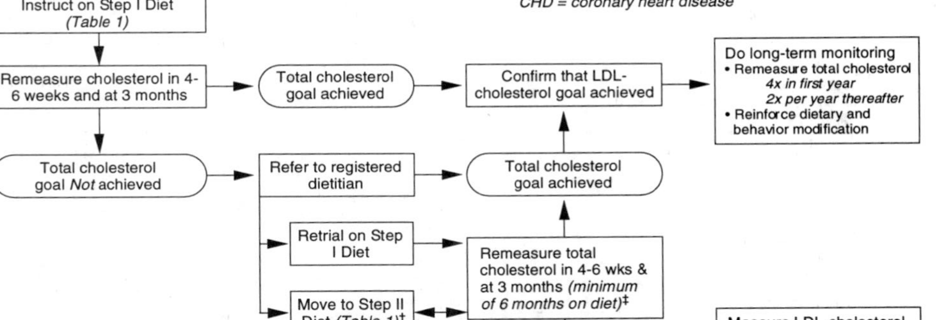


* *See bottom of Figure 1 for CHD risk factors*

† *Drugs may be initiated concurrently with Step II Diet if LDL-cholesterol >160 mg/dL with established CHD or >190-220 mg/dL without CHD but multiple risk factors*

‡ *Drugs may considered after a shorter period of diet in patients with established CHD*

*CHD = coronary heart disease*

*Based on NCEP Adult Treatment Panel II Report (1993)*

# FIGURE 5. DRUG TREATMENT OF HYPERCHOLESTEROLEMIA

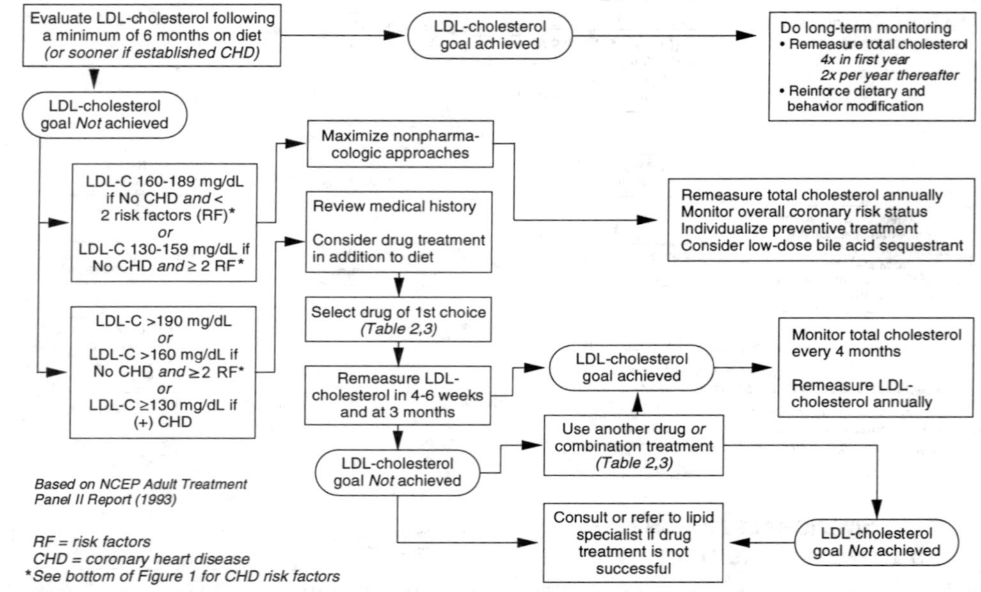


*Based on NCEP Adult Treatment Panel II Report (1993)*

*RF = risk factors*
*CHD = coronary heart disease*
**See bottom of Figure 1 for CHD risk factors*

**Table 1. GUIDELINES FOR DIETARY AND HYGIENIC THERAPY***

| | Step I Diet (% of total calories) | Step II Diet (% of total calories) |
|---|---|---|
| *Total fat* | ≤ 30% | Same |
| *Saturated fat* | 8-10% | < 7% |
| *Polyunsaturated fat* | Up to 10% | Same |
| *Monounsaturated fat* | Up to 15% | Same |
| *Carbohydrates* | 50-60% (mostly from complex carbohydrates ) | Same |
| *Protein* | ≈ 15% | Same |
| *Cholesterol* | < 300 mg/d | < 200 mg/d |
| Physical activity | A regular, moderate exercise regimen that increases heart rate to 70-80% of maximal value for 30-40 min. ≥ 3 times per week is recommended. It is not known what amount and type of exercise have the most beneficial effects on lipids, but HDL cholesterol levels increase over time and with ↑ activity. | |
| Weight control | Weight control is an intrinsic part of dietary therapy as recommended by the NCEP. Total caloric intake should be calculated to achieve and maintain a desirable body weight. | |
| Alcohol | Although moderate alcohol consumption (up to 1 oz ethanol per day) has been associated with a lower risk of CHD, it is not recommended as a therapeutic agent because of possible deleterious effects, such as hypertriglyceridemia, hypertension and the risk for abuse. | |

* The Step I Diet also serves as the dietary recommendations of the National Cholesterol Education Program (NCEP) for the general public. The more intensive Step II Diet is designed for patients with genetic hyperlipidemia, established CHD or atherosclerotic disease, or for whom the Step I Diet has proven insufficient; the assistance of a registered dietician is often useful in maintaining compliance.

## Table 2. DRUG THERAPY BASED ON LIPID PROFILE

The following are guidelines based on the general activity of the drugs. However, drug selection is a highly individualized process, taking into account factors such as tolerance, compliance, and the unique medical condition of the patient.

| Lipid Profile (mg/dL) | | | | |
|---|---|---|---|---|
| LDL-C | HDL-C | Triglyceride | Primary Drug Therapy[1] | Comments |
| ≥ 190 | ≥ 35 | < 200 | Monotherapy: NA, HMG. Combination: BAS + HMG, BAS + NA, HMG + NA[2] | Homozygous familial hypercholesterolemia requires the attention of a lipid specialist. BAS is preferred as monotherapy if liver disease is present. |
| 160-190 | ≥ 35 | < 200 | Monotherapy: BAS, HMG, NA | NA and BAS have proven long-term safety profiles. The Lipid Research Clinics Trial showed a 19% reduction in nonfatal MI with cholestyramine compared to placebo. |
| 160-190 | ≥ 35 | 200-400 | Monotherapy: NA, HMG, (FIB). Combination: HMG + NA[2], HMG + FIB[3], FIB + BAS | The Coronary Drug Project, a secondary-prevention trial, showed a 25% reduction in nonfatal myocardial infarction with NA. |
| 160-190 | < 35 | 200-400 | Monotherapy: NA, HMG, FIB Combination: HMG + NA[2], HMG + FIB[3] | The Helsinki Heart Study showed a decrease in the incidence of CHD with gemfibrozil. FIB is preferred if diabetes or peptic ulcers are present. |
| < 130 | ≥ 35 | > 400 | Monotherapy: NA, FIB | Fish oils may be used as adjunctive therapy. Treat to decrease the risk of pancreatitis. |
| < 130 | < 35 | > 400 | Monotherapy: NA, FIB | NA worsens diabetes control and may activate peptic ulcer disease. Avoid FIB in patients with gallbladder disease. |

BAS = bile-acid sequestrant (cholestyramine, colestipol); FIB = fibric-acid derivative (gemfibrozil); HMG = HMG-CoA reductase inhibitor (lovastatin, simvastatin, fluvastatin, pravastatin); NA = nicotinic acid; (1) Severe elevations may require combination therapy. Avoid all drugs during pregnancy; (2) ↑ risk for myopathy and hepatitis; (3) ↑ risk for myopathy. *See p. 199 for drug information.*

## Table 3. CHARACTERISTICS OF AVAILABLE CHOLESTEROL-LOWERING DRUGS

| Class | Agents | Major Use | Contraindications |
|---|---|---|---|
| HMG-CoA reductase inhibitors | • Fluvastatin<br>• Lovastatin<br>• Pravastatin<br>• Simvastatin | Severe hypercholesterolemia and secondary prevention. Use cautiously in young adults and premenopausal females (long-term safety data not available). | • Absolute: Active or chronic liver disease.<br>• Relative: Concomitant use of cyclosporin, gemfibrizol, or niacin. |
| Bile acid sequestrants | • Cholestyramine<br>• Colestipol | Especially useful in moderate hypercholesterolemia, primary prevention, young adult men, and premenopausal females. | • Absolute: Familial dysbetalipoproteinemia, triglyceride > 500 mg/dL.<br>• Relative: Triglyceride > 200 mg/dL. |
| Nicotinic acid | • Niacin: crystalline form, sustained-release form not yet FDA-approved | Useful in most dyslipidemias. | • Absolute: Active or chronic liver disease.<br>• Relative: NIDDM, severe gout, hyperuricemia, peptic ulcer disease. |
| Fibric acid derivatives | • Gemfibrozil<br>• Clofibrate (rarely used in US) | Severe hypertriglyceridemia, familial dysbetaliproteinemia, combined hyperlipidemia, and diabetes mellitus. Not indicated for LDL lowering in $2^{o}$ prevention. | • Absolute: Hepatic or severe renal dysfunction, primary biliary cirrhosis, gallbladder disease. |
| Probucol | • Probucol | May be used in hypercholesterolemia if other agents ineffective. Has not been shown to reduce CHD rates in a clinical trial. | • Absolute: Evidence of recent or progressive myocardial damage, ventricular arrhythmias, cardiovascular or unexplained syncope, long QT-interval. |

*See p. 1 for abbreviations and p. 199 for drug information.*

# 3. ANGINA PECTORIS

Rose Anton, M.D.
Carl J. Pepine, M.D.

## I. OVERVIEW

Every year almost a million Americans die from coronary artery disease (CAD)-related events; significant morbidity (myocardial ischemia, LV dysfunction, arrhythmias, and hospitalization) occurs in many others. Clinical manifestations of CAD include sudden death, myocardial infarction, heart failure, and angina pectoris. Angina is caused by transient myocardial ischemia due to either atherosclerotic (> 90%) or nonatherosclerotic CAD (e.g., spasm, coronary artery anomalies). It may be classified into one of several clinical syndromes which impact prognosis and therapy. These include chronic stable angina (fixed or variable threshold), new onset angina, or unstable angina (progressive, rest, or post-infarct angina). In addition, CAD may be accompanied by silent ischemia, which can adversely affect clinical outcome.

## II. EVALUATION AND DIAGNOSIS OF CORONARY ARTERY DISEASE

By determining pretest probability according to symptoms, sex, and age, a rational approach to the evaluation of chest pain can be established (Figure 1). Information from functional (stress) testing is of most value in terms of risk stratification for adverse cardiac events; its use as a diagnostic tool has taken a secondary role.

## Figure 1. Evaluation of Chest Pain

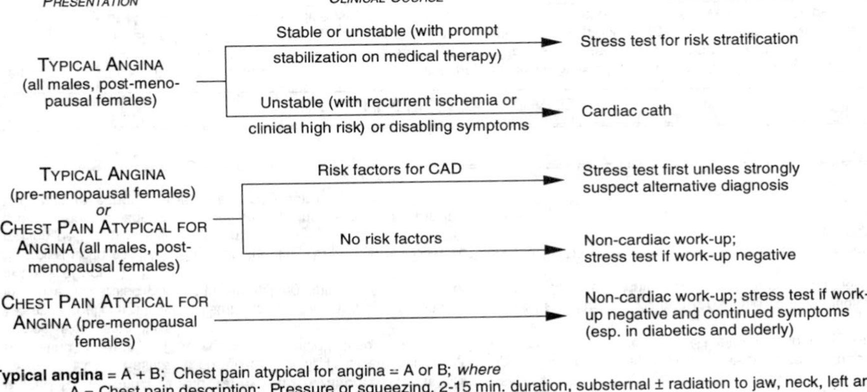


**Typical angina** = A + B; Chest pain atypical for angina = A or B; *where*
A = Chest pain description: Pressure or squeezing, 2-15 min. duration, substernal ± radiation to jaw, neck, left arm
B = Modulating factors: Precipitated by exertion/stress and relieved by rest.

**Stress test** should be performed in absence of antianginals if possible to maximize sensitivity of test. D/C meds and use S.L. nitroglycerin to control symptoms 1d prior to test (3d if long-acting β-blocker used)

**Risk factors:** See bottom p. 22.

**Non-cardiac work-up** based on index of suspicion: Esophageal reflux (Bernstein test, x-ray to detect hiatal hernia, trial of antacids); Esophageal motility disorder (manometry); Peptic ulcer disease (upper GI; trial of $H_2$ blockers); Pancreatitis (amylase/lipase); Gallbladder disease (ultrasound); Musculoskeletal (trial of anti-inflammatory agents); Pulmonary embolus (V/Q scan); Pulmonary hypertension (cardiac echo/cath); Pneumonia (chest x-ray); Pleurisy (chest x-ray, trial of anti-inflammatory agents); Pericarditis (echo, trial of anti-inflammatory agent); MVP (cardiac echo, trial of β-blockers); Psychogenic (trial of anxiolytic, referral to specialist); Cervical radiculopathy (unlikely with normal neurologic exam).

## III. TREATMENT OF CORONARY ATHEROSCLEROSIS: OVERVIEW

- Patients with known or suspected CAD should undergo evaluation to estimate the likelihood of adverse outcome. Subjective complaints of angina do not accurately reflect the true anatomical and functional severity of the atherosclerotic disease process.
- Patients with a **normal or "low risk" stress test result are usually managed medically** based on pathophysiology (i.e., fixed obstruction and/or spasm) and associated conditions (pp. 34-36). Coronary angiography and revascularization are reserved for lifestyle-limiting symptoms refractory to medical therapy.
- Patients with a **"high-risk" stress test result and those with unstable angina refractory to medical therapy are usually referred for coronary angiography and revascularization**. *High-risk findings:*
  - Exercise ECG: Failure to complete 6.5 METs or attain HR > 120 bpm, > 2mm ST depression, post-exercise ST depression persisting > 6 min., ST depression in multiple leads, systolic BP response flat or decreasing, ST elevation in leads without Q waves, exercise-induced VT.
  - Exercise thallium: New redistribution defect at low workload (≤ 6.5 METs or HR ≤ 120 bpm), multiple redistribution defects, increase in cardiac pool of thallium, lung uptake of thallium, redistribution defects remote from infarct zone, redistribution defects in zone of non-Q MI.
  - Exercise echo or RVG: Ejection fraction (EF) ≤ 35%, exercise increase in EF < 5%, multiple new wall motion defects, new wall motion defect(s) at low workload.
  - Dipyridamole or adenosine thallium: Same as exercise thallium.
  - Dobutamine echo: Same as exercise echo.

## A. CHRONIC STABLE ANGINA

| | |
|---|---|
| Overview | One-, two-, and three-vessel disease are each present in 20-30% of patients, while 15% of angiograms are normal. Annual mortality < 4%. Adverse prognostic factors include advanced age, severe angina, abnormal baseline ECG (ST depression, Q waves, LV hypertrophy, intraventricular conduction delay), hypertension, history of MI, peripheral vascular disease, extent of CAD and LV dysfunction, and the severity of inducible ischemia. |

## A. CHRONIC STABLE ANGINA

| | |
|---|---|
| Therapy<br>*General* | • **Identify and control precipitating factors:** PE, GI bleed, sepsis, hyperthyroidism, hypoxemia, anemia, etc.<br>• **Modify risk factors:** Hypertension control, weight reduction, stop cigarette smoking, treat dyslipidemias.<br>• **Modify activity pattern:** Instruct patient to avoid excessive fatigue, take rest periods, modify early morning activities due to an increased tendency for angina to occur in AM (e.g. make bed slowly), minimize exposure to extremes of temperature, eat several smaller meals rather than a few large meals, avoid anxiety-provoking situations, and prophylax against activities known to precipitate angina with nitrates ± an extra dose of a short acting $\beta$-blocker. Consider an individualized exercise prescription based on the results of a symptom-limited exercise test (benefits unproven). |
| *Risk stratify* | **Perform a stress test** off antianginal medications to confirm the diagnosis of ischemic heart disease and to risk stratify. Cardiac catheterization and coronary angiography are indicated for high-risk test results (p. 32). |
| *Stepped-care* | **1) Aspirin:** 160 mg/day or 325 mg every other day (shown to decrease the incidence of death and nonfatal MI).<br>**2) Nitrates:** Sublingual nitroglycerin or inhaled spray to treat episodes or prophylax against activities known to precipitate angina. If angina occurs > 3-4 times/week, longer-acting nitrates (transdermal or oral) should be prescribed. A 10-12 hr nitrate-free interval is needed to minimize nitrate tolerance.<br>**3) Calcium channel blocker (CCB) or $\beta$-blocker** according to the presence of associated conditions (pp. 34-36). In general, $\beta$-blockers are prescribed if an arrhythmia, tachycardia or hypertension is present, while CCB's are prescribed if heart rate is normal or a vasospastic component to the angina is suspected. Monotherapy with nifedipine may cause reflex tachycardia which offsets its beneficial effects, but improves anginal status when added to a $\beta$-blocker. The dose of CCB or $\beta$-blocker should be titrated until the desired response is achieved or side effects develop.<br>**4) Add a CCB when a $\beta$-blocker is chosen initially and visa versa.** Simultaneous use of a $\beta$-blocker (without ISA) and verapamil is not recommended due to the risk of severe bradycardia, AV block, hypotension, and CHF. Some patients benefit from use of more than one CCB (e.g., nifedipine *plus* verapamil or diltiazem). **Be flexible:** As patients develop associated conditions, a change in antianginal strategy may be required (e.g. switch from a $\beta$-blocker to a CCB as peripheral vascular disease progresses).<br>**5)** When ischemic control or lifestyle is unacceptable, refer for **coronary angiography and revascularization**. |

## B. MEDICAL THERAPY OF CHRONIC STABLE ANGINA

| Condition | **β-Blocker vs. CCB†** | Comments |
|---|---|---|
| Arrhythmias, conduction | | |
| *Sinus tachycardia* | **β**-blocker or heart rate slowing CCB (diltiazem or verapamil). | Avoid these agents if tachycardia is due to CHF or hypotension. |
| *Sinus bradycardia* | Dihydropyridine CCB. Alternative: Low dose **β**-blocker with ISA. | If a pacemaker is in place, any **β**-blocker or CCB may be used. |
| *Atrial fibrillation, atrial flutter, or SVT* | **β**-blocker, verapamil, or diltiazem. | **Verapamil is contraindicated when AFIB/flutter conducts over an accessory pathway** |
| *History of ventricular tachycardia (VT)* | **β**-blocker. | **Verapamil may induce fatal hypotension if mistakenly given intravenously during VT.** |
| *AV block* | Dihydropyridine CCB. | Avoid verapamil, diltiazem, and **β**-blockers, all of which may worsen AV block. |
| COPD with bronchospasm, asthma | CCB. Alternative: Low-dose **β**1-selective blocker. | CCB may antagonize hypoxic pulmonary vasoconstriction and worsen gas exchange in severe hypoxic lung disease. |
| Depression, fatigue | CCB. Alternative: Non-lipid soluble **β**-blocker. | Avoid tricyclic antidepressants for at least 6 weeks post MI, and in patients with arrhythmias, heart failure, long QT or resting ST-T changes (↑ risk of proarrhythmia). |
| Diabetes mellitus and hypoglycemia | Diltiazem or verapamil. Alternative: **β**1-selective blocker. | Nonselective **β**-blockers may prevent the recognition of and recovery from hypoglycemia. Nifedipine may exacerbate orthostatic hypotension. Screen for silent ischemia. |
| Heart failure | Dihydropyridine CCB or **β**-blocker with caution. | Second generation CCBs (amlodipine, felodipine) show early promise. |

*† After risk stratification, control of precipitating factors, and nitrates.* *See p. 1 for abbreviations and p. 40 for drug classification.*

## B. MEDICAL THERAPY OF CHRONIC STABLE ANGINA

| Condition | β-Blocker vs. CCB† | Comments |
|---|---|---|
| Hypercholesterolemia | CCB or β-blocker with ISA. | Pindolol may increase HDL-cholesterol levels. |
| Hypertension | β-blocker, labetalol, or CCB. | Nitrates should be used cautiously if diastolic dysfunction is present (may induce hypotension). |
| Hypertrophic obstructive cardiomyopathy | Verapamil and/or β-blockers. Disopyrimide and dual chamber (DDD) pacing may be of value. | Avoid nitrates, nifedipine without β-blockers, and other dihydropyridines (may increase outflow tract obstruction). Angina may be present in the absence of CAD. |
| Peripheral vascular disease | CCB. Alternative: Low-dose β1-selective blocker or β-blocker with ISA. | Nonselective β-blockers may worsen claudication. Screen patients for CAD. |
| Raynaud's phenomenon | Nifedipine. | β-blockers may increase symptoms. |
| Pregnancy | CCB. Alternative: β1-selective blocker. | Warfarin and ACE inhibitors are contraindicated (may cause fetal toxicity). |
| Pulmonary hypertension | CCB. | Preload reduction (nitrates) may precipitate severe hypotension. CCBs may worsen hypoxemia in severe COPD (p. 185). |
| Valvular heart disease<br>*Aortic stenosis* | Mild AS: β-blocker. | If AS is severe, β-blocker and verapamil may cause heart failure, and vasodilators including dihydropyridine CCBs may induce hypotension. Angina may occur in the absence of CAD. |
| *Aortic regurgitation* | Dihydropyridine CCB. | β-blockers may worsen regurgitation. Angina may occur in the absence of CAD. |

*† After risk stratification, control of precipitating factors, and nitrates. See p. 1 for abbreviations and p. 40 for drug classification.*

## B. MEDICAL THERAPY OF CHRONIC STABLE ANGINA

| Condition | β-Blocker vs. CCB† | Comments |
|---|---|---|
| *Mitral stenosis* | β-blocker. Alternative: Verapamil, diltiazem. | Angina does not accurately predict the presence of CAD. |
| *Mitral regurgitation* | Dihydropyridine CCB. | Mitral regurgitation may worsen during angina from episodic papillary muscle dysfunction. |

*† After risk stratification, control of precipitating factors, and nitrates. See p. 40 for drug classification.*

## Figure 2. Evaluation and Management of Chronic Stable Angina or New Onset Angina

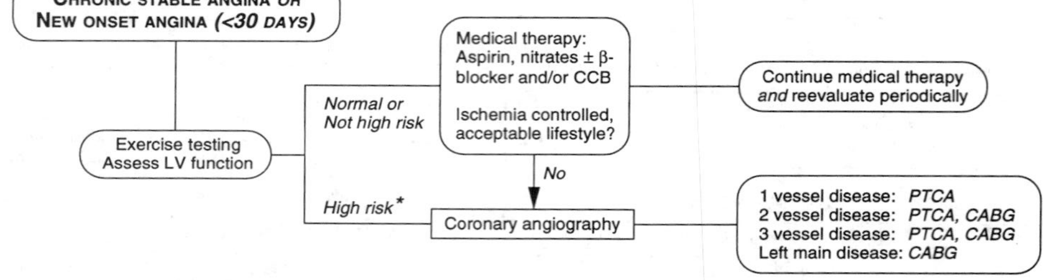


** See p. 32 for high-risk markers*
*CABG = coronary artery bypass grafting; CCB = calcium channel blocker;*
*LV = left ventricular; PTCA = percutaneous transluminal coronary angioplasty*

## C. UNSTABLE ANGINA

| | |
|---|---|
| Overview | • **Pathophysiology:** Ruptured plaque with frequent supervening thromboses and dynamic vasoconstriction.<br>• **Coronary angiography:** Patients without a previous history of MI or angina may have single vessel CAD (40%), 2-vessel CAD (30%), or 3-vessel disease (15%); the angiogram is normal in 10-15%. Among unstable angina patients with previous MI or angina, 50% have 3-vessel disease and 15% have significant left main obstruction.<br>• **Prognosis:** Hospital and one-year mortality ~ 1.5% and < 9% respectively; 5% develop MI within 4-6 weeks and ~ 25% require repeat hospitalization within the first year. |
| Therapy | **Immediate therapy:** Patients with progressive angina without ECG changes or a high-probability of having CAD may be managed as an outpatient according to recent AHCPR Clinical Practice Guidelines (publication no. 94-0602, 1994). Patients with angina at rest, post-infarct angina, or rapidly progressive angina with ECG changes should be managed with hospitalization (in a monitored setting), bed rest, control of precipitating factors, and initiation of medical therapy. The diagnosis is confirmed and MI excluded at this time as well. In-hospital therapy includes:<br>- **Aspirin:** Initiate therapy with 160-325 mg/day of a soluble preparation followed by indefinite therapy with 80-160 mg/day. Shown to ↓ MI and death (Br Med J 1994;308:81).<br>- **Heparin IV:** 5,000-10,000 unit bolus followed by a continuous IV infusion of 10-15 units/kg/hr to maintain ACT at 160-210 seconds or PTT at 1.5-2.5 x control. Shown to ↓ MI and refractory angina (NEJM 1988;319:1105).<br>- **Nitrates IV:** Titrate to prevent recurrent ischemia. Tolerance may develop as early as 24-36 hours.<br>- ***β*-blocker:** Shown to ↓ fatal and nonfatal MI (JAMA 1988;260:2259).<br>• **Nonresponders: Add a calcium channel blocker** (CCB). CCBs have been shown to ↓ recurrent chest pain, although no effect on MI or death has been proven. Avoid monotherapy with nifedipine (Br Heart J 1986;56:400).<br>• **Nonresponders: Urgent coronary angiography and revascularization (PTCA or CABG) ± intra-aortic balloon counterpulsation** (IABP). Efforts should be made to stabilize the patient pharmacologically prior to attempting PTCA. Recent data (TIMI-3B study) suggest that routine cath and PTCA (where appropriate) may improve outcome. Coronary artery bypass grafting has been shown to improve survival for unstable angina patients with 3-vessel disease or significant LV dysfunction (also used for coronary anatomy that is unsuitable for or fails catheter-based intervention). **Thrombolytics should be avoided** (may ↑ bleeding and progression to MI). |

*See p. 1 for abbreviations and p. 40 for drug classification.*

## FIGURE 3. EVALUATION AND MANAGEMENT OF UNSTABLE ANGINA

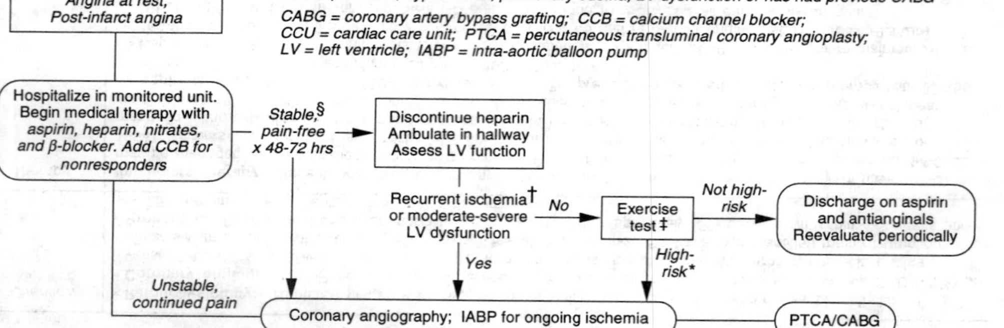


* See p. 32 for high-risk markers

† Thrombolytic therapy of no benefit

§ Routine cath and PTCA/CABG (where appropriate) recently shown to decrease hospital stay, recurrent angina, and rehospitalization days (TIMI-3B trial)

‡ Some advocate triage directly to angioplasty if patient initially presents with marked ST changes in multiple leads, hypotension, pulmonary edema, LV dysfunction or has had previous CABG

CABG = coronary artery bypass grafting; CCB = calcium channel blocker; CCU = cardiac care unit; PTCA = percutaneous transluminal coronary angioplasty; LV = left ventricle; IABP = intra-aortic balloon pump

## D. SILENT ISCHEMIA

| | |
|---|---|
| Overview | While silent ischemia is often uncovered during a screening exercise test or ECG, the first manifestation may be LV dysfunction, arrhythmias or sudden death. Silent ischemia is more common in the morning, in the elderly and in diabetics. At least 15% of Q-wave MIs are totally asymptomatic. Silent ischemia is a risk factor for adverse outcome regardless of whether symptomatic episodes are present. It is currently unknown whether treatment improves prognosis. |
| Therapy | • Prescribe **aspirin** and perform an **exercise stress test** to confirm the diagnosis and risk stratify.<br>• Control precipitating factors, modify risk factors for CAD, and prescribe general activity measures (p. 33).<br>• Consider nitrates, supplemented with calcium channel blockers and/or ***β***-blockers if necessary to prevent recurrent ischemia; exercise testing and/or ambulatory ECG monitoring may be used to assess medical efficacy.<br>• **In the setting of unstable angina or in the post-infarct period, urgent coronary angiography and revascularization** are recommended. Ischemia—either silent or painful—that recurs despite medical therapy identifies the patient at high risk for an adverse clinical outcome. |

## IV. NONATHEROSCLEROTIC CORONARY ARTERY DISEASE

| Etiology | Comments |
|---|---|
| Microvascular angina (Syndrome X) | Syndrome of anginal chest pain and a normal coronary angiogram. Prognosis is excellent. Similar presentation may be found in variant angina, esophageal disorders, mitral valve prolapse, and anxiety (panic) disorder. May respond to nitrates, CCBs, and behavior modification. Aminophylline may be of value for some patients (JACC 1989;14:1450). |
| Variant angina | Anginal pain syndrome caused by transient and unpredictable episodes of epicardial coronary spasm. Most present with **angina at rest and ST elevation**; transient conduction abnormalities and ventricular ectopy/arrhythmia may also occur. Two-thirds of patients have fixed coronary obstruction and exertional angina as well. Recurrent angina and cardiac events occur most often during the first 6 months; MI occurs in up to 20% and death in 10% during this time. A period of stabilization usually occurs |

*See p. 1 for abbreviations and p. 40 for drug classification.*

## IV. NONATHEROSCLEROTIC CORONARY ARTERY DISEASE

| Etiology | Comments |
|---|---|
| Variant angina (cont.) | followed by prolonged or permanent remission (may recur years later). In general, there is an **excellent prognosis for those without significant coronary atherosclerosis.** |
| *Acute severe episode* | **IV nitroglycerin** (100-200 mcg bolus). May require IV verapamil 0.15 mg/kg or diltiazem 0.25 mg/kg, (administered over 2 min.). Antiarrhythmics for ventricular ectopy and atropine/pacemaker for AV block. |
| *Chronic therapy, stepped-care* | **Aspirin and nitrates** (sublingual to treat acute attacks, long-acting preparation to prevent recurrences). For nonresponders, add a **calcium channel blocker** (diltiazem, nifedipine and verapamil appear to be equal in efficacy; treat in maximally tolerated doses). For persistent symptoms, try a different calcium blocker or the combination of 2 or more agents. Prazosin may be of value in some. Consider withdrawing treatment if patient remains asymptomatic for 6 months-1 year. |
| *Additional measures* | Minimize exposure to precipitating factors: cigarettes, cold, emotional distress, and vasoconstrictor drugs (e.g., ephedrine, phenylpropanolamine, amphetamines). Modify cardiovascular risk factors. |
| *If CAD coexists* | **β-blockers** are often of value but should be discontinued if symptoms appear to worsen (may precipitate spasm). In the rare patient with recurrent ischemia refractory to nitrates and calcium blockers who has spasm superimposed on fixed obstruction, **bypass surgery or PTCA** may be considered. Nitrates and calcium blockers should be continued for 6 months after revascularization. |

***Drug classification*** *(see p. 199 for further drug information):*

- **Non-selective β-blockers:** Alprenolol, labetalol, nadolol, oxprenolol, penbutolol, pindolol, propranolol, sotalol, timolol.
- **β-1 selective blockers:** Acebutolol, atenolol, betaxolol, bevantolol, bisoprolol, esmolol, metoprolol, practolol.
- **Lipid-soluble β-blockers:** Propranolol, metoprolol, pindolol.
- **β-blockers with intrinsic sympathomimetic activity (ISA):** Acebutalol, alprenolol, oxprenolol, pindolol, practolol.
- **Non-dihydropyridine calcium channel blockers (CCB):** Verapamil, diltiazem.
- **Dihydropyridine CCB:** Nifedipine, nicardipine, nitrendipine, felodipine, isradipine, amlodipine and others.

# 4. MYOCARDIAL INFARCTION

Cindy L. Grines, M.D.

## I. OVERVIEW

Approximately 1.5 million persons develop myocardial infarction (MI) in the U.S. annually. Complete thrombotic coronary occlusion occurs in 80% of patients with infarction and usually results in transmural myocardial necrosis and Q-waves on ECG (Q-wave MI). Patients with spontaneous reperfusion or well-developed collateral flow are more likely to develop a non-Q-wave (subendocardial) MI, which results in a smaller infarction, better preservation of LV function, and lower in-hospital mortality. However, since non-Q-wave infarctions are "incomplete" (i.e., residual viable myocardium supplied by a diseased coronary artery), reinfarction rates are higher than those observed with Q-wave MI; by 1 year, mortality rates are similar. Therefore, *a more aggressive diagnostic and therapeutic evaluation may be warranted in non-Q-wave MI*. Approximately 15-20% of patients with acute MI expire prior to seeking medical attention and another 15% expire during hospitalization, for an **overall acute mortality rate of 30-35%** (i.e., 140 persons per day). **The majority of in-hospital deaths occur within the first two days; most interventions designed to benefit MI patients are performed acutely**.

## II. TRIAGE BASED ON ECG AND CHEST PAIN DURATION

| ECG† | Lytic | Medical (no lytic) | Acute cath, direct PTCA | Comments |
|---|---|---|---|---|
| ST segment depression | | x | x | Patients who infarct with ST depression have mortality rates of 10-18%, a higher prevalence of multivessel disease, and lower ejection fractions than infarcts without ST elevation. A trend toward ↑ mortality was observed after lytic Rx, which is generally avoided in this setting. |

† If initial ECG does not show ST elevation or LBBB, it should be repeated in 30 minutes.

*See p. 1 for abbreviations and p. 199 for drug information.*

## II. TRIAGE BASED ON ECG AND CHEST PAIN DURATION

| ECG† | Lytic | Medical (no lytic) | Acute cath, direct PTCA | Comments |
|---|---|---|---|---|
| Ischemic T-waves only | | x | | Low risk; no benefit from lytics. Consider echo to screen for regional hypokinesis and cath if a strong clinical suspicion exists. |
| Normal ECG | | x | | If repeated ECGs are entirely normal, the probability of MI is low. |
| ST elevation or LBBB *Less than 6 hours* | x | | x | If lytics are administered within 6 hrs, mortality reduction is 24%. If treated within 1 hr, mortality reduction approaches 50% and MI may actually be aborted. |
| *6-12 hours:* Ongoing pain | x | | x | 17-27% mortality reduction with lytics, regardless of pain status. |
| No pain | x | x | x | Reperfusion therapy is generally reserved for large infarcts (anterior MI or ST elevation in 5 or more leads). If small infarct or patient has ↑ risk of bleeding (elderly, hypertensive, etc.), medical therapy may be appropriate. |
| *12-24 hours:* Ongoing pain | | | x | Ongoing pain suggests viable myocardium. Reperfusion rates with lytics are inversely proportional to time delay; PTCA reperfusion rates are independent of time. |
| No pain | | x | | No proven benefit of lytics. |
| *> 24 hours* | | x | | No proven benefit of lytics but limited data available. |

† If initial ECG does not show ST elevation or LBBB, it should be repeated in 30 minutes.

*See p. 1 for abbreviations and p. 199 for drug information.*

## Figure 1. Triage of Acute Myocardial Infarction

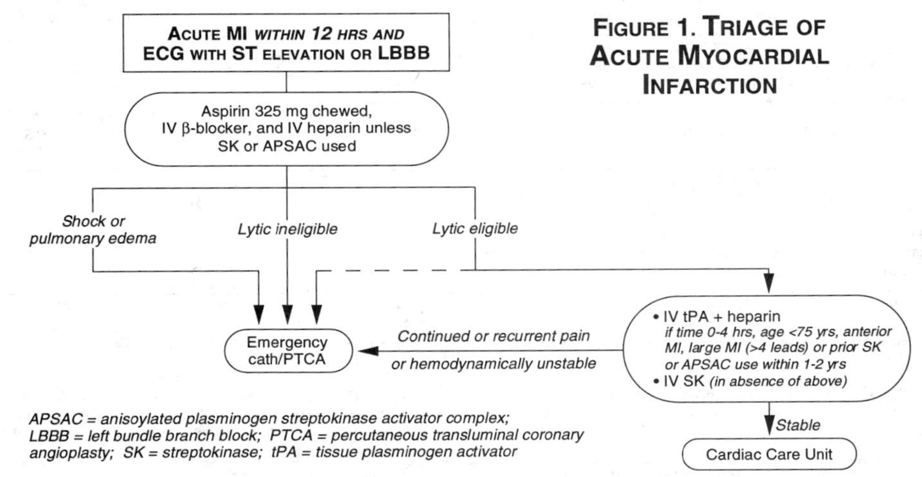


*APSAC = anisoylated plasminogen streptokinase activator complex; LBBB = left bundle branch block; PTCA = percutaneous transluminal coronary angioplasty; SK = streptokinase; tPA = tissue plasminogen activator*

## III. TRIAGE BASED ON ASSOCIATED CONDITIONS IF TIME ≤ 12 HOURS AND ECG DEMONSTRATES ST ELEVATION OR LBBB

Recent trials have shed insight into the preferred method of reperfusion (thrombolytics or angioplasty) for certain patient subgroups, although a consensus of opinion is lacking. Based on available data and personal experience, triage recommendations for acute MI are proposed; in many situations, either thrombolytics or angioplasty may be used. It should be noted that limited or no data exist on the use of thrombolytic therapy for many patient subsets.

| Condition | Lytic | Medical (no lytic) | Acute Cath/ Direct PTCA | Comments |
|---|---|---|---|---|
| Age > 70 years | x | | x | Elderly high in-hospital mortality from MI (20-25%). Despite an increased risk of intracranial bleed following lytics, reperfusion improves overall survival. If lytics are indicated, streptokinase (SK) is preferred over tPA (lower risk of intracranial bleed). Primary PTCA may be preferred to further reduce the risk of intracranial bleeding and to improve survival benefit. |
| Blood pressure<br>*Systolic >200 or diastolic >120 mmHg* | | | x | Avoid lytics--high-risk of intracranial bleed. Limited data. |
| *BP >200/120 to <200/120 with meds* | x | | x | PTCA is preferred. If hypertension can be controlled, SK is acceptable but the risk of intracranial bleed is increased 2-fold. Avoid tPA (highest risk of intracranial bleed). |
| *Systolic < 90 mmHg despite fluids* | x | | x | Hypotensive patients (BP < 100 mmHg) benefit from thrombolysis. Patients with frank cardiogenic shock should undergo direct PTCA; lytics are of no proven benefit. |

*See p. 1 for abbreviations and p. 199 for drug information.*

| Condition | Lytic | Medical (no lytic) | Acute Cath/ Direct PTCA | Comments |
|---|---|---|---|---|
| Previous CABG | x | | x | Poor reperfusion with IV lytics if vein graft is occluded. If cath lab is available, perform acute cath/PTCA; if not, lytics are acceptable since native coronary occlusion may be responsible. |
| Infarct location<br>*Anterior* | x | | x | Early mortality is reduced with lytics compared to placebo. If cath lab is available, acute PTCA may be preferred. |
| *Lateral* | x | | x | Circumflex coronary artery occlusion may present as inferior, lateral, or posterior MI but is electrocardiographically silent in 50% |
| *Inferior, limited* | x | | x | Mortality reduction with reperfusion. |
| *RV infarct* | x | | x | Hypotension is common. Treat as outlined on p. 94. |
| Prior MI | x | | x | High in-hospital mortality (15%). If lytics are used, routine cath and PTCA improve outcome. |
| Pulmonary edema | x | | x | High mortality. Acute cath/PTCA to facilitate reperfusion. Optimize hemodynamics with Swan-Ganz catheter and exclude mechanical defects (acute mitral regurgitation, VSD). |
| Streptokinase, APSAC allergy or prior use | x | | x | Streptokinase antibodies appear within 5 days of treatment and persist 1-2 years; use tPA during this time interval. |
| Bleeding & others<br>*Acute pancreatitis* | | x | x | PTCA is recommended for large MIs. While pancreatitis is an absolute contraindication for lytics, cath may be considered if the diagnosis of pancreatitis vs. MI is uncertain. (Pancreatitis may cause inferior ST elevation). Obtain amylase levels in patients with epigastric pain. |

*See p. 1 for abbreviations and p. 199 for drug information.*

| Condition | Lytic | Medical (no lytic) | Acute Cath/ Direct PTCA | Comments |
|---|---|---|---|---|
| *Aortic dissection suspected* | | | x | Absolute contraindication to lytic therapy. Catheterization may be performed if dissection is suspected to involve the coronaries, thus resulting in MI. Aortic dissection should be suspected if pain radiates to the back, arm BPs are unequal, or mediastinum is widened on chest x-ray. Obtain MRI, CT scan or transesophageal echo to confirm the diagnosis. |
| *Blood dyscrasia* | | | x | Excluded from all lytic trials due to risk of bleeding. |
| *Cerebral aneurysm or neoplasm* | | | x | Absolute contraindication to lytic therapy due to high risk of intracranial bleed. |
| *CPR* | x | | x | Lytics acceptable if CPR is less than 10 min. in duration, neurologic status is intact, and no rib fractures are present. |
| *Diabetic retinopathy* no hemorrhage | x | | x | Fundoscopic examinations not reported in any lytic trials. |
| ⊕ hemorrhage | | | x | PTCA is the preferred approach. Rare cases of retinal bleed with lytics, but not an absolute contraindication in high risk patients. |
| *Head trauma* | | | x | Recent (< 6 months) head trauma resulting in loss of consciousness or skull fracture is an absolute contraindication to lytic therapy. |
| *Hematuria* | x | | x | Avoid lytics if gross hematuria is present. |

*See p. 1 for abbreviations and p. 199 for drug information.*

| Condition | Lytic | Medical (no lytic) | Acute Cath/ Direct PTCA | Comments |
|---|---|---|---|---|
| *Heme ⊕ stool* | | | x | Active bleeding is an absolute contraindication to lytics. Unless there is a history of GI bleeding, rectal exams are usually deferred to avoid vagal reactions and hypotension. |
| *Hemoptysis* | | | x | Avoid lytics unless hemoptysis is due to CHF or pulmonary embolism. |
| *LA or LV thrombus* | | | x | Lytics theoretically should be avoided to prevent partial lysis and embolization of thrombus (note: lytics have been used in some cases of prosthetic valve thrombosis, however). Limited data. |
| *Lumbar puncture* | | | x | Lytics should probably be avoided although no data available. If CSF is bloody, acute cath/PTCA should be avoided due to the need for anticoagulation (unless MI is large). |
| *Menstruating female* | x | | x | No increase in serious bleeding with lytics. |
| *Mitral valve disease with AFIB* | x | | x | Lytics theoretically should be avoided to prevent partial lysis and embolization of clot. Limited data available. |
| *Oral anticoagulation, chronic* | | | x | Lytics may ↑ the risk of intracranial bleeding. Limited data available. |
| *Pericardial friction rub* | | x | | Implies pericarditis is responsible for ST elevation. If MI is still a consideration, cath to confirm and perform PTCA if appropriate. Avoid lytics to ↓ risk of pericardial hemorrhage and tamponade. |
| *Pregnant* | | | x | Shield abdomen and pelvis from radiation. Avoid lytics (possible fetal damage). |

*See p. 1 for abbreviations and p. 199 for drug information.*

| Condition | Lytic | Medical (no lytic) | Acute Cath/ Direct PTCA | Comments |
|---|---|---|---|---|
| *Pregnancy status unknown* | | | x | If there is a high probability of pregnancy, avoid lytics until pregnancy test results are available. |
| Peptic ulcer disease *Active symptoms, ⊖h/o bleed, heme⊖* | x | | x | No data available for patients with active symptoms. |
| *Asymptomatic, h/o bleed, heme ⊖* | x | | x | Generally recommended to avoid lytics if GI bleed has occurred within the last 2 months (not enrolled in any lytic trial). |
| Stroke history *Cerebral infarct* | x | | x | Lytics are acceptable if the stroke is more than 6 months old, however, the risk of intracranial bleeding is increased. |
| *Intracerebral bleed* | | | x | Absolute contraindication to lytics. PTCA is probably acceptable if bleed is more than 6 months old and the MI is large. |
| *Subarachnoid hemorrhage* | | | x | No available data. PTCA may be attempted if the bleed is more than 2 months old, the MI is large, and the source of subarachnoid hemorrhage has been surgically corrected. |
| *Type unknown* | | | x | PTCA is preferred. Lytics are acceptable if the stroke is remote. Do not delay reperfusion therapy awaiting CT scan. |
| Surgery (major) *< 2 weeks* | | | x | Increased risk of major bleed with lytics. |
| *> 2 weeks* | x | | x | PTCA is preferred if surgery has occurred within the past month, but lytics are acceptable if the MI is large. |

*See p. 1 for abbreviations and p. 199 for drug information.*

## IV. THROMBOLYTIC THERAPY

Although acute (90-minute) patency rates differ between agents, 3-hour patency rates are similar among all lytic drugs. Until recently, large randomized trials suggested that all agents were similar at improving LV function and reducing mortality. Recent data using a new accelerated dosing regimen of tPA with concomitant IV heparin suggested a 1% mortality benefit for tPA as compared to streptokinase (SK). However, in 3 separate trials, tPA had a significantly higher rate of intracranial bleeding compared to SK. Based on the available data, I believe **tPA should be used if any of the following circumstances are present:**

- **Early presentation (< 4 hrs)**
- **MI is either large (> 4 ECG leads with ST elevation) or anterior MI in location**
- **Age under 75 years**
- **History of prior SK or APSAC use in the past 1-2 years**

### A. THROMBOLYTIC REGIMENS

| Thrombolytic Agent | Dosage | Acute patency | Systemic lysis | Need for heparin | Allergy | Cost† |
|---|---|---|---|---|---|---|
| Streptokinase (SK) | 1.5 million units (MU) IV over 30-60 min. | 50% | Yes | No | Yes | $300 |
| Urokinase (UK) | 1.5 MU IV bolus & 1.5 MU IV over 1 hr | 70% | Yes | ? | No | $2000 |
| Anistreplase (anisoylated plasminogen streptokinase activator complex; APSAC) | 30 U IV bolus over 3-5 min | 70% | Yes | No | Yes | $1700 |
| Tissue plasminogen activator (tPA) | 100 mg maximum: 15 mg bolus *and* 0.75 mg/kg over 30 min *and* 0.5 mg/kg over next 60 min | 80% | No | Yes | No | $2300 |

† Pharmacy cost at William Beaumont Hospital

*See p. 1 for abbreviations and p. 199 for drug information.*

## B. MANAGEMENT OF LYTIC COMPLICATIONS

| Complication | Therapy |
|---|---|
| Bleeding, minor | Local compression (puncture site, oral, nasal). |
| Bleeding, major (GI, intracranial) | *Any focal neurological deficit or significant deterioration in mental status should be presumed to be an intracranial hemorrhage until CT scan results are available.* Order STAT hemoglobin, hematocrit, platelets, PT/PTT and fibrinogen. Treat before results are available: Discontinue lytic, heparin, and aspirin. **Administer protamine sulfate** (50 mg IV over 1-3 min) to reverse heparin's effects, **packed RBCs** for hypotension or a hematocrit < 25%, and **cryoprecipitate** (10 units IV) if the fibrinogen is suspected to be low (within 6-8 hrs after tPA, 30 hrs after SK or urokinase, 36 hrs after APSAC). If bleeding persists, repeat IV cryoprecipitate, give 2 units of **fresh frozen plasma**, and consider use of epsilon-**aminocaproic acid** (5 gm over 1 hr). For refractory bleeding, consider platelet transfusions even if the platelet count is normal. |
| Fever | Aspirin or acetaminophen. |
| Hypotension | IV fluids. Slow or temporarily discontinue SK or APSAC; resume when BP > 90 mmHg. Not an allergic reaction unless associated with anaphylaxis. |
| Rash | Stop SK or APSAC. Administer benadryl (50 mg IV or PO). Add steroids if severe (hydrocortisone 100 mg IV q 6 hrs). If full lytic dose was not received, consider 50 mg tPA or acute cath/PTCA. |
| Anaphylaxis | See pp. 97-98. |
| Rigors | Demerol (25 mg IV). |
| Arrhythmias | • **Bradycardia, 3°AV block**: Occurs most commonly with reperfusion of inferior MI. Usually resolves within minutes. Treat with atropine and fluids. Transcutaneous pacer is rarely needed.<br>• **Bezold-Jarish reflex**: Bradycardia & hypotension (usually in response to sudden reperfusion of RCA). Treat with atropine and fluids. May require temporary pacer. Vasopressors for persistent hypotension/bradycardia: Metaraminol (0.5-5 mg IV bolus), norepinephrine (0.5-30 mcg/min IV), phenylephrine (0.2 mg slow IV push). |

*See p. 1 for abbreviations and p. 199 for drug information.*

## B. MANAGEMENT OF LYTIC COMPLICATIONS

| Complication | Therapy |
|---|---|
| Arrhythmias (cont.) | • **Idioventricular rhythm**: No treatment necessary if rate < 120 bpm and no hypotension.<br>• **Ventricular tachycardia**: Nonsustained VT: Runs are common and usually subside with time; observe for 10 min. before starting lidocaine. Sustained VT or VF: Defibrillation and start IV lidocaine. |

## V. ACUTE MI: MEDICAL THERAPY

| ACUTE TREATMENT (beneficial) | ACUTE TREATMENT (potentially detrimental) |
|---|---|
| • Thrombolytic agents<br>• Aspirin<br>• Heparin: intravenous if tPA used or anterior MI; low dose subcutaneous heparin in others<br>• Intravenous nitrates<br>• Intravenous $\beta$-blockers | • Nifedipine<br>• Prophylactic lidocaine |
| **CHRONIC TREATMENT (beneficial)** | **CHRONIC TREATMENT (potentially detrimental)** |
| • Aspirin<br>• Warfarin, if aspirin is not used or LV thrombus present<br>• ß-blockers<br>• ACE inhibition if ejection fraction < 40%<br>• Diltiazem or verapamil if non Q-wave MI without heart failure | • Calcium channel blockers if pulmonary congestion is present<br>• Prophylactic antiarrhythmics (Class I agents) |

*See p. 1 for abbreviations and p. 199 for drug information.*

## V. ACUTE MI: MEDICAL THERAPY

| Agent | Dosage | Comments |
|---|---|---|
| ACE inhibitor | Captopril (initial dose: 6.25, titrate to 50 mg po bid-tid as tolerated), ramipril (2.5-5 mg po bid), lisinopril (10 mg po qd); others are probably as effective. Start at low-dose within a few days of MI, titrate up, continue indefinitely. | Indications: Clinical evidence of heart failure; asymptomatic patients post-MI with ejection fractions < 40%. Shown to reduce short and long term mortality. |
| Anticoagulation<br>*Acute* | • SQ heparin: 5,000-12,500 units q 12 hrs.<br>• IV heparin: Bolus 100 units/kg followed by an infusion of 1,000-1,300 units/hr (adjust to achieve PTT 2-2.5 x normal). | • Indications for IV heparin: Concurrently with tPA; continue for 5-7 days to reduce reocclusion rates. Also for patients with anterior MI, low cardiac output, AFIB or LV thrombus.<br>• All other patients should receive low-dose SQ heparin during periods of immobilization to reduce the risk of DVT and PE.<br>• Contraindications: Active bleeding. |
| *Chronic* | Warfarin (INR 2.5-4.5). | Indications: Patients with LV thrombus or chronic risk of thromboembolic complications (AFIB, low cardiac output, prolonged immobilization). Contraindications: Active bleeding. Longterm anticoagulation has been shown to reduce the rate of recurrent MI & death (NEJM 1990;323:147), however, its role compared to aspirin alone awaits definition. |
| Antiarrhythmics<br>*Acute*<br>*(Lidocaine)* | Loading dose (IV bolus 1 mg/kg followed by 0.5 mg/kg bolus 10 min later); infusion rate 1-4 mg/min; ↓ dose for the elderly and patients with CHF. | Indications: Sustained VT or recurrent, hemodynamically-significant nonsustained VT. ***Prophylactic* lidocaine is not recommended** due to a 38% increase in mortality, which is primarily due to asystole (Circulation 1990;82:II-117). |

*See p. 1 for abbreviations and p. 199 for drug information.*

## V. ACUTE MI: MEDICAL THERAPY

| Agent | Dosage | Comments |
|---|---|---|
| Antiarrhythmics *Chronic* | Not recommended unless sustained VT develops more than 48 hours after MI. | Suppression of chronic PVCs following acute MI with encainide or flecainide has been shown to increase mortality (NEJM 1989;321:406). Amiodarone may be of benefit to patients ineligible for ß-blockers (JACC 1992;20:1056) and for those with complex ectopy (JACC 1990;16:1711). Defibrillator trials in progress. |
| Aspirin | 160-324 mg chewed acutely then po daily: start immediately and continue indefinitely. | Indications: All MI patients. Contraindications: Active bleeding. Acute therapy shown to reduce reinfarction, stroke and death (Lancet 1988;II-349); longterm therapy shown to decrease reinfarction and death (Br Med J 1988;296:320). |
| **β**-blocker *Acute* | Metoprolol (5 mg IV q 2 min x 3, followed in 15 min by 50 mg po bid x 2, and then 100 mg po bid if tolerated), atenolol (5-10 mg IV followed by 100 mg po qd) or other IV ß-blockers without ISA. | Indications: All MI patients except those with hypotension, AV block, bradycardia, severe heart failure, or a history of bronchospasm. Shown to reduce infarct size and mortality by 13% (Prog Cardiovasc Dis 1985;27:335), VF and cardiac rupture (Lancet 1984;2:883). Also shown to reduce reinfarction and intracranial hemorrhage after lytics (Circulation 1991;83:422). |
| *Chronic* ***β*****-** *blocker* | Start acutely and continue at least 2 yrs: Propranolol 60 mg tid-qid, timolol 20 mg qd, or others (no difference between nonselective and selective agents, although **β**-blockers without ISA appear to be more effective than those with ISA. | Indications: All MI patients unless low risk subset. Longterm **β**-blockade reduces the rate of reinfarction and death (primarily sudden death) up to 6 years after MI (JAMA 1982;247:1707). If the patient is revascularized, asymptomatic, and does not have exercise-induced ischemia, some cardiologists withhold **β**-blockers. Contraindications: Symptomatic bradycardia, heart block, asthma. |

*See p. 1 for abbreviations and p. 199 for drug information.*

## V. ACUTE MI: MEDICAL THERAPY

| Agent | Dosage | Comments |
|---|---|---|
| Calcium channel blocker | Diltiazem 90 mg q 6 hrs or verapamil 120 mg tid; start early (2-5 days) and continue for 1 year. | **Indications**: **Non-Q-wave MI**. **Contraindications: Heart failure or severe LV dysfunction**. Studies: *Diltiazem* decreased early reinfarction and recurrent angina in non-Q-wave MI but increased mortality if CHF or severe LV dysfunction was present (NEJM 1988;319:385); *Verapamil* showed a trend toward decreased reinfarction but had a marginal effect on mortality (Am J Cardiol 1990;66:33); *Nifedipine* increased recurrent infarction and death (Circulation 1990;82:II-117) and is contraindicated in all MI patients unless a ß-blocker is also given. |
| Magnesium sulfate | Not recommended. | May ↓ ventricular arrhythmias (Circulation 1992;86:774) but no impact on mortality (ISIS-4, unpublished) despite earlier suggestive studies. |
| Morphine | 2-5 mg IV q 5-30 min for pain. | In addition to its analgesic properties, morphine dilates peripheral venous and arterial beds, thereby reducing both preload and afterload. Avoid in COPD due to the risk of respiratory depression. Adverse effects can be reversed with *naloxone* (0.4-2.0 mg IV). |
| Nitroglycerin *Acute* | 10-20 mcg/min IV, increase by 5-10 mcg/min q 5 min until BP falls by 10% (30% if hypertensive). | IV nitroglycerin may decrease infarct size and mortality if given within 4 hrs of anterior MI (Lancet 1988;1:1088). Avoid in hypotension or RV infarction. **Tolerance may occur after 1 day** of continuous therapy. |
| *Chronic* | Oral/topical nitrates are not routinely recommended. | Oral nitrates given at day 1 post-MI did not alter mortality at 1 month (ISIS-4 & GISSI-3, unpublished). |
| Oxygen | 1-4 liters nasal cannula. | Given by convention but no clear data to support routine use. May actually increase coronary vascular resistance. Pulse oximetry to determine need. |

*See p. 1 for abbreviations and p. 199 for drug information.*

## VI. ACUTE MI: NON-MEDICAL THERAPIES

| Modality | Indications | Comments |
|---|---|---|
| Transfer to facility equipped for PTCA and CABG | • Persistent chest pain after thrombolysis<br>• Recurrent chest pain<br>• Hemodynamic instability: CHF, hypotension, shock<br>• Suspected mechanical defects (VSD, acute MR)<br>• Recurrent VT/VF which is difficult to control | Arrhythmias, hypotension, and bleeding that develop during transfer have been effectively treated with low mortality rates. |
| Pulmonary artery (Swan-Ganz) catheterization | • Hypotension unresponsive to fluids<br>• Unexplained tachycardia, tachypnea, hypoxemia or acidosis<br>• Moderate LV failure (rales 1/3 up lung fields)<br>• Suspicion of VSD or acute mitral regurgitation | Swan-Ganz catheter allows determination of wedge pressure, cardiac output and systemic vascular resistance, which can be used to distinguish the etiology of hypotension (See Ch. 7) and guide therapy. |
| Temporary pacemaker<br>*Prophylactic* | • New LBBB<br>• Bifascicular block: RBBB with left anterior or left posterior fascicular block<br>• Alternating LBBB and RBBB | Usually left in place for 48-72 hrs to prevent hemodynamic collapse should 3° AV block develop. Transcutaneous leads are quickly placed and avoid bleeding complications if thrombolytics or anticoagulants are given. |
| *Therapeutic* | • Asystole<br>• Mobitz II 2° AV block<br>• 3° AV block<br>• Bradycardia with hypotension<br>Exception: Pacing may not be required if bradycardia or 3° AV block occurs with inferior MI and resolves with atropine. | If hemodynamically unstable, a transcutaneous lead may be needed until a transvenous lead can be placed. **AV sequential pacing may be preferred** over ventricular pacing in severe LV diastolic dysfunction and RV infarction; optimization of AV synchrony may increase cardiac output. |

*See p. 1 for abbreviations and p. 199 for drug information.*

## VI. ACUTE MI: NON-MEDICAL THERAPIES

| Modality | Indications | Comments |
|---|---|---|
| Primary PTCA (instead of thrombolysis) | • Indications based on ECG, chest pain duration, and associated conditions: See pp. 41-48.<br>• Thrombolytic exclusion due to bleeding risk<br>• Cardiogenic shock<br>• Patients with prior CABG if vein graft is suspected culprit | In *lytic eligible* patients, use of primary PTCA reduces recurrent ischemia, reinfarction, stroke, shortens length of hospital stay, and reduces mortality in high risk subsets (elderly, anterior MI) (NEJM 1993;328:673). For patients with cardiogenic shock, primary PTCA improves survival from 20% (medical therapy alone) to 50% |
| PTCA post-lytic<br>*Immediate PTCA (vessel patent)* | • Continued or recurrent ischemia<br>• Hemodynamic instability or shock | Routine immediate PTCA should not be performed if thrombolytics restore vessel patency unless there is evidence of ongoing ischemia. |
| *Rescue PTCA (vessel occluded - failed thrombolysis)* | Continued pain and ECG changes 90-120 minutes after starting thrombolytic, particularly if:<br>- Large MI, especially anterior<br>- Hemodynamic instability<br>- Prior MI or impaired non-infarct zone function | Rescue PTCA improves clinical outcome and regional LV function. Vigorous anticoagulation, adjunctive urokinase or streptokinase, and/or IABP is recommended to reduce high reocclusion rates. |
| *Delayed PTCA (2-7 days after thrombolysis)* | • Spontaneous or provokable ischemia<br>• History of prior MI | Routine performance of delayed PTCA for patent vessels is not recommended. However, delayed PTCA reduces mortality if there is a history of prior MI (Circulation 1992;85:1254). |

*See p. 1 for abbreviations and p. 199 for drug information.*

## VI. ACUTE MI: NON-MEDICAL THERAPIES

| Modality | Indications | Comments |
|---|---|---|
| Intra-aortic balloon pump (IABP) | Cardiogenic shock or CHF not responding promptly to therapy; refractory post-MI angina; mechanical defects (MR, VSD); failed thrombolysis; suboptimal flow post-PTCA; critical 3-vessel or left main disease with LV dysfunction. | IABP improves coronary perfusion (augmentation of diastolic BP) and improves cardiac output and filling pressures (afterload reduction of LV). IABP may reduce reocclusion of infarct vessel and may enhance coronary patency following thrombolysis. |
| Surgery | Failed PTCA with persistent pain or hemodynamic instability (if surgery can be performed within 6-8 hrs); left main disease; proximal 3-vessel disease with a patent infarct vessel, especially if unsuitable for PTCA; acute mitral regurgitation or ventricular septal rupture. | Perioperative mortality: CABG alone 4-5%, CABG in setting of acute MR 10%, CABG + VSD repair from anterior MI 20% and from posterior MI 70% (more difficult operation). When surgery is performed during a lytic state, there is a 4% risk of reoperation for bleeding. |

## VII. RISK STRATIFICATION POST-MI

- The identification of high risk patients and aggressive utilization of revascularization strategies has improved clinical outcomes. Poor prognostic features include *clinical variables* (advanced age, diabetes, hypotension, heart rate > 100 bpm, CHF, large infarction [> 4 leads with ST elevation], frequent PVCs or VT > 48 hrs from MI) and *angiographic variables* (ejection fraction < 40%, LV hypokinesis in areas remote from current infarction, LV aneurysm, persistent occlusion or suboptimal flow in the infarct vessel, saphenous vein graft occlusion, and mechanical defects such as VSD, acute MR, and cardiac rupture).
- Stress testing (exercise or pharmacologic) and electrophysiology studies have further identified high-risk patients. The most appropriate methods for risk stratification post-MI have not been well tested and many physicians use different approaches. Suggested approaches to the management of patients post-MI are outlined in Figures 2 and 3.

*See p. 1 for abbreviations and p. 199 for drug information.*

## Figure 2. Risk Stratification of MI Survivors: *Cath vs Non-Invasive Evaluation for Coronary Disease**

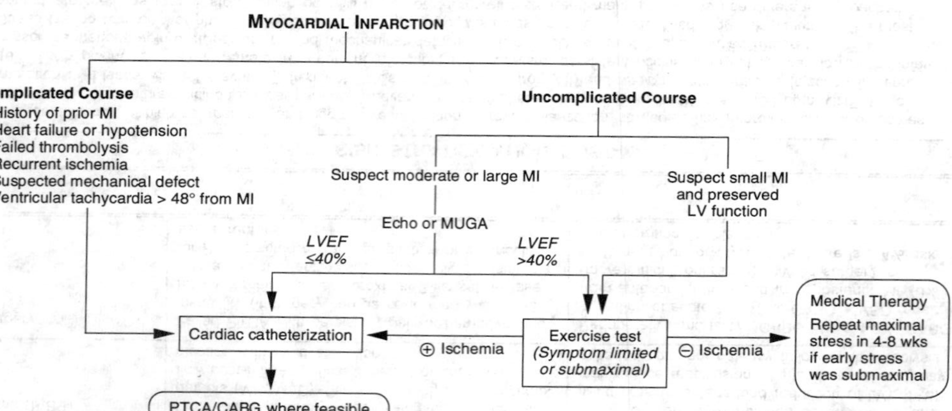


** Some would advocate routine performance of cath to eliminate repetitive, costly, non-invasive testing.*
*CABG = coronary artery bypass grafting; MUGA; multigated acquisition scan; MI = myocardial infarction;*
*PTCA = percutaneous transluminal coronary angioplasty*

**Figure 3. Risk Stratification of MI Survivors:** ***Screening and Evaluation for Arrhythmias***

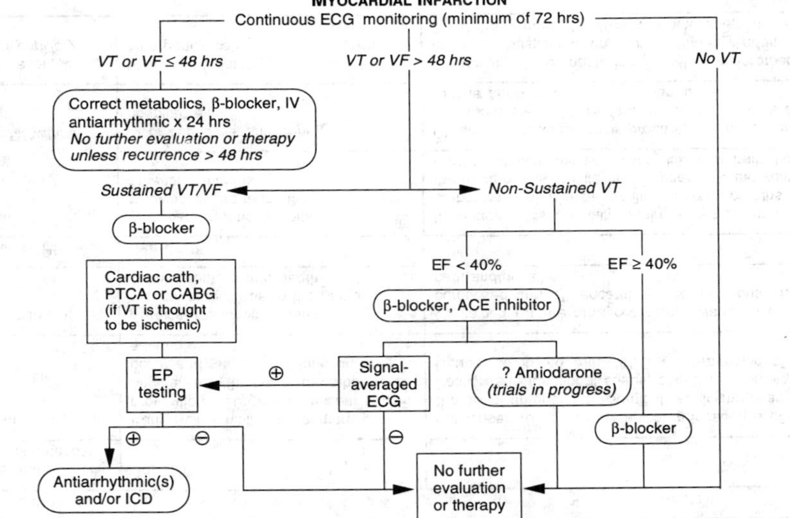


*MI = myocardial infarction; VT = ventricular tachycardia; VF = ventricular fibrillation; ACE = angiotensin converting enzyme; EP = electrophysiology; ICD = internal cardioverter-defibrillator; EF = ejection fraction*

## VIII. COMPLICATIONS OF ACUTE MI

| Complication | Therapy | Comments |
|---|---|---|
| Arrhythmias and conduction disturbances | See Ch. 5. | |
| LV aneurysm | Early ACE inhibitor for primary prevention. Surgical resection if CHF, angina, arrhythmias or thromboemboli occur and residual LV function is adequate. | Incidence: 10%. Usually apical in location & develops within 3 mos. of anterior MI. Surgical repair improves ejection fraction and functional status; operative mortality 10%. Usually combined with CABG ± EP-mapping of arrhythmia. |
| LV pseudoaneurysm | Surgical resection is usually recommended due to the risk of cardiac rupture and death. | Contained rupture of myocardium: Narrow base; wall composed only of pericardium and thrombus. Diagnosed by cath and/or echo. |
| LV dysfunction/CHF | See Ch. 8. | |
| LV thrombus | IV heparin during hospitalization followed by warfarin (INR 2.0-3.0) for at least 3 months. | Incidence: 20%. Usually within 5 days of anterior MI. Risk of embolization is highest within the first 3 months, especially if the thrombus is mobile or protrudes into the ventricle. Anticoagulation decreases the risk of embolization. |
| *Anterior MI without thrombus* | IV or sub-Q heparin during hospitalization. | Chronic anticoagulation is probably not necessary unless the EF is less than 30% or AFIB is present. Some advocate routine anticoagulation for 3 months. |
| Mitral regurgitation, acute *Ruptured papillary muscle* | IABP, vasodilators, inotropes, emergency cath and surgery (see p. 95). | Incidence: 1%, primarily inferior MI's (posteromedial papillary muscle). Suspect when acute pulmonary edema develops at 2-7 d. Early mortality: 70% with medicine, 10% with surgery. |

*See p. 1 for abbreviations and p. 199 for drug information.*

## VIII. COMPLICATIONS OF ACUTE MI

| Complication | Therapy | Comments |
|---|---|---|
| Mitral regurgitation (cont.)<br>*Papillary muscle dysfunction* | Vasodilators followed by PTCA or CABG. | More common in inferior MI. May be persistent or transient due to intermittent ischemia. If MR is due to papillary muscle ischemia without rupture, PTCA may be of benefit. |
| Pericarditis<br>*Acute* | Aspirin + analgesics. Use nonsteroidal anti-inflammatory agents sparingly (may impair MI healing and ↑ coronary vascular resistance). | Incidence: ≤ 10%. Most common 2-4 days after Q-wave MI. Tamponade infrequent. *Relative* contraindication for anticoagulation and an *absolute* contraindication for thrombolysis. |
| *Dresslers syndrome* | Nonsteroidal anti-inflammatory agents. Steroids (tapered over 2-4 weeks) if nonsteroidal agents fail. | Immunologic reaction occuring 1-12 wks after MI. Incidence: 1%. Symptoms include fever, chest pain, polyserositis, pericardial and pleural effusions. Recurrences common. May progress to constriction. |
| Post-infarct angina | IV heparin (if resting angina) + **β**-blocker followed by catheterization and PTCA or CABG. | Post-infarct angina occurs more frequently after thrombolysis (30%) than after primary PTCA (10%). Associated with increased reinfarction and death. |
| Reinfarction | Resume IV heparin followed by acute PTCA. Consider second dose of lytics if first dose given > 48 hrs earlier. Avoid SK or APSAC if administered previously. | Occurs more frequently after lytic therapy and in non-Q-wave MI. Associated with increased mortality. Preventive therapy includes aspirin and/or **β**-blocker. |
| Right ventricular (RV) infarct | See p. 94. | May produce hypotension and shock despite preserved LV function. Diagnosis: ECG (ST elevation in right precordial leads), echo (hypokinetic or akinetic RV). |

*See p. 1 for abbreviations and p. 199 for drug information.*

## VIII. COMPLICATIONS OF ACUTE MI

| Complication | Therapy | Comments |
|---|---|---|
| Rupture, free wall | Emergency pericardiocentesis followed by thoracotomy and surgical repair. | Incidence: 1-3%. Most common several days after a large anterior Q-wave infarction. Shock, electromechanical dissociation, and signs of tamponade occur suddenly; death is often immediate. Early reperfusion and the use of ***β***-blockers decrease the risk of rupture, whereas the risk is increased following late (> 12 hrs) lytic therapy. Mortality rates, even with surgery, are extremely high. |
| Shock | See p. 94. | Incidence 5-8% within the first days. Mortality rates range from 65%-90%. |
| Ventricular septal rupture | IABP, vasodilators; emergency cardiac catheterization and surgical repair. See p. 96. | Incidence: 0.5-2%, usually 3-5 days post MI. Suspect in all MI patients who develop a new systolic murmur. Mortality with medical therapy alone is 90%. Surgical mortality is 30% for VSD and anterior MI, 70% for VSD and inferior MI (technically more difficult operation). Early surgical intervention is recommended for patients with unstable hemodynamics or end-organ dysfunction. If the patient is stable, optimal timing of surgery is controversial: some surgeons advocate delaying surgical repair ≥ 3 weeks. |

*See p. 1 for abbreviations and p. 199 for drug information.*

# 5. CARDIAC ARRHYTHMIAS AND CONDUCTION DISTURBANCES

John P. DiMarco, M.D., Ph.D.

## I. ATRIAL ARRHYTHMIAS

| Arrhythmia | Therapy |
|---|---|
| Sinus tachycardia | Therapy is directed at the underlying cause (e.g., hypovolemia, anemia, fever, hyperthyroidism). If heart rate itself is deleterious (e.g., angina), **$\beta$**-blockers are usually the best form of therapy. However, if **drug therapy** is used to slow *reflex* tachycardia (hypovolemia) or *compensatory* tachycardia (LV dysfunction), it **may precipitate severe hypotension and heart failure**, respectively. |
| Sinus bradycardia | Should not be treated unless it produces hypotension, is clearly associated with symptoms (angina, syncope, heart failure), or provokes ventricular arrhythmias. Treatment: See bradycardia algorithm, p. 85. |
| Atrial premature depolarization | Therapy is usually not required. If highly symptomatic, use a **$\beta$**-blocker. Class IA antiarrhythmics may suppress APD's, but side effects are common. If APD's triggers AFIB or SVT, use a Class IA agent ± AV nodal blocker. |
| Multifocal atrial tachycardia | Optimize cardiopulmonary status. Rate control is very difficult; metoprolol, verapamil and amiodarone may be effective but data are inconclusive. **Cardioversion is of no value.** |
| SVT<br>*AV node re-entry* | • Most common type of SVT (60%). ECG shows a narrow QRS, a rate of 150-250 bpm (usually 180-200 bpm), and a P-wave that is either buried in or immediately follows the QRS (i.e., RP interval < 90 msec).<br>• Acute treatment: *Stepped-care*: (1) Vagal maneuvers (valsalva, carotid sinus massage); (2) IV adenosine, verapamil, or diltiazem (if heart failure is evident, IV digoxin should be used instead of a calcium channel blocker); and (3) procainamide or propafenone.<br>• Chronic prevention: Vagal maneuvers alone are usually sufficient if episodes are infrequent, well-tolerated, and short-lived. Catheter ablation (curative in 95%) or drug therapy (AV nodal blocker) is required if SVT occurs at very fast rates, results in syncope, requires cardioversion, occurs frequently, or is of long duration. A Class IA or IC agent is usually added for persistent symptoms. |

*See p. 1 for abbreviations, p. 75 for classification of antiarrhythmics, and p. 199 for drug information.*

| Arrhythmia | Therapy |
|---|---|
| SVT (cont.) | |
| *AV re-entry* | See Wolff-Parkinson-White Syndrome (pp. 72-73). |
| *Sinus node re-entry* | Rare type of SVT. ECG looks identical to sinus tachycardia.<br>• Acute treatment: Vagal maneuvers, adenosine, verapamil or diltiazem.<br>• Chronic prevention: Verapamil. The role of catheter ablation awaits definition. |
| *Intra-atrial re-entry* | 5% of SVTs. ECG looks identical to automatic atrial tachycardia.<br>• Acute treatment: Procainamide, pacing, or cardioversion.<br>• Chronic prevention: Amiodarone. The role of catheter ablation is unknown. |
| *Automatic atrial tach* | Rare type of SVT in adults.<br>• Acute treatment is directed at the underlying cause. ***β***-blocker may be of value.<br>• Chronic prevention: Role of catheter ablation is unknown. |
| Atrial flutter | Any narrow QRS tachycardia at a rate of 150 bpm should be assumed to be atrial flutter. In response to carotid sinus massage, a gradual increase in AV block and flutter waves are often evident.<br>• Acute therapy: **Cardioversion** using 50-100-200-360 joules (stable rate control is usually difficult to maintain with drugs). **Rapid atrial pacing** is of value especially when cardioversion is contraindicated (e.g., digitalis intoxication). Drug therapy (AV nodal blocker followed by either a Class IA, IC or III agent) is primarily used *in conjunction* with DC shock or rapid atrial pacing to increase conversion rates and maintain sinus rhythm. When drug therapy is used, monitor for an increase in ventricular rate as atrial rate slows (1:1 conduction).<br>**Anticoagulation is not required** prior to electrical or chemical cardioversion, pacing, or drugs. Consider insertion of a temporary pacemaker prior to cardioversion when > 2:1 block is present; these patients may have underlying sick sinus syndrome (p. 72) and manifest high-grade sinus or AV nodal block immediately after successful cardioversion.<br>• **Chronic prevention: Class IA, IC, or III antiarrhythmic**. For nonresponders with severe symptoms, either permanent antitachycardia pacing alone or catheter ablation ± permanent ventricular pacing is recommended. Surgical therapy is considered investigational. |

*See p. 1 for abbreviations, p. 75 for classification of antiarrhythmics, and p. 199 for drug information.*

## ATRIAL FIBRILLATION (AFIB)

| | |
|---|---|
| Overview | More than 1 million people in the U.S. have AFIB, which is associated with a 5-7 fold increase in stroke rate, a decrease in functional capacity (owing to the loss of atrial kick), and an increase in the risk of bleeding (from chronic anticoagulation). Common associations include rheumatic mitral disease, hypertension, ischemic heart disease, and thyrotoxicosis; others conditions include MI, COPD, pulmonary embolism, hypokalemia, pericarditis, atrial septal defect, heart failure, alcohol binging, and idiopathic. |
| Special subsets | • AFIB with a **slow ventricular response:** May have **sick sinus syndrome**. Severe bradyarrhythmias, sinoatrial and/or AV nodal block may occur during cardioversion; a temporary pacemaker should therefore be kept on standby.<br>• AFIB with **regular ventricular response:** Usually due to **digitalis toxicity** where it actually represents complete AV block with junctional tachycardia. Cardioversion with DC shock is contraindicated.<br>• AFIB with **wide QRS:** Due to the presence of either a bundle branch block (preexistent or rate-dependent), aberrancy, or a preexcited QRS (**Wolff-Parkinson-White syndrome**). |
| Outpatient management | May be considered for patients with absent or mild symptoms, especially when LV function is normal. If episodes are short-lived and well-tolerated, rest and sedation may be all that is required. Otherwise, treatment is based on *ventricular rate*:<br>• Rate > 100 bpm: Oral AV nodal blocker, anticoagulation with warfarin X 3 weeks (INR 2.0-3.0), and then hospitalization for elective cardioversion (p. 66).<br>• Rate < 100 bpm: Anticoagulation with warfarin x 3 weeks (INR 2.0-3.0) followed by hospitalization for elective cardioversion. |
| Inpatient management | Required for all patients with moderate-to-severe symptoms. Should also be considered for patients with mild symptoms when significant LV dysfunction or other serious medical conditions exist.<br>• AFIB < 2 days old: Rate control and cardioversion during the same admission.<br>• AFIB > 2 days old: Rate control and anticoagulation during the initial hospitalization, continue medications at home for at least 3 weeks, and then rehospitalize for elective cardioversion. |

*See p. 1 for abbreviations, p. 75 for classification of antiarrhythmics, and p. 199 for drug information.*

## ATRIAL FIBRILLATION (AFIB)

| | |
|---|---|
| Acute therapy<br>*Rate control* | *Continuous ECG monitoring* is recommended while **digoxin, β-blocker, verapamil, or diltiazem** is titrated to a ventricular rate of 60-90 bpm. Advantages of β-blockers and calcium blockers over digoxin include faster rate control when IV preparations are used (15-30 minutes vs. hours), safer cardioversion, and better rate control during exercise and stress. When digoxin is used, higher-than-usual doses and serum levels are often required. For **nonresponders, combine 2 AV nodal agents** (monitor for AV block or bradyarrhythmias upon conversion to sinus rhythm) **or use a Class IC** antiarrhythmic. |
| *Anticoagulation* | • AFIB < 2 days old: Cardioversion may be attempted *without* prior anticoagulation.<br>• AFIB > 2 days old: Requires at least 3 weeks of warfarin (INR 2.0-3.0) *prior to and following* elective chemical or electrical cardioversion to minimize systemic embolization. If transesophageal echocardiography demonstrates the absence of atrial clot, one report suggested that prolonged anticoagulation may not be necessary prior to cardioversion (NEJM 1993;328:750). |
| *Elective cardioversion* | **Requires hospitalization**. While the likelihood of successful cardioversion decreases as the duration of AFIB increases, the effect of left atrial enlargement is controversial; while some reports suggest that left atrial diameters > 45-50 mm decrease the likelihood of success, others do not.<br>• **Chemical conversion: Class IA or IC agent is preferred**. .Propafenone, sotalol, and amiodarone may be successful in 50% of Class IA failures. If AFIB is less than 2 days old, conversion rates are 70-90% for Class IA and IC drugs (unknown for amiodarone). If AFIB is more than 2 days old, conversion rates are 20-30% for all drugs.<br>• **Electrical conversion (100-200-360 joules)** is usually performed *after* a trial of chemical cardioversion. However, if a reversible cause is corrected (e.g., hypokalemia, hyperthyroidism, resolving PE or pericarditis), electrical conversion may be performed without prior attempts at chemical conversion. For **nonresponders**, administer **IV procainamide** (500-750 mg; rate not to exceed 30-50 mg/min) and **reattempt cardioversion** using 360 joules. Consider internal cardioversion for refractory cases (Circulation 1992;86:1415). |
| *Once in sinus rhythm* | When initially used, antiarrhythmics and AV nodal blockers should be continued longterm unless a correctable cause has been reversed. Warfarin is usually discontinued after 3 weeks. Despite continuous therapy with a Class IA, IC, or amiodarone, only 50% of patients remain in sinus rhythm at 1 year . |

*See p. 1 for abbreviations, p. 75 for classification of antiarrhythmics, and p. 199 for drug information.*

## ATRIAL FIBRILLATION (AFIB)

| | |
|---|---|
| *Options for nonresponders* | (1) Chronic rate control with an AV nodal blocker (diltiazem, verapamil, **β**-blockers, and combination therapy with digoxin + diltiazem afford better rate control during periods of stress than digoxin alone); (2) His-Bundle ablation plus VVIR pacing; (3) AFIB surgery (investigational). |
| Prophylaxis | • First episode: Combination therapy with an AV nodal blocker + Class IA drug or monotherapy with a Class IC drug. Prophylaxis may not be required if a reversible cause is corrected, or the initial episode was not accompanied by heart failure, angina, hypotension, or very fast rates.<br>• History of paroxysmal AFIB: If episodes occur infrequently and are self-limited, prophylaxis may not be required. If symptomatic due to rapid rates, consider prophylaxis with an AV nodal blocker alone.<br>• Frequent or highly symptomatic recurrences: Treat with an AV nodal blocker, a Class IA or IC agent, and longterm anticoagulation with warfarin (INR 2.0-3.0; with prosthetic valve, INR 3.0-4.5). Patients less than 60 years old with "lone AFIB" (no organic heart disease, hypertension, or previous embolism) may be adequately prophylaxed with aspirin instead of warfarin. |

## II. JUNCTIONAL AND BENIGN VENTRICULAR ARRHYTHMIAS

| Arrhythmia | Therapy |
|---|---|
| Junctional premature depolarization | No therapy is required. |
| Junctional tachycardia (non-paroxysmal) | No therapy is usually required. Most episodes are self-limited and clinically unimportant unless caused by digitalis toxicity. If symptoms develop due to the loss of AV synchrony, overdrive suppression with atrial pacing is often of value. If rates are very fast, consider use of an AV nodal blocker. |
| Premature ventricular contractions | No therapy is usually required. Suppression of chronic asymptomatic PVC's neither improves survival nor is recommended. Attempts to suppress PVC's following acute MI has been shown to increase mortality (NEJM 1991;324:781). |

*See p. 1 for abbreviations, p. 75 for classification of antiarrhythmics, and p. 199 for drug information.*

| Arrhythmia | Therapy |
|---|---|
| Non-sustained VT (NSVT) | No therapy is usually required. When NSVT complicates hypertrophic cardiomyopathy, there is an increased risk of sudden death (5-8% per year), but the role of therapy is controversial. |
| Accelerated idioventricular rhythm (AIVR) | The majority of episodes are self-limited, asymptomatic, and do not require therapy. Overdrive atrial or AV sequential pacing may be of value when clinical or hemodynamic instability occurs from the loss of AV synchrony. |

## III. SUSTAINED VENTRICULAR TACHYCARDIA

| Subset | Comments |
|---|---|
| Prior MI | Internal cardioverter-defibrillator (ICD) ± drug therapy can usually control symptoms. Among antiarrhythmics, sotalol and amiodarone appear to be the most effective agents. Catheter ablation is possible but usually does not eliminate all inducible VT's. If a discrete aneurysm is present, mapping and resection is often effective. |
| Idiopathic dilated cardiomyopathy | Bundle branch reentry should be suspected. If right bundle branch reentry is found, catheter ablation should be performed. The efficacy of catheter ablation or surgery for other VT's has not been clearly established, therefore, most cardiologists prefer ICD therapy if the patient is not yet a transplant candidate. |
| RV dysplasia | Sotalol appears to be the most effective agent, however, disease progression over time limits drug efficacy. |
| Tetralogy of Fallot | VT usually originates from the site of a surgical scar and may be eliminated with either map-guided surgery or catheter ablation. |
| No structural heart disease | VT often arises from the RV outflow tract (i.e., LBBB morphology on ECG) and may be effectively treated by catheter ablation. Drug therapy: $\beta$-blockers are often effective; Class IC agents are the most likely to work when $\beta$-blockers fail. Note: If VT is catecholamine related, it may respond to verapamil or adenosine and thus mimick SVT with aberrancy. |

*See p. 1 for abbreviations, p. 75 for classification of antiarrhythmics, and p. 199 for drug information.*

## IV. CARDIAC ARREST SURVIVORS

| Subset | Comments |
|---|---|
| All patients | Suspect reversible causes such as electrolyte imbalance, drug toxicity, ischemia. |
| CAD with prior MI | Suspect acute ischemia if monomorphic VT cannot be induced at EP study; revascularization alone is often effective in this case. Current treatments of choice for inducible VT include **internal cardioverter defibrillator (ICD), sotalol, and amiodarone**. |
| CAD without prior MI | Acute ischemia is the usual cause and **revascularization** the usual therapy. EP study demonstrates either no inducible VT or only VF. |
| Dilated or hypertrophic cardiomyopathy | Less than 30% have inducible monomorphic VT at EP study. **ICD** is considered the therapy of choice due to the progressive nature of the disease. |
| No structural heart disease | Suspect spasm, occult repolarization abnormalities (long QT syndrome), drug toxicity, etc. Usually unable to induce VT at EP study. **$\beta$-blockers and/or ICD are usual therapies.** |

## V. TREATMENT OF CONDUCTION ABNORMALITIES

| Type | Therapy |
|---|---|
| $1^{o}$ AV block | Therapy is not indicated unless the PR interval is very long (> 400 msec) and is accompanied by symptoms. |
| $2^{o}$ AV block<br>*Type I* | • Asymptomatic: No therapy is required.<br>• Symptomatic: Atropine (0.5-2.0 mg) followed by ventricualar pacing. If block develops in the setting of ischemia, tissue adenosine may be the cause and aminophylline may be of value.<br>• In inferior MI, Type I block may precede the development of complete heart block, which is usually well-tolerated, stable, and does not require pacing. |

*See p. 1 for abbreviations, p. 75 for classification of antiarrhythmics, and p. 199 for drug information.*

## V. TREATMENT OF CONDUCTION ABNORMALITIES

| Type | Therapy |
|---|---|
| $2^{o}$ AV block (cont.)<br>*Type II* | Temporary followed by permanent pacing, regardless of symptomatic status, due to the high risk of progression to complete heart block (ventricular escape rate is usually inadequate to maintain BP). |
| 2:1 AV block, type unknown | • Asymptomatic and AV nodal site of block suspected (narrow QRS): Observation only.<br>• Symptoms or infranodal site of block suspected (wide QRS): Temporary followed by permanent pacing.<br>His-Bundle recordings may be required to identify the level of block. In general, carotid sinus massage worsens AV nodal and improves infranodal block, while the opposite effects are seen with atropine. |
| $3^{o}$ AV block (complete heart block) | • Temporary followed by permanent pacing is usually required.<br>• Temporary pacing alone may be indicated if block is due to a reversible etiology (e.g., hyperkalemia) or occurs in the early post-op setting. Temporary pacing is not usually necessary during acute inferior MI if there is a narrow complex escape rhythm and the patient is stable. |
| Fascicular block | No therapy is required for isolated left anterior or posterior fascicular block. |
| Bundle branch block<br>*Left (LBBB)* | No therapy is usually required. However, if LBBB develops during acute MI, temporary pacing x 48-72 hours is recommended. A temporary pacemaker should be immediately available for all patients with LBBB undergoing right heart cath due to the increased risk of complete heart block. |
| *Right (RBBB)* | No therapy is required. |
| Bifascicular block (RBBB with left anterior or posterior fascicular block) | • New onset with MI: Temporary pacing. If even transient $3^{o}$ block develops, permanent pacing is required.<br>• Chronic block: If asymptomatic, no therapy is required. If symptoms of cerebral hypoperfusion occur (e.g., lightheadedness, syncope), consider an EP study with pacemaker implantation for infranodal block or marked prolongation of HV interval (> 80-100 msec). Management is unaffected by PR interval. |
| Alternating LBBB & RBBB | Temporary followed by permanent pacing due to the high risk of progression to complete heart block. |

*See p. 1 for abbreviations, p. 75 for classification of antiarrhythmics, and p. 199 for drug information.*

## VI. SELECTED TOPICS: DIFFERENTIATION OF WIDE-COMPLEX TACHYCARDIA

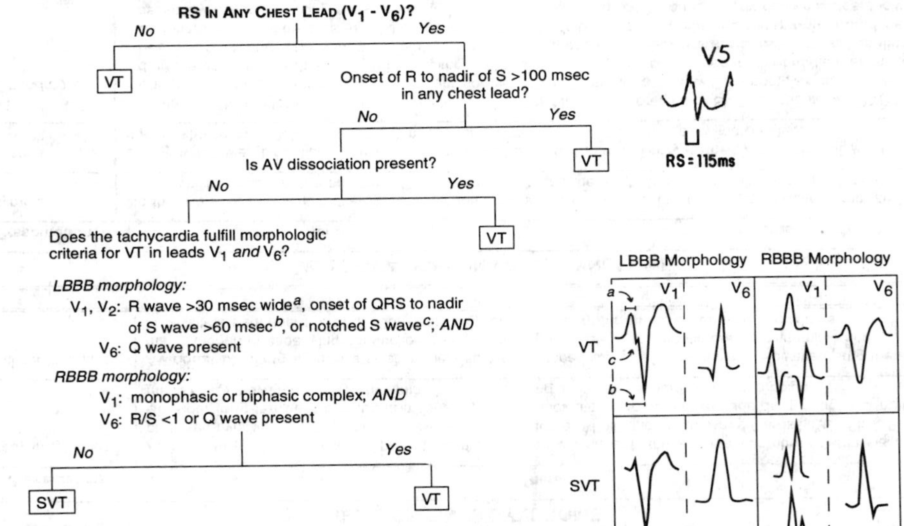


SVT = *Supraventricular tachycardia*; VT = *Ventricular tachycardia*

## B. SICK SINUS SYNDROME

| Presentation | Therapy |
|---|---|
| Bradyarrhythmias | **Permanent pacing** is indicated patients with symptomatic bradyarrhythmias; dual chamber or atrial pacing is preferred over ventricular pacing (lower incidence of stroke, AFIB, and death; Am J Cardiol 1990;65:729). Consider **long-term anticoagulation** for acceptable candidates. Be sure to exclude drug-induced or neurally-mediated (vasovagal) bradyarrhythmias before assigning sick sinus syndrome as the etiology. |
| Tachyarrhythmias | **AV nodal blocking agents** are recommended for accompanying atrial arrhythmias. However, drug therapy may exaggerate underlying conduction abnormalities, precipitate symptomatic bradyarrhythmias, and necessitate permanent pacing. Consider **long-term anticoagulation** for acceptable candidates. |

## C. WOLFF-PARKINSON-WHITE SYNDROME

| Presentation | Therapy | Comments |
|---|---|---|
| Asymptomatic | No therapy is usually required. High-risk occupations (e.g. pilots, divers, bus drivers) may benefit from an EP study, which is used to characterize AP refractory period and the ability to sustain malignant arrhythmias. | |
| Syncope | EP study followed by antiarrhythmics or **catheter ablation of the accessory pathway**, the latter of which **is successful in over 95%** of cases and has a complication rate of < 1% in healthy individuals. | |
| SVT<br>*Orthodromic* | • Acute Rx: IV adenosine, verapamil, or diltiazem.<br>• Chronic prevention: Accessory pathway ablation vs. drug therapy either with an AV nodal blocker (± Class IA or IC) or monotherapy with a Class III agent. Catheter ablation is curative in > 90% and is especially useful for young patients and those refractory to or intolerant of drugs. | Most common type of SVT in patients with WPW. ECG shows a narrow QRS complex during SVT unless a preexistent or rate-dependent bundle branch block is present. **If preexcitation is evident on baseline ECG** (delta-wave), **digoxin and verapamil should be avoided** unless an EP study demonstrates a low-risk for life-threatening arrhythmias during AFIB. |

*See p. 1 for abbreviations, p. 75 for classification of antiarrhythmics, and p. 199 for drug information.*

## C. WOLFF-PARKINSON-WHITE SYNDROME

| Presentation | Therapy | Comments |
|---|---|---|
| *Antidromic SVT* | Same as for orthodromic SVT. | **ECG:** Wide QRS complex during SVT **simulates VT**. |
| Atrial fibrillation (AFIB) | • Acute treatment: Procainamide (IV 10-12 mg/kg, rate ≤ 50 mg/min) or cardioversion. **Avoid acute therapy with IV verapamil, digoxin, lidocaine and probably adenosine**, which may result in fatal hypotension, increased ventricular rate, or VF.<br>• Chronic prevention: Catheter ablation vs. EP-guided drug therapy usually with a Class IA or IC agent. | • If AFIB conducts over an accessory pathway (manifest AP), an irregular *wide* QRS tachycardia will be evident, which may degenerate into VF.<br>• If the AP is concealed (i.e., unable to conduct antegradely), AFIB will manifest as an irregular *narrow* QRS tachycardia. These pts are not at ↑ risk of sudden death. Treat as routine AFIB (pp. 65-67). |

## D. DIGITALIS TOXICITY

| | |
|---|---|
| Contributing factors | The risk of clinical toxicity increases as digoxin levels rise. For any given level, the risk of toxicity is increased if any of the following are present: hypokalemia, hypomagnesemia, hypothyroidism, hypercalcemia, advanced age, renal insufficiency, hypoxemia, ischemia, or amyloid. Drugs that increase digoxin levels include quinidine, amiodarone, verapamil, propafenone, and spironolactone. |
| Manifestations | • GI symptoms: anorexia, nausea, vomiting, diarrhea.<br>• CNS abnormalities: fatigue, headache, agitation, lethargy, seizures.<br>• Visual disturbances: scotoma, color perception changes, halos.<br>• Others: gynecomastia, hyperkalemia, cardiac arrhythmias (see below). |
| Arrhythmias | Atrial premature depolarizations (APD's), atrial tachycardia ± block, junctional tachycardia, premature ventricular contractions (PVC's; bigeminal or trigeminal pattern), ventricular tachycardia (monomorphic, bidirectional), sinoatrial block, AV nodal block, AFIB with a regular ventricular response, and Type I second degree AV block (Wenckebach). |

*See p. 1 for abbreviations, p. 75 for classification of antiarrhythmics, and p. 199 for drug information.*

## D. DIGITALIS TOXICITY

| Manifestation | Therapy | Comments |
|---|---|---|
| Non-life threatening | • Observation if stable.<br>• Bradyarrhythmias: Atropine and/or pacemaker.<br>• Ventricular tachyarrhythmias: Lidocaine or phenytoin. | Correct electrolyte abnormalities. **Potassium administration may cause or worsen AV block.** |
| Life-threatening | Digoxin-specific antibody (administered over 30 min; each vial is reconstituted in 4 cc's of sterile water):<br>• *Acute ingestion:*<br>No. of vials = [ingested dose (mg) x 0.8] / 0.6<br>• *Chronic intoxication:*<br>No. of vials = [serum level (ng/ml) x weight (kg)] / 100<br>• *If the ingested amount and serum level are unknown,* 20 vials (12 mg) should be administered<br>It may be necessary to repeat the dose if toxicity has not been reversed after several hours. | Indications for digoxin antibody: Life-threatening heart block, ventricular arrhythmias, bradyarrhythmias, hyperkalemia. Clinical improvement begins within 30-60 min. **Recurrence of digoxin toxicity may occur ≥24 hrs later** and require repeat dosing. Monitor potassium carefully; hypokalemia usually develops during therapy. |

## E. TORSADE DE POINTES

| Presentation | Therapy | Comments |
|---|---|---|
| Torsade de Pointes (TdP) | • Stop offending drug (Class IA and III antiarrhythmics, phenothiazines, tricyclic antidepressants) and correct low serum potassium, magnesium, and calcium.<br>• **Cardioversion** for patients who are clinically or hemodynamically unstable.<br>• If TdP is bradycardia- or pause-dependent, use **isoproterenol or pacing** to increase heart rate to 100-120 bpm.<br>• **Magnesium sulfate** (2 gm IV over 1 min [10 cc of 20% solution] followed by an infusion of 3-20 mg/min) can be of benefit even when the serum magnesium is | Polymorphic VT (rate 200-250 bpm) with prolonged QT interval (usually > 500 msec). Tachycardia is usually nonsustained but **may deteriorate into VF** or terminate with sinus arrest or |

*See p. 1 for abbreviations, p. 75 for classification of antiarrhythmics, and p. 199 for drug information.*

## E. TORSADE DE POINTES

| Presentation | Therapy | Comments |
|---|---|---|
| Torsade de Pointes (TdP) (cont.) | normal (Circulation 1988;77:392). May need to repeat initial bolus after 5 min.<br>• **Lidocaine** is occasionally of value.<br>• Avoid longterm therapy with Class IA, IC, and III agents except amiodarone. | slow ventricular escape before returning to baseline rhythm. |

## F. SYNCOPE

| | |
|---|---|
| Evaluation | See p. 76. Tilt test can be used to diagnose neurally-mediated (vasovagal) syncope. |
| Prognosis | One-year mortality: cardiac etiology 18-33%, non-cardiac etiology 12%, unknown etiology 6%. |
| Treatment | **Positive tilt test: β-blocker** is considered the drug of choice. Increased salt intake and fludrocortisone (Florinef 0.05-0.2 mg po qd) are often useful adjuncts. Other potential therapies include transdermal scopolamine, ephedrine, disopyramide, and theophylline. For patients with symptomatic recurrences despite medical therapy, permanent pacing may be helpful. |

***Drug classification*** (see p. 199 for further drug information):
**AV nodal blocker:** Digoxin, ***β***-blocker, verapamil, diltiazem.
**Class IA**: Quinidine (oral, IV), procainamide (oral, IV), disopyramide (oral).
**Class IB:** Lidocaine (IV), mexilitine (oral), tocainide (oral).
**Class IC**: Flecainide (oral), propafenone (oral).
**Class II:** ***β***-blockers (oral, IV).
**Class III**: Amiodarone (oral, IV), sotalol (oral).
**Class IV:** Calcium blocker (oral, IV).

# Figure 1. Evaluation of Syncope

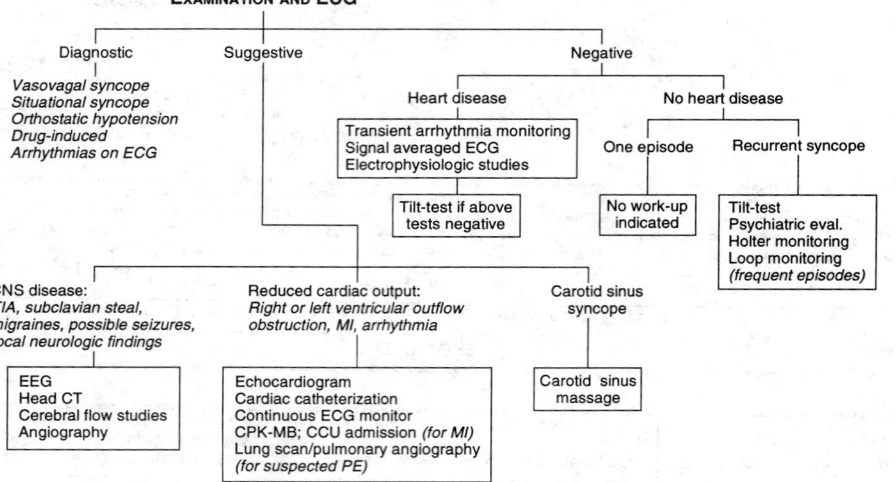


*CCU = coronary care unit; CNS = central nervous system; CPK-MB = creatine phosphokinase-MB; CT = computed tomography; EEG = electroencephalography; MI = myocardial infarction; PE = pulmonary embolism; TIA = transient ischemic attack. Adapted from Kapoor WN. Am J Med. 1991;90:91-106.*

# 6. TREATMENT OF CARDIAC ARREST AND LIFE-THREATENING ARRHYTHMIAS

William A. Murray, M.D.
W. Douglas Weaver, M.D.

## I. OVERVIEW

The various treatment algorithms in this chapter provide an acceptable initial recipe to follow but are not intended as a substitute for thinking about the individual patient, the etiology of the arrhythmia, and more directed therapy. Limited data are available to prove that many accepted ACLS interventions are beneficial. The following clinical recommendations apply to all treatment algorithms:

- Treat the patient, not the monitor.
- Algorithms for cardiac arrest presume that the condition under discussion continually persists, that the patient remains in cardiac arrest, and that CPR is always performed.
- **Adequate airway, ventilation, oxygenation, chest compressions and defibrillation** are more important than administration of medications and take precedence over initiating an intravenous (IV) line or injecting pharmacologic agents. Endotracheal intubation by skilled personnel should be performed as soon as practical; intubation attempts should not exceed 30 seconds.
- Several medications (**epinephrine, lidocaine and atropine**) can be administered via the endotracheal tube, but clinicians must use an **endotracheal dose 2-2.5 times the IV dose**.
- With few exceptions, IV medications should be administered as a rapid bolus followed by a 20-30 mL bolus of IV fluid and immediate elevation of the extremity. This will enhance drug delivery into the central circulation, which may take 1-2 minutes. IV access should be obtained via an antecubital vein whenever possible.
- IV fluids for volume expansion are not recommended during routine resuscitation from cardiac arrest unless there is an obvious indication (hemorrhage, RV infarct, trauma, etc.).

## II. BASIC LIFE SUPPORT IN THE ADULT*

| | |
|---|---|
| General approach | **Call for help first:** Activate the emergency medical service (EMS) in cases of pre-hospital arrest and call a "code" for hospitalized patients. Once help and a defibrillator are on the way, assess and support the patient's airway, breathing and circulation ("ABCs"). |
| Airway | • **Position victim supine** on a firm, flat surface.<br>• **Move lower jaw forward**. If no head or neck trauma evident, tilt forehead back and lift chin forward.<br>• **Remove foreign material** or vomitus from mouth. |
| Breathing | • Assess for spontaneous respirations: Observe chest; listen and feel for air during exhalation<br>• Rescue breathing should be performed in the absence of spontaneous effective respiration. The mouth-to-mouth technique is a quick way to provide oxygen to the victim. The **nose should be pinched closed, 2 slow breaths given followed by 10-12 breaths/minute. Enough breath should be given to see the chest rise and hear air escape during exhalation**. Avoid rapid flow and excess volume to prevent gastric distension. |
| Circulation | • Cardiac arrest is recognized by pulselessness in carotid/femoral arteries ≥ 5 sec. in an unconscious victim.<br>• **If the patient is in bed, a board--preferably the full width of the bed--should be placed under the patient's back**. The heel of one hand is placed on the lower half of the sternum, the 2nd hand placed on top of the first, and chest compressions performed with shoulders positioned directly over the arms. **The sternum should be depressed 1.5 - 2 inches for normal adults; if the carotid/femoral pulses cannot be felt during compression, greater downward force is required**. The duration of compression should be 50% of the compression-release cycle. Compression should generate systolic pressure peaks of 60-80 mmHg., but diastolic pressures are low and cardiac output is only 1/3 of normal. **Chest compression rate should be 80-100 per minute**. Single rescuers should perform cycles of 15 compressions followed by 2 ventilations; 2 rescuers should perform 5 compressions followed by one ventilation.<br>• CPR should only be interrupted briefly for endotracheal intubation, defibrillation and quick assessment of rhythm. |

* JAMA 1992;268:2184

## III. ADVANCED CARDIAC LIFE SUPPORT (ACLS) DRUGS†

| Drug | Dose | Comments |
|---|---|---|
| Epinephrine | 1 mg IV (10 mL of 1:10,000 solution) or 2 mg via the endotracheal tube and repeated at 3-5 minute intervals as needed. A higher dose (5 mg or 0.1 mg/kg) may be considered if the initial dose is ineffective or if given via the endotracheal tube. | Indicated for asystole, pulseless electrical activity, and VF or pulseless VT that persists after defibrillation. Pressor effect may be inactivated if mixed with bicarbonate. Tissue necrosis may develop if drug extravasates. |
| Sodium bicarbonate | 1 meq/kg IV initially, followed by one-half the original dose at 10-minute intervals (44.6 or 50 meq per ampule). If possible, the dosage should be based on arterial blood gas results. | May be especially beneficial in the setting of pre-existing metabolic acidosis, hyperkalemia, or tricyclic antidepressant overdose, although in most cases of cardiac arrest, it **should be used -- if at all -- only after other therapies have proved ineffective**. If used, monitor closely for metabolic alkalosis, volume overload, and $CO_2$ retention. Catecholamines and calcium salts may be inactivated if added to the bicarbonate infusion. |
| Atropine | 0.5 mg (1 mg for asystole) repeated every 3-5 minutes to a maximum of 3 mg. | Indicated for symptomatic bradyarrhythmias, especially if accompanied by hypotension, ventricular ectopy, or asystole. Atropine may cause sinus tachycardia--and rarely--VT or VF. |
| Isoproterenol | 1 mg in 500 mL of $D_5W$ (2 mcg/mL) at an infusion rate of 2-10 mcg/min titrated according to heart rate and rhythm. | Indicated for the temporary control of refractory Torsades de Pointes and hemodynamically significant bradycardia while awaiting pacemaker therapy. Contraindications: Acute MI and ventricular arrhythmias, especially if digitalis toxicity is suspected. Use with extreme caution in hypokalemic patients (↑ risk of proarrhythmia). |

† *Modified from JAMA 1992;268:2199*

## III. ADVANCED CARDIAC LIFE SUPPORT (ACLS) DRUGS†

| Drug | Dose | Comments |
|---|---|---|
| Calcium | 10% calcium chloride is the preferred preparation and is given as an IV bolus of 2-4 mg/kg. | Not been shown to improve survival. May exacerbate post-resuscitation cerebral/myocardial ischemia and digitalis toxicity. **Use should be limited** to situations in which definite indications exist (e.g., hyperkalemia, hypocalcemia, calcium channel blocker toxicity). |
| Lidocaine | Initial dose: 1 mg/kg (50-100 mg) by IV bolus injection, followed by a second bolus of one-half dose 5 min later and IV infusion of 2-4 mg/min (1 g in 250 mL of $D_5W$). | Used to treat VT, VF, and wide-complex tachycardias of uncertain etiology. Main side effect is CNS toxicity (drowsiness, disorientation, ↓ hearing, paresthesias, muscle twitching, agitation, seizures). Use cautiously in the elderly, and those with impaired liver function or low cardiac output states. |
| Procainamide HCl | Loading dose: Infusion rate is 30-50 mg/min until any of the following occurs: (1) the dysrhythmia is suppressed; (2) hypotension occurs; (3) the QRS interval widens by 50%; or (4) a total of 17 mg/kg of procainamide has been given. Maintenance therapy may be given as a continuous IV infusion at a rate of 1-4 mg/min. The dosage should be reduced in the presence of renal failure. | Indicated for VT refractory to lidocaine and WPW tachycardias. Procainamide may cause hypotension, conduction disturbances, or cardiac arrest; therefore, blood pressure and cardiac rhythm must be closely monitored when the drug is being used. Procainamide should not be used in the setting of pre-existing QT prolongation or Torsades de Pointes (↑ risk of proarrhythmia). |
| Bretylium tosylate | The dose for VF is 5 mg/kg (~ 500 mg) given as an undiluted bolus injection followed by defibrillation. The dose may be increased to 10 mg/kg (or 1 g) and repeated as necessary every 5 minutes up to a maximum of 35 mg/kg. | May be of value for refractory VF and VT, although some reports (and a growing number of cardiologists) question its utility for monomorphic VT (Am Heart J 1983;105:973). May cause hypotension and, in the awake patient, nausea and vomiting after rapid injection. |

*† Modified from JAMA 1992;268:2199*

## III. ADVANCED CARDIAC LIFE SUPPORT (ACLS) DRUGS†

| Drug | Dose | Comments |
|---|---|---|
| Dopamine | Initial IV infusion rate of 2.5-5 mcg/kg/min (400 mg or 800 mg in 500 mL of $D_5W$; 800-1600 mcg/mL). Titrate to blood pressure, using the lowest infusion rate possible to control hypotension. A norepinephrine infusion may be added if > 20 mcg/kg/min of dopamine is required to maintain BP. | Indicated for cardiogenic shock and refractory hypotension not responding to intravenous fluid replacement. Dopamine may cause tachyarrhythmias, ectopic beats, nausea, vomiting, and significant vasoconstriction. Avoid mixing dopamine with bicarbonate since it may be inactivated. |
| Norepinephrine | Initial IV infusion rate of 0.5-1 mcg/min (8 mg in 500 mL D5W; 16 mcg/mL) with subsequent titration to blood pressure. May be inactivated if administered in the same IV line as alkaline solutions. | Indicated for severe hypotension not caused by hypovolemia or cardiogenic shock. Adverse effects include an increase in myocardial oxygen requirements, soft tissue necrosis if extravasation occurs, and renal/mesenteric vasoconstriction. |

† *Modified from JAMA 1992;268:2199*

## IV. ADVANCED CARDIAC LIFE SUPPORT: DEFIBRILLATION

Immediately defibrillation is mandatory; do not allow intubation, attempts at IV access, or drug treatment to delay the life-saving potential of early defibrillation. The standard placement is **one electrode just to the right of the upper sternum below the clavicle and the other at the level of the left nipple**, with the center of the electrode in the left mid-axillary line. Transdermal medication patches should be removed before defibrillation. The operator should **announce "stand clear"** and ensure that personnel have no contact with patient, stretcher or equipment. Defibrillation for pulseless VT or VF should be administered as three stacked shocks in sequence; the rescuer should *not* pause during the initial stacked sequence to check for pulse or administer medications as long as the monitor displays VF or VT.

# Figure 1. Ventricular Fibrillation and Pulseless Ventricular Tachycardia

- ABC's (p. 78)
- Precordial thump in witnessed arrest if no pulse and a defibrillator is not immediately available
- Perform CPR until defibrillator attached; continue if VF/VT is confirmed

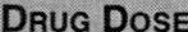

Defibrillate up to 3 times for persistent VF/VT (200 J, 300 J, 360 J)

→ Persistent or recurrent VF/VT

→ PEA (go to figure 2)

→ Return of pulse
- Support airway
- Support breathing
- Provide medications appropriate for blood pressure, heart rate and rhythm

→ Asystole (go to figure 3)

Persistent or recurrent VF/VT:

- Continue CPR
- Intubate at once
- Obtain IV access

**Epinephrine** 1 mg IV push, repeat every 3-5 min

Defibrillate 360 J (multiple sequenced shocks are acceptable, especially when medications are delayed)

Administer **antiarrhythmics, magnesium, sodium bicarbonate** (if indicated) for persistent or recurrent VF/VT

- Defibrillate 360 J, 30-60 sec after each dose of medication
- Pattern should be drug-shock, drug-shock

## Drug Doses

- **Epinephrine** 1 mg IV push every 3-5 min. If this approach fails, several dosing regimens can be considered:
  - *Immediate:* **epinephrine** 2-5 mg IV push, every 3-5 min
  - *Escalating:* **epinephrine** 1 mg - 3 mg - 5 mg IV push (3 min apart)
  - *High:* **epinephrine** 0.1 mg/kg IV push every 3-5 min
- **Antiarrhythmics:**
  1. **Lidocaine** 1.5 mg/kg IV push. Repeat in 3-5 min to total loading dose of 3 mg/kg; then use:
  2. **Procainamide** 30 mg/min in refractory VF (max. total 17 mg/kg)
  3. **Bretylium** 5 mg/kg IV push. Repeat in 5 min at 10 mg/kg
  - **Magnesium sulfate** 1-2 g IV in Torsades de Pointes, suspected hypomagnesemic state, or severe refractory VF
- **Sodium bicarbonate** (1 mEq/kg IV):
  - *If known preexisting hyperkalemia*
  - *If known preexisting bicarbonate-responsive acidosis*
  - *If overdose with tricyclic antidepressants*
  - *To alkalinize the urine in drug overdoses*
  - *If intubated and continued long arrest interval*
  - *If hypoxic lactic acidosis*

*Modified with permission: JAMA 1992, Vol. 268, No. 16*

# FIGURE 2. PULSELESS ELECTRICAL ACTIVITY

- Continue CPR
- Intubate at once
- IV fluid (normal saline, lactated ringers)
- Confirm absent pulse using Doppler ultrasound

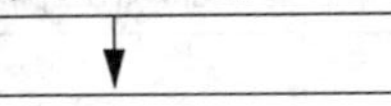

*Consider Reversible Causes:*

- Hypovolemia
- Hypoxia
- Tamponade
- Tension pneumothorax
- Hypothermia
- Massive PE
- Drug toxicity
- Hyperkalemia
- Acidosis
- Massive MI / Shock

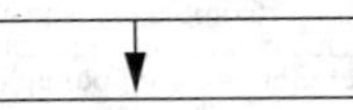

**Epinephrine** 1 mg IV push, repeat every 3-5 min

If absolute bradycardia (<60 beats/min) or relative bradycardia, give **atropine** 1 mg IV; Repeat as needed every 3-5 min up to a total of 0.04 mg/kg

## DRUG DOSES

- **Epinephrine** 1 mg IV push every 3-5 min. If this approach fails, several dosing regimens can be considered:
  - *Intermediate:* **epinephrine** 2-5 mg IV push, every 3-5 min
  - *Escalating:* **epinephrine** 1 mg - 3 mg - 5 mg IV push (3 min apart)
  - *High:* **epinephrine** 0.1 mg/kg IV push every 3-5 min
- **Atropine**
  - 1 mg IV, repeat every 3-5 min up to a total of 0.04 mg/kg
  - Shortening dosing intervals may be helpful
- **Sodium bicarbonate** (1 mEq/kg IV):
  - *If known preexisting hyperkalemia*
  - *If known preexisting bicarbonate-responsive acidosis*
  - *If overdose with tricyclic antidepressants*
  - *To alkalinize the urine in drug overdoses*
  - *If intubated and continued long arrest interval*
  - *Upon return of spontaneous circulation after long arrest interval*
  - *If hypoxic lactic acidosis*

*Modified with permission: JAMA 1992, Vol. 268, No. 16*

# FIGURE 3. ASYSTOLE

- Continue CPR
- Intubate at once
- Obtain IV access
- Confirm asystole in more than one lead and proper monitor gain

↓

Consider reversible causes*

↓

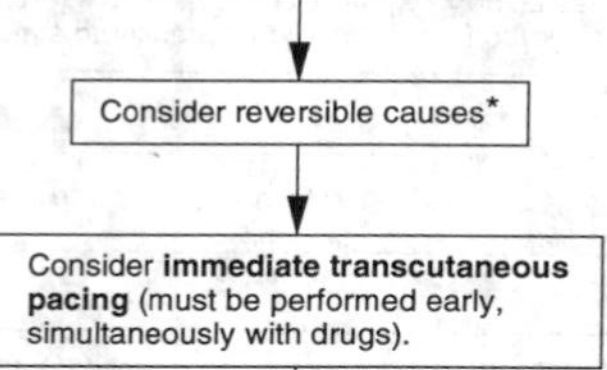

Consider **immediate transcutaneous pacing** (must be performed early, simultaneously with drugs).

↓

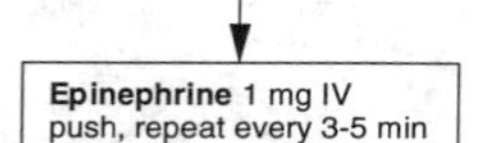

**Epinephrine** 1 mg IV push, repeat every 3-5 min

↓

**Atropine** 1 mg IV, repeat every 3-5 min up to a total of 0.04 mg/kg

↓

If patient remains in asystole or other agonal rhythms after successful intubation and above measures, and no reversible causes are identified, consider termination of resuscitative efforts by a physician.

### DRUG DOSES

- **Epinephrine** 1 mg IV push every 3-5 min. If this approach fails, several dosing regimens can be considered:
  - *Immediate:* **epinephrine** 2-5 mg IV push, every 3-5 min
  - *Escalating:* **epinephrine** 1 mg - 3 mg - 5 mg IV push (3 min apart)
  - *High:* **epinephrine** 0.1 mg/kg IV push every 3-5 min
- **Atropine** 1 mg IV, repeat every 3-5 min up to a total of 0.04 mg/kg
- **Sodium bicarbonate** (1 mEq/kg IV):
  - *If known preexisting hyperkalemia*
  - *If known preexisting bicarbonate-responsive acidosis*
  - *If overdose with tricyclic antidepressants*
  - *To alkalinize the urine in drug overdoses*
  - *If intubated and continued long arrest interval*
  - *Upon return of spontaneous circulation after long arrest interval*
  - *If hypoxic lactic acidosis*

* Reversible causes of Asystole:

- *Hypoxia*
- *Hypercalcemia*
- *Hypokalemia, hyperkalemia*
- *Preexisting acidosis*
- *Drug overdose*
- *Hypothermia*
- *Acidosis*

*Modified with permission: JAMA 1992, Vol. 268, No. 16*

# Figure 4. Bradycardia

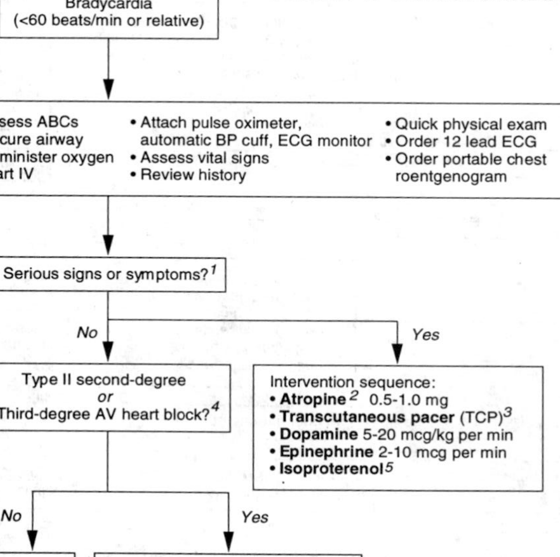


## Comments

1. Clinical manifestations include: *Symptoms:* Chest pain, shortness of breath, decreased level of consciousness. *Signs:* Low BP, shock, CHF, acute MI.
2. **Atropine** should be given in repeat doses in 3-5 min up to total of 0.04 mg/kg. Consider shorter dosing intervals in severe clinical conditions. *Note:* Denervated transplanted hearts will not respond to atropine. Go at once to pacing, catecholamine infusion, or both.
3. **Do not delay TCP** while awaiting IV access or for atropine to take effect if patient is symptomatic. Verify patient tolerance and mechanical capture. Use analgesia and sedation as needed.
4. **Never treat third-degree heart block plus ventricular escape beats with lidocaine.**
5. Isoproterenol should be used, if at all, with extreme caution. At low doses it is possibly helpful; at higher doses it is harmful.

*Modified with permission: JAMA 1992, Vol. 268, No. 16*

FIGURE 5. TACHYCARDIA (HEMODYNAMICALLY STABLE)

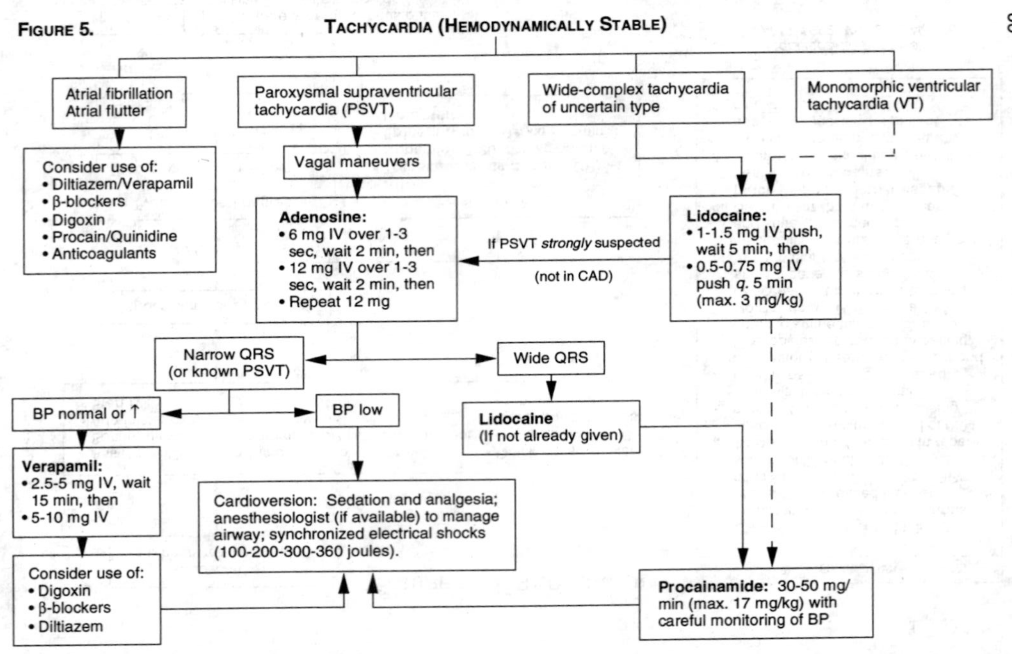

# 7. SHOCK

Mark Freed, M.D.

## I. OVERVIEW

Shock is a syndrome in which the delivery of oxygen is inadequate to maintain proper end-organ function. Manifestations include those common to the shock state (hypotension, oliguria, mental status changes, lactic acidosis) and those of the underlying disorder (e.g., hematemesis in upper GI bleed, urticaria and wheezing in anaphylaxis). Disseminated intravascular coagulation (DIC), adult respiratory distress syndrome (ARDS), mesenteric ischemia, myocardial ischemia/dysfunction, and hepatic/renal failure may complicate the clinical course. Prognosis depends on the type and severity of shock, the time elapsed until the initiation of treatment, the presence of co-morbid conditions, and the development of complications. Untreated, shock is uniformly fatal: even with early therapy, septic and cardiogenic shock are associated with mortality rates in excess of 50%.

## II. STABILIZING THE PATIENT AND MANAGING THE SHOCK STATE

| | |
|---|---|
| Airway | • **Endotracheal intubation** is required to maintain a patent airway (e.g., laryngeal edema or trauma), when mechanical ventilation is necessary (see below), and to prevent aspiration in high-risk patients (e.g., mental obtundation or massive hematemesis). |
| Breathing | • Supplemental $0_2$ for all.<br>• Indications for **mechanical ventilation** include respiratory rate > 30/min, use of accessory muscles of respiration, $p0_2 < 40$ mmHg, and severe respiratory acidosis. Consider use in cardiogenic shock even when not required for oxygenation/ventilation due to salutary effects on work of breathing and myocardial $0_2$ consumption. |
| Circulation | • Secure at least two IV lines (16 gauge or larger).<br>• If lungs are clear to auscultation, administer IV fluids (crystalloids, colloids, blood) ± vasopressors (dopamine 10-50 mcg/kg/min and/or norepinephrine 0.5-30 mcg/min). If hypotension persists and pulmonary edema is absent, a MAST suit should be applied until more definitive measures can be employed (p. 91). |

*See p. 1 for abbreviations and p. 199 for drug information.*

## II. STABILIZING THE PATIENT AND MANAGING THE SHOCK STATE

| | |
|---|---|
| **Circulation** (cont.) | • If pulmonary edema is present, therapy depends on etiology and associated hemodynamics:<br>- BP < 60 mmHg: Norepinephrine (0.5-30 mcg/min) and/or dopamine (10-20 mcg/kg/min). Once systolic BP is 70-80 mmHg, add dobutamine (5-20 mcg/kg/min), discontinue norepinephrine, and try to wean dopamine to "renal dose" (2-4 mcg/kg/min).<br>- Ongoing myocardial ischemia: Emergency intraaortic balloon pumping (IABP), cardiac cath, and PTCA or CABG when feasible. Cardiac transplantation should be considered for refractory shock or severe LV dysfunction.<br>- Acute valvular stenosis/regurgitation: Emergency cardiac cath and balloon valvuloplasty, valve replacement or repair. IABP is often of value for mitral regurgitation and aortic stenosis, but is contraindicated in moderate-severe aortic regurgitation.<br>• Correct acidosis, hypoxemia and hypothermia; inotropes and vasopressors are less effective in these settings.<br>• **If the patient has been receiving β-blockers, glucagon** (5-10 mg IV bolus; maintenance infusion 2-5 mg/hr) may increase inotropicity via non-adrenergic mechanism. **If the patient has been receiving calcium channel blockers** and hypotension persists despite above measures, **10% calcium chloride** (5-10 mL IV over 5-10 min) may improve ventricular function.<br>• Arrhythmias: See Ch. 5,6. |
| Goals of therapy | $0_2$ saturation > 90%, mean arterial pressure > 60 mmHg, urine output > 20 cc/hr, alert and oriented, clearing of metabolic acidosis (pH 7.3-7.5), and temperature > 35°C. |
| Monitoring | Intra-arterial line for monitoring of BP; bladder catheter for monitoring of urine output; and a thermodilution pulmonary artery catheter with an $O_2$ saturation thermistor for monitoring of central venous pressure (CVP), pulmonary artery pressure, pulmonary capillary wedge pressure (PCWP), cardiac output (CO), pulmonary vascular resistance (PVR), systemic vascular resistance (SVR), mixed venous oxygen saturation ($MVO_2$), and arterial oxygen saturation. |

*See p. 1 for abbreviations and p. 199 for drug information.*

## II. STABILIZING THE PATIENT AND MANAGING THE SHOCK STATE

| | |
|---|---|
| Others | Draw 30 cc of blood for emergency laboratory analysis and obtain arterial blood gas. Treat conditions:<br>• **Hypoglycemia: Thiamine** 100 mg IM (to prevent Wernicke's encephalopathy) followed by 1 amp **D50** IV.<br>• **Narcotic overdose** (e.g., morphine, meperidine): **Naloxone** (Narcan) 0.4-2.0 mg IV every 5 minutes until awake up to 10 mg. Repeat dosing may be necessary to treat late relapses.<br>• **Benzodiazipine overdose** (e.g., diazepam, chlordiazepoxide): **Flumazenil** (Romazicon) 0.2 mg IV every 5-10 minutes until pt awakens or up to 3 mg in one hour. Repeat dosing may be necessary to treat late relapses.<br>• **Adrenal insufficiency** or patients receiving steroids: **Hydrocortisone** 100-200 mg IV every 4-6 hrs. (p. 97).<br>• Drug overdose: Removal of ingested drug (gastric lavage, activated charcoal, bowel irrigation and/or hemodialysis depending on specific agent), administer specific antidote (p. 99), and contact Poison Control Center.<br>• **Seizures: Diazepam** 0.1-0.2 mg/kg IV at rate of 1-2 mg/min; may require repeat doses. Be prepared for endotracheal intubation and mechanical ventilation if respiratory depression develops. Once controlled, phenytoin and/or phenobarbital should be administered to prevent recurrences (15 mg/kg at a rate not to exceed 25-50 mg/min; follow levels). |
| Remember | • **Shock may have more than one cause** (e.g. GI bleed (hypovolemic shock) → acute MI (cardiogenic shock); Septic shock → acute adrenal insufficiency (distributive shock) → stress-induced gastritis (hypovolemic shock)). Therefore, it is essential to perform a complete history and physical, ECG, chest x-ray, and complete blood chemistries on *all* patients.<br>• **Even if an obvious cause is present, ask yourself**:<br>Is sepsis present? Is there GI bleeding? Is there myocardial ischemia, arrhythmias, conduction abnormalities? Is adrenal insufficiency contributing to the shock state? Is a drug overdose possible?<br>• **Anticipate complications:**<br>Lactic acidosis, myocardial ischemia, arrhythmias and conduction disturbances (continuous ECG monitoring required), hepatic dysfunction, disseminated intravascular coagulation, stress-induced GI bleeding, adrenal insufficiency, sepsis, renal failure, adult respiratory distress syndrome. |

*See p. 1 for abbreviations and p. 199 for drug information.*

**FIGURE 1. INITIAL MANAGEMENT AND DIFFERENTIAL DIAGNOSIS OF SHOCK***

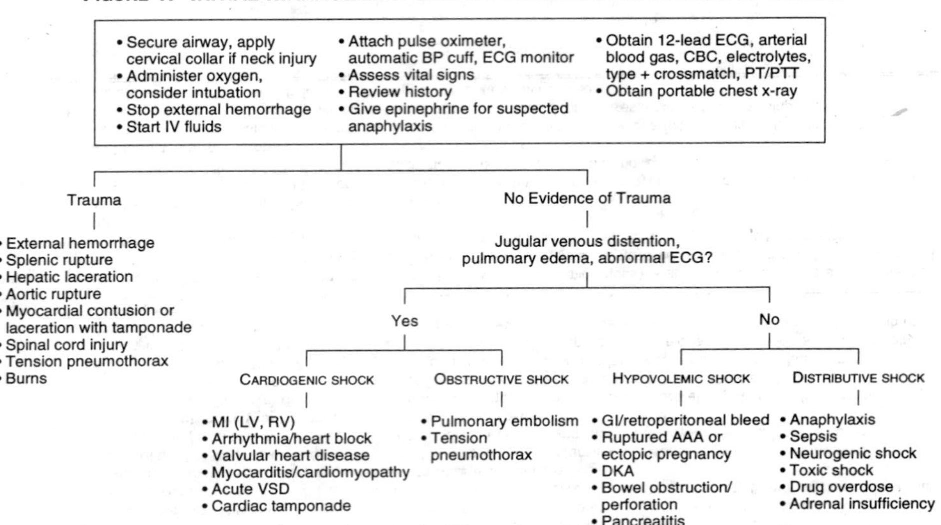


**Remember: More than one cause may be present (e.g. GI bleed→ hypotension→ MI).*
*MI = myocardial infarction; L(R)V = left (right) ventricle; VSD = ventricular septal defect; GI = gastrointestinal; DKA = diabetic ketoacidosis; AAA = abdominal aortic aneurysm*

| III. HYPOVOLEMIC SHOCK: GENERAL MANAGEMENT | |
|---|---|
| General | Use large peripheral veins for IV access. Draw blood for hematocrit, Type & Cross (≥ 6 units of packed RBCs), platelets, PT/PTT, electrolytes, BUN, creatinine, and liver function tests. Insert NG tube if cause is unknown (may diagnose UGI bleed); lavage with room temperature saline to remove clots and food. If GI bleeding is identified, obtain GI and surgical consultation early. |
| Fluids | Normal saline or Lactated Ringers through 2 or more IV lines until hypotension resolves, or if hemorrhagic shock is present, until packed RBCs are available. **Pressurized IV bags and hand-injections** using 50 cc syringes facilitate large volume fluid administration for severe shock. |
| Transfusion | Packed RBCs require use of an 18-gauge catheter or larger, 0.9 NaCl to prevent RBC lysis, a 170-$\mu$m filter to entrap microaggregates and fibrin, and a blood warmer to prevent hypothermia. Each unit (~ 350 mL) should raise recipient's hemoglobin by 1 gm/dL (hematocrit by 3%). **Group O (universal donor)** RBCs may be given to group A, B, O or AB patients and **group AB patients (universal recipient)** may receive group A, B, AB, or O RBCs. Leukocyte-reduced RBCs will frequently alleviate non-hemolytic febrile reactions. Patients with a history of severe allergic reactions should be premedicated with an antihistamine. |
| Drug Therapy (Pressors) | • Dopamine: 10-20 mcg/kg/min IV infusion.<br>• Norepinephrine: 0.5-30 mcg/min IV infusion.<br>• Phenylephrine: 0.1-0.18 mg/min IV infusion; once stabilized, decrease rate to 0.04-0.06 mg/min. |
| Mechanical Support | **Military antishock trousers (MAST):** Temporizing measure for the treatment of hypovolemic or distributive shock until more definitive measures are instituted. **Absolute contraindications** include heart failure, cardiogenic shock and body temperatures less than 32°C (may induce cardiac arrest). |
| Cause-specific therapy | For definitive therapy of peptic ulcer disease, varices, Mallory-Weiss tear, diverticulosis, angiodysplasia, Meckel's diverticulum, retroperitoneal bleed, pancreatitis, and diabetic ketoacidosis, refer to Essentials of Cardiovascular Medicine, unabridged version, pp. 234-238. |

*See p. 1 for abbreviations and p. 199 for drug information.*

## Figure 2. Initial Evaluation of Cardiogenic Shock

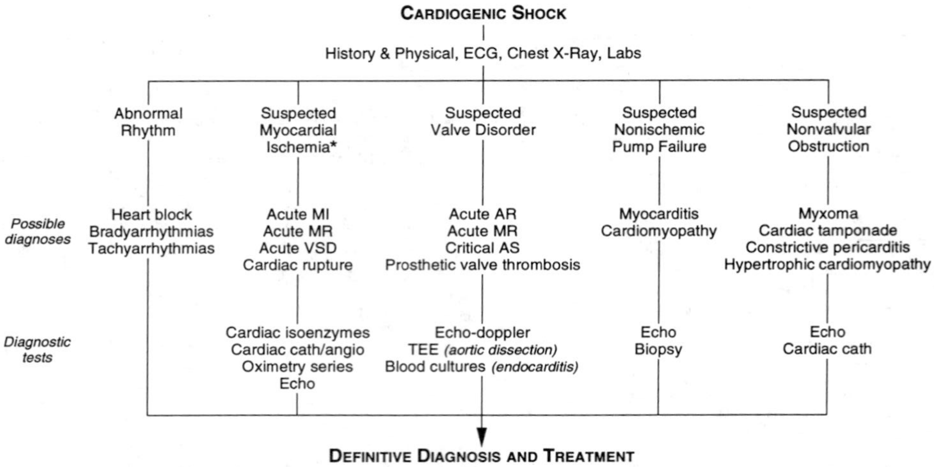

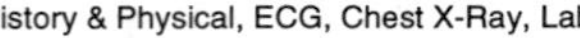

**Cardiogenic Shock**

History & Physical, ECG, Chest X-Ray, Labs

| | Abnormal Rhythm | Suspected Myocardial Ischemia* | Suspected Valve Disorder | Suspected Nonischemic Pump Failure | Suspected Nonvalvular Obstruction |
|---|---|---|---|---|---|
| *Possible diagnoses* | Heart block<br>Bradyarrhythmias<br>Tachyarrhythmias | Acute MI<br>Acute MR<br>Acute VSD<br>Cardiac rupture | Acute AR<br>Acute MR<br>Critical AS<br>Prosthetic valve thrombosis | Myocarditis<br>Cardiomyopathy | Myxoma<br>Cardiac tamponade<br>Constrictive pericarditis<br>Hypertrophic cardiomyopathy |
| *Diagnostic tests* | | Cardiac isoenzymes<br>Cardiac cath/angio<br>Oximetry series<br>Echo | Echo-doppler<br>TEE *(aortic dissection)*<br>Blood cultures *(endocarditis)* | Echo<br>Biopsy | Echo<br>Cardiac cath |

**Definitive Diagnosis and Treatment**

**Remember:* Myocardial ischemia may be a *complication of shock* (e.g. GI bleed→ hypotension→ myocardial ischemia) *rather than the primary cause.*

*MI = myocardial infarction; MR = mitral valve regurgitation; AR = aortic valve regurgitation; AS = aortic valve stenosis; TEE = transesophageal echo; VSD = ventricular septal defect*

## Figure 3. Management of Low Output Based on Hemodynamics

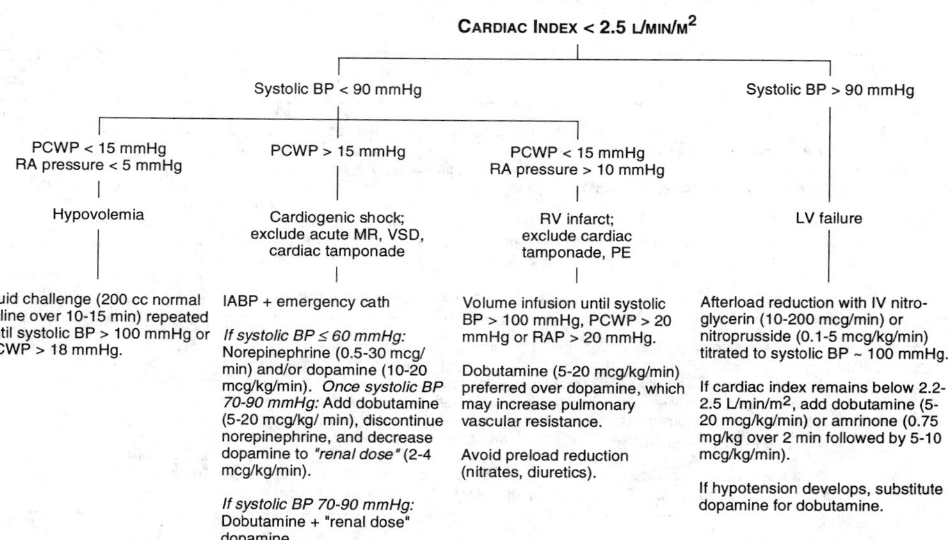


*L(R)V = left (right) ventricle; MR = mitral regurgitation; PCWP = pulmonary capillary wedge pressure; RA = right atrial; VSD = ventricular septal defect; PE = pulmonary embolus; IABP = intra-aortic balloon pump*

## IV. CARDIOGENIC SHOCK: CAUSE-SPECIFIC THERAPY

| Etiology | Therapy |
|---|---|
| Acute myocardial infarction (MI) | • **Chewable aspirin (325 mg), IV heparin (10,000 unit bolus), emergency cardiac cath, and direct angioplasty supported by intraaortic balloon pumping (IABP)**. Exclude acute mitral regurgitation (MR) and ventricular septal rupture at time of cath (or by echo).<br>• Parenteral inotropes, vasopressors, and afterload reduction as guided by hemodynamics (p. 93).<br>• Consider early mechanical ventilation to decrease the work of breathing and myocardial oxygen consumption.<br>• **Emergency bypass surgery** for failed angioplasty, left main or severe 3-vessel CAD.<br>• Refractory shock: IABP or left ventricular assist device as a bridge to **cardiac transplantation**.<br>• Treat complications: In addition to severe LV dysfunction, acute mechanical complications (RV infarction, MR, VSD, LV free-wall rupture with tamponade) and electrical complications (arrhythmia, AV block) may contribute to the shock state. |
| Right ventricular (RV) infarction | **Primary angioplasty or thrombolytic therapy followed by stepwise therapy until hypotension and low output resolve**:<br>1) Volume load until BP > 100 mmHg, LV filling pressure > 20 mmHg, or right atrial pressure > 20 mmHg. High filling pressures are required for optimal RV function; preload reducing agents such as nitrates and diuretics should be avoided acutely.<br>2) Dobutamine 5-20 mcg/kg/min.<br>3) Dopamine 5-20 mcg/kg/min (caution: may ↑ pulmonary vascular resistance and RV afterload).<br>4) IABP, especially if significant LV dysfunction is present. AV sequential pacing to maintain AV synchrony ("atrial kick") during bradyarrhythmias or heart block. The roles of right ventricular assist device and pulmonary artery balloon counterpulsation are unresolved.<br>5) Cardiac transplantation for refractory shock. |
| Myocarditis/ cardiomyopathy | See p. 153. |

*See p. 1 for abbreviations and p. 199 for drug information.*

## IV. CARDIOGENIC SHOCK: CAUSE-SPECIFIC THERAPY

| Etiology | Therapy |
|---|---|
| Hypertrophic cardiomyopathy crisis | • **Phenylephrine** to ↑ systemic vascular resistance and ↓ outflow obstruction (initial dose: 0.1-0.18 mg/min IV).<br>• $\beta$-blocker (IV) to ↓ contractility, heart rate, and outflow obstruction.<br>• IV fluids to ↑ LV cavity size and ↓ outflow obstruction.<br>• Emergency cardioversion for AFIB.<br>• AV sequential pacing to maintain AV synchrony ("atrial kick") during heart block.<br>• Avoid nitrates, diuretics, and vasodilators (may ↑ outflow tract obstruction). |
| Acute mitral regurgitation (MR) | • **Intra-aortic balloon pump** (to decrease regurgitant volume and increase forward stroke volume, cardiac output, and coronary perfusion pressure) ***followed by*** **nitroprusside (0.3-10 mcg/kg/min)**. Dobutamine (5-20 mcg/kg/min) may be of adjunctive value.<br>• **Emergency** cardiac cath followed by mitral **valve repair or replacement** for papillary muscle rupture. Operative mortality 35%. Ischemic MR without papillary muscle rupture may improve after urgent PTCA. |
| Acute aortic regurgitation | • Nitroprusside (0.3-10 mcg/kg/min) to maintain systolic BP ≈ 100 mmHg and **emergency valve replacement.**<br>• $\beta$-blocker *before* nitroprusside if caused by aortic dissection (p. 172); $\beta$-blockers may increase the regurgitant fraction but are necessary to offset the increase in shear force caused by nitroprusside.<br>• Antibiotics for infectious endocarditis (Ch. 11).<br>• Percutaneous cardiopulmonary support if cardiac arrest is imminent.<br>• Intra-aortic balloon pumping is contraindicated (increases regurgitant fraction). |
| Critical aortic stenosis | Either **emergency valve replacement** or balloon valvuloplasty *followed by* elective valve replacement. IV vasopressors and IABP to support BP; gentle use of diuretics may improve pulmonary congestion (caution: aggressive preload reduction may induce severe hypotension); inotropes often of limited value (relatively fixed cardiac output). |
| Atrial myxoma | **Emergency surgical excision**. Change in body position may temporarily relieve obstruction. |

*See p. 1 for abbreviations and p. 199 for drug information.*

## IV. CARDIOGENIC SHOCK: CAUSE-SPECIFIC THERAPY

| Etiology | Therapy |
|---|---|
| Prosthetic valve thrombosis | Thrombolytic therapy vs surgical excision of clot. Thrombolytic therapy has been successfully employed to lyse clot and improve valve function in the non-shock state; definitive recommendations await further testing. |
| Ventricular septal rupture | • **Intra-aortic balloon pumping followed by vasodilators** (hydralazine or nitroprusside) ± inotropes. Note: Nitroprusside may increase vascular resistance and left-to-right shunting; should this occur, hydralazine is often a useful substitute.<br>• **Emergency surgical repair** is required; coronary bypass grafting, aneurysectomy, and mitral valve replacement (posterior septal ruptures) may also be necessary.<br>• Transcatheter VSD closure has been successfully performed for nonoperative candidates. |
| Cardiac rupture, free wall | See p. 62. |
| Cardiac tamponade | IV fluids (rapid infusion), inotropes, and vasopressors as needed to support BP during preparation for **emergency pericardiocentesis** (see pp. 157-158). |

## V. OBSTRUCTIVE SHOCK

| Etiology | Therapy |
|---|---|
| Pulmonary embolus | Thrombolytic therapy or pulmonary embolectomy for lytic-ineligible patients. See Ch. 16. |
| Tension pneumothorax | **Emergency chest tube** placement. If not immediately available, insert a large (16-gauge or larger) needle or angiocath into the pleural space at 3rd or 4th intercostal space along the anterior axillary line. If penetrating wound present, keep wound open with insertion of gloved finger or clamp. Unless immediately corrected, respiratory failure and cardiovascular collapse ensue. |

*See p. 1 for abbreviations and p. 199 for drug information.*

## VI. DISTRIBUTIVE SHOCK

| Etiology | Therapy |
|---|---|
| Acute adrenal insufficiency | • Aggressive search for and treatment of precipitating factor; correct electrolyte, glucose abnormalities, hypothyroidism and panhypopituitarism when present.<br>• **IV fluid resuscitation**: May need > 500 cc/hr of 0.9 NaCl x 2-4 hrs. IV vasopressors and inotropes may be required for temporary support of BP.<br>• **IV corticosteroids**: Hydrocortisone 100-200 mg IV bolus every 4-6 hrs x 24 hrs followed by 50 mg every 6 hrs x 24 hrs if response is satisfactory. Begin oral steroids on day 3 with prednisone (20-30 mg/d in divided doses) ± fludrocortisone (Florinef, 0.05-0.2 mg/d). **If the diagnosis is in doubt**, substitute dexamethasone (5-10 mg IV bolus) for the first dose of hydrocortisone and perform **ACTH (Cortrosyn) stimulation test**: Obtain baseline cortisol, give $ACTH_{1-24}$ (0.25 mg IV over 2 min), and draw repeat cortisol levels at 30 and 60 minutes. Failure to stimulate cortisol by 5-8 mcg/dL to > 15-18 mcg/dL suggests adrenal insufficiency. Hydrocortisone interferes with the test, dexamethasone does not. |
| Anaphylactic shock | 1) **Remove offending agent**: Stop drug infusion or remove insect stinger. To delay absorption of insect antigen, infiltrate epinephrine (0.2-0.3 cc of 1:1,000 solution) around sting site; proximal tourniquet may also be of value.<br>2) **Secure airway:** Endotracheal intubation, cricothyroidotomy, tracheostomy as necessary.<br>3) **Epinephrine:** *Hypotension*: 1-5 cc of 1:10,000 solution via IV or endotracheal tube; an IV drip (1-4 mcg/min) may be required to prevent relapses. *Skin or pulmonary manifestations without hypotension*: 0.3-0.5 cc of 1:1,000 solution (0.3-0.5 mg) subcutaneously every 10-20 min as needed.<br>4) **Fluid resuscitation:** Aggressive IV fluids to replete extracellular volume deficit (up to 1 liter of 0.9 NaCl with dextrose 10-15 min).<br>5) **Vasopressors:** Dopamine (5-20 mcg/kg/min) or norepinephrine (0.5-30 mcg/min) if hypotension persists.<br>6) **MAST trousers** should be considered in cases of persistent shock.<br>7) **Steroids:** Hydrocortisone 100-200 mg every 4-6 hrs x 24 hrs. Increased responsiveness to adrenergic agents may be evident within 2 hrs, but no direct effects for 6-12 hrs.<br>8) **Antihistamines:** Diphenhydramine HCl (25-50 mg) and $H_2$ blocker (e.g., cimetidine 300 mg) IV/PO q 6-8 hrs.<br>9) **For bronchospasm:** Albuterol (0.5 cc of 0.5% solution in 2-5 cc of normal saline) as aerosolized mist every |

*See p. 1 for abbreviations and p. 199 for drug information.*

## VI. DISTRIBUTIVE SHOCK

| Etiology | Therapy |
|---|---|
| Anaphylactic shock (cont.) | 15-30 min. Aminophylline: loading dose 5-6 mg/kg over 20 min followed by 0.2-0.9 mg/kg/hr to maintain serum levels of 10-20 mcg/dL.<br>• Prophylaxis: Desensitization for drug allergy or insect sting. For radiocontrast allergy, no regimen is fully protective: One approach includes the administration of prednisone 60 mg, diphenhydramine HCl 50 mg, and cimetidine 300 mg every 6 hrs starting one day prior to exposure (last dose ≈ 1 hr before case). May give supplemental IV hydrocortisone (100-200 mg) and diphenhydramine HCl (50 mg) immediately prior to the procedure, especially for emergency cases without prior prophylaxis.<br>• Be prepared to treat relapses, which, although uncommon, may occur 1-2 days later. |
| Septic shock | **1) Identify and eradicate the infection** including cultures of sputum, urine, and blood. Chest x-ray, urinalysis, antibiotic therapy, and surgical drainage as needed.<br>**2) Fluid resuscitation:** 200 cc of normal saline or lactated ringers over 5 min. If unresponsive, give an additional 1-1.5 L over 20 min. If still unresponsive, consider invasive monitoring and infuse an additional 2-4 L over 1 hr. If shock is severe at onset, persistent, or is complicated by pulmonary edema, use vasopressors to support BP.<br>**3) Vasopressors:** Dopamine 5-20 mcg/kg/min. Nonresponders: Norepinephrine (0.5-30 mcg/min) and attempt to wean dopamine to renal dose (2-4 mcg/kg/min).<br>**4) Inotropes:** Dobutamine 5-20 mcg/kg/min (for low cardiac output) in combination with dopamine or norepinephrine. Intra-aortic balloon pumping may be of adjunctive value.<br>**5) Prevention of nosocomial infections:** Aseptic technique for IV catheters, intra-arterial catheters, and mechanical support devices (ventilator, intraaortic balloon pump), handwashing, isolation techniques for patients shedding virulent organisms, and hospital surveillance program.<br>When the source of infection escapes early detection, **search typical sites of occult infection** including the urinary tract, biliary system, pelvis, and retroperitoneum. Cause of death: Multiple organ system failure (50%), unresponsive hypotension (40%), and severe cardiac failure (10%). **Steroids of no value**. |

*See p. 1 for abbreviations and p. 199 for drug information.*

## VII. DRUG OVERDOSE

| Drug | COMMENTS |
|---|---|
| **β**-blockers | • Features: Hypotension, bradycardia, hypoglycemia (impaired glycogenolysis), hyperkalemia, bronchospasm, heart failure, seizures (lipid-soluble agents), AV block, asystole.<br>• Treatment: **Glucagon** may improve inotropicity and electrical conduction via non-adrenergic mechanisms (increased cAMP). Dose: 5-10 mg IV bolus; maintenance infusion of 2-5 mg/hr. |
| Calcium channel blockers | • Features: Hypotension, bradycardia, AV block.<br>• Treatment: If hypotension persists despite general measures (fluids, pressors, etc.), **10% calcium chloride** (5-10 mL IV over 5-10 min) may improve cardiac contractility. Effect on heart block is usually less pronounced. |
| Sedative-hypnotics | • Features: Hypotension with deep coma. Decreased muscle tone and hypothermia may be present as well.<br>• Treatment: Hemodialysis or hemoperfusion for refractory hypotension due to selected agents (e.g. phenobarbital, meprobamate). **Flumazenil (Mazicon),** a benzodiazipine antagonist, may be of value. Dose: 0.2 mg IV q 5-10 min up to 3-4 mg. |
| Theophylline | • Features: Hypotension, tachycardia, seizures, tachyarrhythmias, hypokalemia.<br>• Treatment: IV **β**-blocker (Esmolol) may be of value for hypotension and atrial/ventricular tachyarrhythmias; activated charcoal; hemoperfusion for severe intoxication. |
| Tricyclic antidepressant | • Features: Mydriasis, dry mouth, tachycardia, agitation, seizures, coma. Cardiovascular manifestations: Widened QRS (> 100 msec), prolonged QT and PR intervals (due to quinidine-like properties), AV block, Torsade de Pointes, ventricular tachycardia, profound hypotension.<br>• Treatment is controversial. Contact regional poison control center. |

*See p. 1 for abbreviations and p. 199 for drug information.*

## VIII. MANAGEMENT OF COMPLICATIONS

| Complication | Therapy |
|---|---|
| Acidosis (lactic) | • Treat underlying condition.<br>• Endotracheal intubation and mechanical hyperventilation.<br>• If pH < 7.1-7.2 and serum $HCO_3$ < 10 meq/L, consider raising serum $HCO_3$ to 12 meq/L: No. amps $NaHCO_3 = \frac{(12 - \text{serum } HCO_3) \times 0.5 \times (\text{weight, kg})}{44}$<br>• As acidosis resolves, monitor closely for the development of hypokalemia and low ionized $Ca^{++}$ (tetany, parasthesias). Acidosis may temporarily worsen as lactate is washed out of previously hypoxic tissues. |
| Adult respiratory distress syndrome (ARDS) | • **Mechanical ventilation**: Required in the vast majority of cases to maintain oxygenation ($p0_2 \geq 55$ mmHg), ventilation ($pCO_2 \leq 40\text{-}45$ mmHg), and to decrease the work of breathing. Initial ventilator settings: Assist-controlled ventilation, tidal volume 10-15 cc/kg, rate 10-12 per minute, $FIO_2$ 100%, PEEP 5-7.5 cm of $H_20$, I/E ratio 1:1 or greater. Once an adequate $pO_2$ is confirmed, begin to dial the $FI0_2$ down to ≤ 50%; if unable to maintain oxygenation, increase PEEP and/or minute ventilation. Obtain ABGs 15 minutes after every change in ventilator setting and q 6 hours thereafter. **Weaning from mechanical ventilatory support** can be attempted as the disease process nears resolution, as manifested by clinical stability, minute ventilation < 10 L/min, vital capacity of 10-15 cc/kg, maximum inspiratory pressure more negative than minus 20 $cmH_20$, a ratio of dead space-to-tidal volume < 0.6, and a $pO_2$ > 60 mmHg on $FI0_2$ ≤ 40%. If unable to wean from ventilator by 2 weeks, consider tracheostomy.<br>• Obtain daily chest x-rays to assess progress, ensure proper positioning of ET tube, and exclude barotrauma.<br>• **Thermodilution pulmonary artery catheter** is used to assess cardiac function, filling pressures (i.e., volume status), systemic and pulmonary vascular resistances. Goal is to maintain the lowest wedge pressure consistent with adequate organ perfusion. Continued... |

| Complication | Therapy |
|---|---|
| ARDS (cont.) | • High index of suspicion and early therapy of superinfection (bronchopneumonia). Common pathogens include gram negatives (especially pseudomonas) and S. aureus. Empiric therapy: Vancomycin and either 1) ceftazidine *or* 2) ticarcillin/clavulinate + an aminoglycoside. Definitive therapy based on culture and sensitivity.<br>• **Frequent (q 2 hrs) nasotracheal suction**/lavage with small volumes of normal saline **and chest physiotherapy** to mobilize secretions and decrease mucous plugging and atelectasis.<br>• **Sedation** with valium, hypnotics, and/or narcotics to keep the patient comfortable and from fighting the ventilator.<br>• **Aggressive nutritional support**.<br>• Unless the cause is rapidly reversed, a prolonged and complicated clinical course is the rule with mortality in excess of 60%. |
| Aspiration | • **Prevention is the key: Intubate** patients with impaired mentation or frequent emesis (e.g. large UGI bleed), administer small-volume tube **feedings only if evidence of gastric emptying is present**, and provide **prophylaxis against stress gastritis** with sulcralfate (1 gm via NG tube or po q 6 hrs) or $H_2$ blockers (to maintain gastric pH >3.5). *Empiric antibiotics and steroids are of no benefit and may be detrimental.*<br>• Laryngoscopy or nasopharyngoscopy for relief of upper airway obstruction (stridor), bronchoscopy to remove particulate matter, and positive pressure ventilation for severe lung injury.<br>• Manage complications including bacterial superinfection, lung abscess, empyema, and ARDS. **Superinfection** is usually polymicrobial and may be treated with clindamycin, cefoxitin, or ampicillin-sulbactam. If superinfection develops in the hospital, add coverage for gram negative organisms with gentamicin, a broad-spectrum penicillin (piperacillin), a cephalosporin (ceftazidine), or a monobactam (aztreonam). |

## VIII. MANAGEMENT OF COMPLICATIONS

| Complication | Therapy |
|---|---|
| Disseminated intravascular coagulation (DIC) | • Eliminate the cause.<br>• If fibrinogen level < 50 mg/dL or < 100 mg/dL with bleeding, give **cryoprecipitate** (10 units) to maintain fibrinogen > 100 mg/dL. If platelet count < 5,000-20,000/mcL or < 50,000/mcL with bleeding, transfuse 1 unit of **platelets** per 10 kg of body weight.<br>• Overwhelming microthrombosis: **Antithrombin III or fresh frozen plasma**. Use of heparin is controversial.<br>• Labs: Prolonged PT, thrombocytopenia, hypofibrinogenemia, increased fibrin degradation products; PTT and thrombin time lack sensitivity for the diagnosis. |
| Nutritional deficiency | • In the early acute setting, provide calories with D5.45 NaCl. Monitor for hyperglycemia (insulin resistant state frequently exists).<br>• **If shock persists beyond 48 hrs**, replete protein stores (1.5 gm/kg/d) with **total parenteral nutrition**. If hepatic dysfunction with encephalopathy is present, restrict protein intake to 0.6 gm/kg/d using branched-chain amino acids; advance as tolerated.<br>• Monitor $K^+$, phosphorus, $Ca^{++}$ and glucose. |
| Mesenteric ischemia | • High index of suspicion and early surgical consultation. Early pain--often acute, severe and colicky--is frequently out of proportion to the physical examination, which is relatively benign early on. Non-occlusive mesenteric ischemia usually manifests as periumbilical cramping. Labs are nonspecific; metabolic acidosis and leukocytosis usually indicate bowel infarction.<br>• **Urgent laparotomy:** Attempt to revascularize ischemic segments and resect infarcted intestine. Second look laparotomy (24-48 hours later) is controversial. |
| Myocardial dysfunction | • IV diuretics, vasopressors, and inotropes to maintain systolic BP > 80 mmHg and cardiac index ≥ 2.5 L/min/$m^2$ (p. 93).<br>• Predisposes to multiple organ system failure syndrome. |
| Sepsis | • Regular microbial surveillance; aggressive diagnosis and treatment of suspected infection. |

*See p. 1 for abbreviations and p. 199 for drug information.*

## VIII. MANAGEMENT OF COMPLICATIONS

| Complication | Therapy |
|---|---|
| Stress gastritis | • **Prevention is the key**: High-risk patients should be treated with either sucralfate (1 gm via NG tube or orally q 6 hrs), a continuous IV infusion of $H_2$ receptor antagonist (cimetidine 50 mg/hr, ranitidine 6.25 mg/hr; ↓ dose by 50% if GFR < 30 cc/min) or hourly antacids via NG tube to maintain gastric pH > 3.5.<br>• Bleeding may be overt or occult, and is usually difficult to control. High-risk patients include those with burns over 50% of body, sepsis, respiratory failure, fulminant hepatic failure, hypotension, and renal failure. Mortality exceeds 30%. |

| Renal failure | Therapy |
|---|---|
| *General measures* | • **Identify and eliminate the cause:** Discontinue nephrotoxic drugs, reverse hypotension (pressors, antibiotics, transfusions), and improve cardiac output (inotropes for pump failure, pericardiocentesis for tamponade, surgery for ventricular septal rupture or severe valve dysfunction, antianginals/PTCA/CABG for ischemia).<br>• **Administer renal-dose dopamine** (2-4 mcg/kg/min) to increase renal blood flow.<br>• **Convert oliguric to nonoliguric** renal failure: Consider mannitol (12.5-25 gm IV over 30 min.) ± high-dose furosemide (up to 200 mg IV over 2-5 min q 8 hrs), bumetadine drip (1-2 mg/hr), or metolazone (10-20 mg po qd). If urine output improves (> 30-40 cc/hr), support with periodic diuretics.<br>• **Adjust dosage of drugs** excreted by the kidneys.<br>• **Aggressive nutritional support**. Goal: Maintain positive nitrogen balance despite hypercatebolic state. Enteral feeding are preferred over parenteral feedings. Restrict protein intake to 0.7-1.0 gm/kg/d using essential amino acids. Ensure a daily caloric intake of 25-40 kcal/kg.<br>• **Institute dialysis early.** Indications include $K^+$ > 6.5 mEq/L after treatment, serum bicarbonate < 10 mEq/L after therapy, refractory pulmonary edema, BUN > 100 and creatinine > 10 mg/dL, encephalopathy, bleeding diathesis, pericarditis, GI bleeding due to uremic enteropathy, and nutritional requirements that would precipitate volume overload or uremia. |

*See p. 1 for abbreviations and p. 199 for drug information.*

| Renal failure | Therapy |
|---|---|
| *Complications* | |
| Fluid overload | Hemofiltration or dialysis. |
| Bleeding | Desmopressin (0.3-0.4 mcg/kg over 15-30 min) to increase von Willibrand factor. Cryoprecipitate (10 units q 12-24 hrs) may also be of value. Dialysis is often required to control GI bleeding from uremic enteropathy and platelet dysfunction. GI bleeding is a major cause of death in these patients. |
| Infection | Requires a high index of suspicion, early diagnosis, and prompt therapy. Common sites of infection: lungs and surgical wounds. Fever and leukocytosis may be absent. Like GI bleeding, infection is a major cause of death in these patients. |
| Hyperkalemia | • **Regular insulin** (5-10 units IV) and glucose (1 amp. D50; 25 gm) over 5 min.<br>• **$NaHCO_3$:** 1 amp [44.6 meq] of 7.5% solution IV over 5 min repeated x 2 as needed over 30 min.<br>• **Kayexalate**: For acute severe hyperkalemia, 100 gm in 200cc's of 20% sorbitol as an enema. For moderate or subacute cases, 15-30 gm in 50-100cc's of 10% sorbitol po tid-qid (may cause volume overload and hypernatremia).<br>• **Dialysis** for refractory cases.<br>• **Calcium**: For life-threatening arrhythmias or conduction abnormalities, 10-20 cc of 10% calcium gluconate is given IV over 5-10 min. Caution: may induce digitalis toxicity; will precipitate if given in IV solutions containing bicarbonate. |
| Hyperphosphatemia | Dietary restriction (720 mg/d) + $PO_4$-binding antacids (e.g. Amphogel 15-30 cc po tid with meals). |
| Hypermagnesemia | For severe neuromuscular or cardiac complications (paralysis, respiratory failure, heart block, asystole), 10-20cc's of 10% calcium gluconate over 5-10 min (see hyperkalemia for precautions) ± dialysis. |

*See p. 1 for abbreviations and p. 199 for drug information.*

# 8. HEART FAILURE

Kanu Chatterjee, M.B, F.R.C.P.

## I. OVERVIEW

Congestive heart failure (CHF) affects 1% of the U.S. population (2.5 million patients) and accounts for more than 500,000 hospital admissions annually. Coronary artery disease (CAD) and myocardial infarction (MI) have replaced hypertension as the most frequent causes of heart failure. Common presenting symptoms include dyspnea and fatigue; others include paroxysmal nocturnal dyspnea (severe attacks of dyspnea ± bronchospasm that awaken the patient from sleep), orthopnea (dyspnea that occurs in the recumbent position and is relieved by elevation of the upper body), unexplained confusion and altered mental status, chest pain, palpitations and syncope. The most common signs include a third heart sound, pulmonary rales, increased jugular venous pressure (JVP), and peripheral edema, which is typically symmetrical, pitting, at first dependant and later generalized; other signs include pulsus alternans (alternating strong and weak peripheral pulsations), Cheyne-Stokes respiration (cyclical alternations of apnea and tachypnea during sleep), a sustained LV apical impulse, those due to heightened adrenergic tone (tachycardia, diaphoresis, cool pale extremities), and those due to right heart failure (hepatomegaly, ascites, and hepatojugular reflux [increase in jugular venous pulse after compression of right upper quadrant]). **One year mortality: Mild-moderate heart failure 20%** (NEJM 1986;314:1547); **severe heart failure 50%** (NEJM 1987;316:1429). Death may result from progressive heart failure or may occur suddenly, presumably due to ventricular tachyarrhythmias; bradyarrhythmias and heart block are much less common. Adaptive changes to severe chronic elevations of pulmonary capillary pressure often lead to an **underestimation of the severity of the hemodynamic abnormalities as assessed from the physical examination**.

Management:

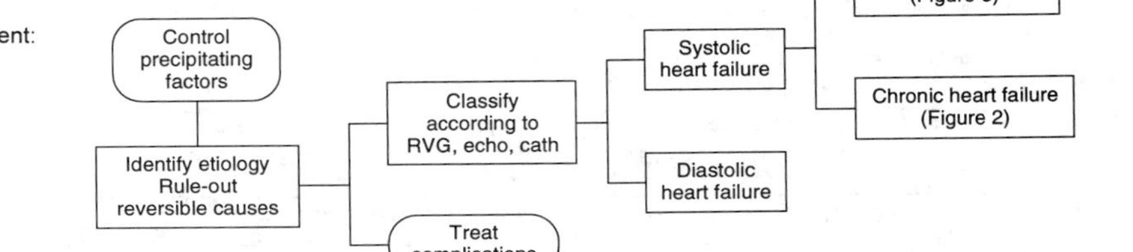


*RVG = radionuclide ventriculography*

# II. MANAGEMENT OF CHRONIC HEART FAILURE

## A. TREATMENT OF PRECIPITATING FACTORS

| | |
|---|---|
| Arrhythmias | Inappropriate bradycardia (sinus node or AV node disease) or tachycardia (AFIB, flutter, SVT, VT). |
| Drugs | Agents causing water retention including estrogens, androgens, chlorpropamide; nonsteroidal anti-inflammatory agents including ibuprofen, phenylbutazone, indomethacin; calcium channel blocking agents, especially verapamil and occasionally diltiazem; cardiac antiarrhythmic agents such as disopyramide, procainamide, flecainide; adriamycin; radiation therapy (> 4000 rads to the mediastinum); digitalis (in patients with hypertrophic obstructive cardiomyopathy); propranolol and other *β*-adrenergic blocking agents; **steroids**; minoxidil; certain tricyclic psychotropic agents, (e.g., amitriptyline). |
| Non-compliance with meds, diet | Many patients vehemently deny noncompliance despite overt dietary and medical indiscretion. High salt diet may precipitate heart failure. |
| Ischemia, MI | See Ch. 4 |
| Stress | Noncardiac medical conditions may precipitate heart failure in moderate-severe but compensated LV dysfunction. Examples include infection, PE, anemia, hypoxemia, hyperthyroidism, pregnancy, etc. |

## B. TREATMENT OF REVERSIBLE CAUSES

| Etiology | Therapy | Comments |
|---|---|---|
| Alcohol | Abstinence (See Beriberi, p. 107). | May cause a dilated cardiomyopathy or precipitate acute CHF. |
| Atrial myxoma | Surgical excision. | May cause "acute mitral stenosis" due to tumor prolapse. |
| Cardiac tamponade | Pericardiocentesis (p. 157). | Inability to fill right heart chambers due to external compression from pericardial fluid. |
| Cocaine | Abstinence. Cath & PTCA or lytic therapy for acute MI. | May also induce subendocardial necrosis, acute coronary thrombosis, and myocarditis. |

## B. TREATMENT OF REVERSIBLE CAUSES

| Etiology | Therapy | Comments |
|---|---|---|
| Congenital heart disease | Surgical correction. | Obstruction or regurgitant lesions, shunts, and hypoplastic heart chambers may cause heart failure (see Ch. 14). |
| Constrictive pericarditis | Diuretics and surgical stripping of pericardium. | Restricted filling of cardiac chambers (see p. 158). |
| Coronary artery disease | Revascularization with PTCA or coronary bypass surgery. | Myocardial ischemia may induce **systolic, diastolic, and papillary muscle dysfunction** with mitral regurgitation. |
| Endocardial fibrosis, hypereosinophilic syndrome, Loefflers | Endocardial resection ± valve replacement. Loefflers: corticosteroids ± cytotoxic agents. | **LV cavity obliteration** due to eosinophil infiltration, fibrosis, and thrombus formation. Eosinophilia in peripheral blood. |
| High-output failure | | Usually requires the presence of underlying heart muscle disease. |
| *Anemia* | Bed rest, oxygen, slow blood transfusions with diuretics. Iron, folate, $B_{12}$ replacement. | Obtain diagnostic studies (iron, ferritin, folate, etc.) prior to transfusion. |
| *AV fistula* | Surgical ligation/excision vs. embolization with gelfoam pellets. | Cardiac output is directly proportional to the size of the fistula and inversely proportional to systemic vascular resistance. |
| *Beriberi* | Thiamine (100 mg IV; 25 mg po daily x 2 wks), diuretics, nitrates. | In alcoholics on high carbohydrate diets. Increased serum pyruvate and lactate levels with low red blood cell transketolase levels. |
| *Pagets disease* | Diuretics and nitrates. | Diagnosis: Increased alkaline phosphatase, bone x-rays. |
| *Thyrotoxicosis* | Correct hyperthyroidism. Digoxin for CHF, $\beta$-blockade for AFIB. | Heart failure or AFIB may be the first sign of hyperthyroidism in the elderly ("apathetic" hyperthyroidism). |

## B. TREATMENT OF REVERSIBLE CAUSES

| Etiology | Therapy | Comments |
|---|---|---|
| Hemochromatosis | Repeated phlebotomy ± chelation therapy with desferoxamine. | Increased cardiac deposition of iron. Diabetes, cirrhosis, and hyperpigmentation may be present. |
| Hypertension | Control blood pressure (Ch. 1). | Diastolic dysfunction that may progress to systolic dysfunction. |
| Hypothyroidism | Cautious thyroid replacement; may precipitate myocardial ischemia. | Rare cause of dilated congestive cardiomyopathy. Usually requires coexistent organic heart disease. Pericardial effusion common. |
| Hypertrophic cardiomyopathy | See pp. 112-113. | Idiopathic, hypertrophic, nondilated LV results in diastolic dysfunction and is associated with sudden death. |
| Infective endocarditis | See Ch. 11. | Causes of acute heart failure include valvular insufficiency (most common), coronary artery embolism, purulent pericarditis with tamponade, heart block, and tachyarrhythmias. |
| Metabolic | Replacement therapy. | Hypophosphatemia and hypocalcemia may impair inotropicity. |
| Myocarditis | See p. 152-153. | Can mimic acute MI (chest pain, ECG changes, ↑ CPK-MB). |
| Peripartum | See p. 164. | |
| Pheochromocytoma | See p. 16. | Chronic elevated catecholamines results in dilated cardiomyopathy. |
| Sarcoidosis | Steroids. Amiodarone or internal cardioverter/defibrillator for VT | Dilated or restrictive cardiomyopathy. Arrhythmias and heart block are common with severe cardiac involvement; **sudden death** may occur. |
| Valve disease | See Ch. 9. | May produce diastolic and systolic LV dysfunction. |
| Ventricular aneurysm | Surgical resection or plication when LV function is adequate. | Most common after anterior Q-wave MI. Arrhythmias may also occur. Rupture occurs infrequently and is especially uncommon late. |

## FIGURE 2. MANAGEMENT OF CHRONIC OR REFRACTORY HEART FAILURE (SYSTOLIC)

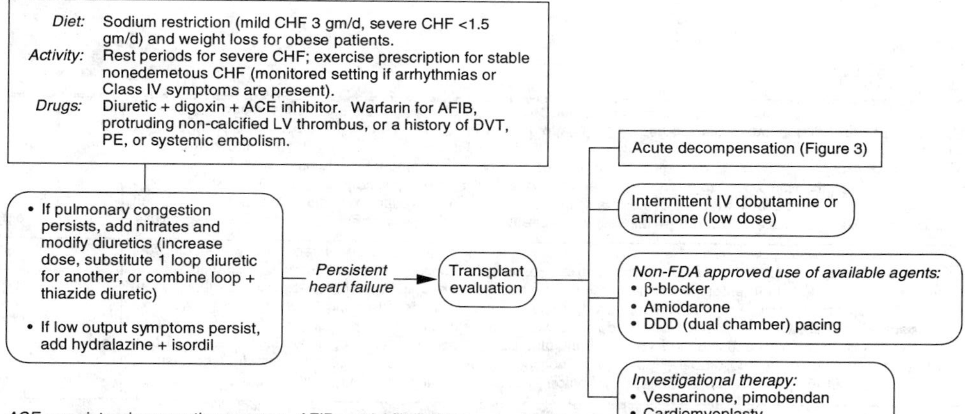


*ACE = angiotensin converting enzyme; AFIB = atrial fibrillation; DVT = deep venous thrombosis; PE = pulmonary embolism*

## III. ACUTE HEART FAILURE

| | |
|---|---|
| Overview | Myocardial infarction (MI) is the most common cause of acute heart failure and is due to both systolic dysfunction (impaired contractility) and diastolic dysfunction (decreased LV compliance). Symptoms vary from mild pulmonary congestion to severe low output and cardiogenic shock depending on the extent of nonfunctioning myocardium. **Cardiogenic shock** usually develops when the extent of myocardial necrosis exceeds 40% of LV mass, but may also result from a relatively smaller infarct when the RV is involved, mechanical complications are present (papillary muscle infarction, ventricular septal rupture), or when sustained bradyarrhythmias or tachyarrhythmias occur. In-hospital mortality ranges from 6% for those with normal LV function to 80% for patients with cardiogenic shock. |
| Killip classification | Clinical and radiologic examinations during acute MI allow assessment of heart failure severity, prognosis, and the need for hemodynamic monitoring. Quoted mortality rates are lower if reperfusion occurs:<br>• Class I: No signs of LV dysfunction; hospital mortality 6%; hemodynamic monitoring not required.<br>• Class II: $S_3$ gallop and/or mild-moderate pulmonary congestion; hospital mortality 30%; hemodynamic monitoring required.<br>• Class III: Acute severe pulmonary edema; hospital mortality 40%; hemodynamic monitoring required.<br>• Class IV: Shock syndrome; hospital mortality 80-90%; hemodynamic monitoring required. |

*See p. 1 for abbreviations and p. 199 for drug information.*

## FIGURE 3. MANAGEMENT OF ACUTE HEART FAILURE (SYSTOLIC)*

*ACE = angiotensin converting enzyme*
*AR = aortic regurgitation*
*BP = blood pressure*
*CBC = complete blood count*
*IABP = intra-aortic balloon pump (counterpulsation)*
*MR = mitral regurgitation*
*VAD = ventricular assist device*

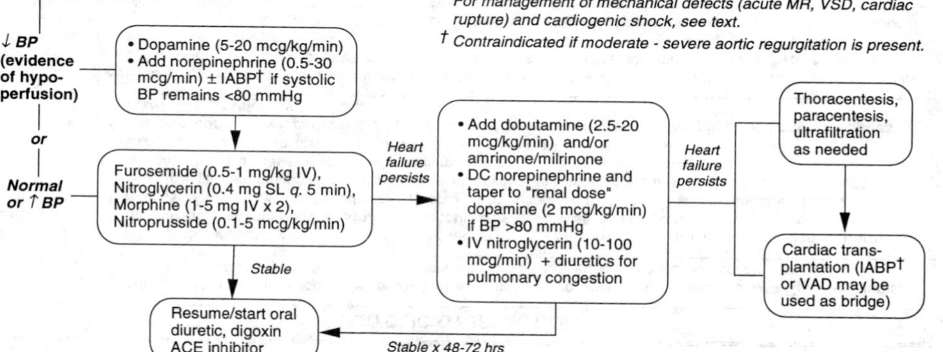


* *For management of mechanical defects (acute MR, VSD, cardiac rupture) and cardiogenic shock, see text.*

† *Contraindicated if moderate - severe aortic regurgitation is present.*

## IV DIASTOLIC DYSFUNCTION

| | |
|---|---|
| Overview | Diastolic dysfunction is responsible for **20% of all heart failure episodes**. It presents with CHF symptoms, relatively normal systolic function, and the absence of valve disease or pericardial constriction. |
| Work-up of CHF symptoms | • Assess LV function by echocardiography or radionuclide ventriculography. **If ejection fraction is normal or near-normal, suspect diastolic dysfunction as the cause of congestive heart failure**.<br>• Assess LV wall thickness by echocardiography. If considerably increased, the differential diagnosis includes hypertrophic cardiomyopathy and infiltrative diseases such as amyloid. If wall motion is normal, suspect ischemic heart disease or restrictive cardiomyopathy.<br>• Exclude valvular heart disease by echo Doppler evaluation.<br>• **Exclude constrictive pericarditis by CT scan, MRI, or cardiac cath if the physical findings suggest restrictive physiology** (p. 113). |
| Therapy<br>*General* | • Careful titration of diuretics and venodilators (e.g., nitroglycerin) are often of value for the relief of congestive symptoms. However, excessive administration may result in decreased cardiac output, hypotension, and prerenal azotemia.<br>• Hypertension and LV hypertrophy should be treated with calcium channel blockers, ACE inhibitors, and/or ***β***-blockers; these agents often improve diastolic function and decrease LV mass.<br>• Ischemia should be treated with nitrates, calcium channel blockers, ***β***-blockers, and revascularization.<br>• Atrial tachyarrhythmias (AFIB/flutter, SVT) should be treated with ***β***-blockers, verapamil, diltiazem, or digoxin (especially when systolic dysfunction coexists). Reductions in heart rate often improves diastolic filling and cardiac performance.<br>• AV sequential pacing may improve ventricular filling during bradycardia or AV block by optimizing and maintaining timed atrial contraction.<br>• **Positive inotropes such as digoxin should be avoided unless systolic failure coexists**. |
| *Hypertrophic cardiomyopathy (HCM)* | • **Asymptomatic patients should avoid strenuous physical activity and underwater sports**.<br>• Antibiotic prophylaxis for bacterial endocarditis is recommended for all patients (p. 150).<br>• Medical therapy: Symptomatic patients with *normal or hyperdynamic systolic function* should be considered for treatment with verapamil, diltiazem, or a ***β***-blocker; these agents improve diastolic relaxation, |

## IV DIASTOLIC DYSFUNCTION

| | |
|---|---|
| *Hypertrophic cardiomyopathy* *(cont.)* | LV filling and symptoms, although high doses may be required. Diuretics may further improve symptoms, although overdiuresis may ↑ outflow obstruction and cause clinical deterioration. Symptoms caused by poor systolic function are treated in the usual fashion (diuretics, digoxin, ACE inhibitor).<br>• Nonresponders: **Combination therapy with a calcium channel and β-blocker; disopyramide; dual chamber pacing** with a short AV interval.<br>• Surgery: For refractory symptoms in obstructive HCM, **myomectomy and/or mitral valve replacement** improves longterm symptomatic status in > 70%, although its effect on prognosis is unknown.<br>• **Empiric amiodarone:** May be of benefit for patients with atrial and/or ventricular arrhythmias, although its effect on longterm survival awaits definition. |

## V RESTRICTIVE CARDIOMYOPATHY

| | |
|---|---|
| Overview | Restrictive cardiomyopathy comprises only 5% of all cardiomyopathies and results from **increased stiffness of either or both ventricles** due to myocardial or endomyocardial fibrosis. Systolic function remains normal, at least initially. The **pericardium is normal**. Involvement of the AV valves is common and may cause mitral and tricuspid regurgitation. Pulmonary hypertension is common. Symptoms are nonspecific (dyspnea, atypical chest pain, fatigue, poor exercise tolerance, lower extremity swelling, palpitations due to AFIB or ventricular arrhythmias; in infiltrative disease such as amyloidosis and hemochromatosis, dizziness and syncope may occur due to involvement of the sinoatrial and/or AV node). Physical exam: Elevation of jugular venous pressure with further rise during inspiration (**positive Kussmaul's sign**) **and a sharp Y-descent** (early diastolic ventricular filling) is usually observed. The LV apical impulse is usually not markedly displaced and may be normal. Murmurs of mitral regurgitation, tricuspid regurgitation and signs of pulmonary hypertension are common. Diagnosis: Cardiac catheterization; endomyocardial biopsy in some; exclude constrictive pericarditis. |
| Therapy | No specific treatment is available for restrictive cardiomyopathy. Diuretics and nitrates may be used to control congestive symptoms, although excessive therapy may be associated with low output and hypotension. **Cardiac transplantation is the only definitive treatment**. |

*See p. 1 for abbreviations and p. 517 for drug information.*

# 9. VALVULAR HEART DISEASE

James A. Goldstein, M.D.

| I. AORTIC STENOSIS (AS) | |
|---|---|
| Etiology | Congenital: Unicuspid or bicuspid valve (prevalence 2%; presents as AS late [age 50]; responsible for 50% of aortic valve replacements [AVR]). Acquired: Rheumatic (mitral valve also involed), degenerative calcific (most common cause of AS; account for 90% of AVRs in 7th & 8th decades). Less common causes: Hyperlipidemia, rheumatoid arthritis, Pagets disease, end-stage renal failure, infective endocarditis (Candida, H. Parainfluenza). |
| Presentation | • Dyspnea, angina (50% without CAD), reduced exercise capacity (relatively late presentation), syncope (increased risk of sudden death). Complications include infective endocarditis, embolization (single episode not an indication for valve replacement), arrhythmias (uncommon until late in course), GI bleed (right-sided angiodysplasia; AVR prevents recurrence; when AS is mild-moderate, angiodysplasia can be managed by electrocautery or colonic resection).<br>• Course typified by a long latent period during which progressive obstruction and LV hypertrophy (LVH) occur. Even when severe, **aortic stenosis may be asymptomatic for many years**. Once symptoms develop, morbidity and mortality are increased; life expectancy for those with angina, syncope, and heart failure due to systolic dysfunction are 5, 3, and 2 years, respectively. |
| Diagnosis | Echocardiography, cardiac catheterization. |

*See p. 1 for abbreviations and p. 199 for drug information.*

## SUMMARY: PHYSICAL EXAM FINDINGS IN AORTIC STENOSIS

| | MILD AS AVA 1.2-2.0 $cm^2$ | MODERATE AS AVA 0.75-1.2 $cm^2$ | SEVERE AS (AVA < 0.75 $cm^2$) | |
|---|---|---|---|---|
| | | | **Compensated, NL LVEF** | **Decompensated, LVEF ↓** |
| Carotid upstroke and amplitude | N or slight ↓ upstroke | ↓ Upstroke and amplitude | ↓↓↓ Upstroke & amplitude; shudder & thrill | ↓↓↓ Upstroke & amplitude; shudder & thrill |
| Precordium | N | Sustained PMI; palpable $S_4$ | Sustained ± displaced PMI; palpable thrill | Enlarged, displaced & sustained PMI; palpable S4, S3, thrill |
| Auscultation: *S1* | N | N | N | ↓ |
| *S2* | N | N or single | Single, ↓ intensity | Single or paradoxically split, ↓ intensity |
| *S4* | -- | + | + | + |
| *S3* | -- | -- | -- | + |
| Murmur | Moderate pitch; mid-peak | High pitch; mid-to-late peak | Harsh quality, late peak; may radiate to axilla and mimic MR (Gallavardins) | Harsh quality, late peak; may hear functional MR |

PMI = point of maximal impulse; AVA = aortic valve area; LVEF = left ventricular ejection fraction; N = normal; -- = absent; + = present; MR = mitral regurgitation; ↓ = decreased

*See p. 1 for abbreviations and p. 199 for drug information.*

# Figure 1. Management of Aortic Stenosis (AS)

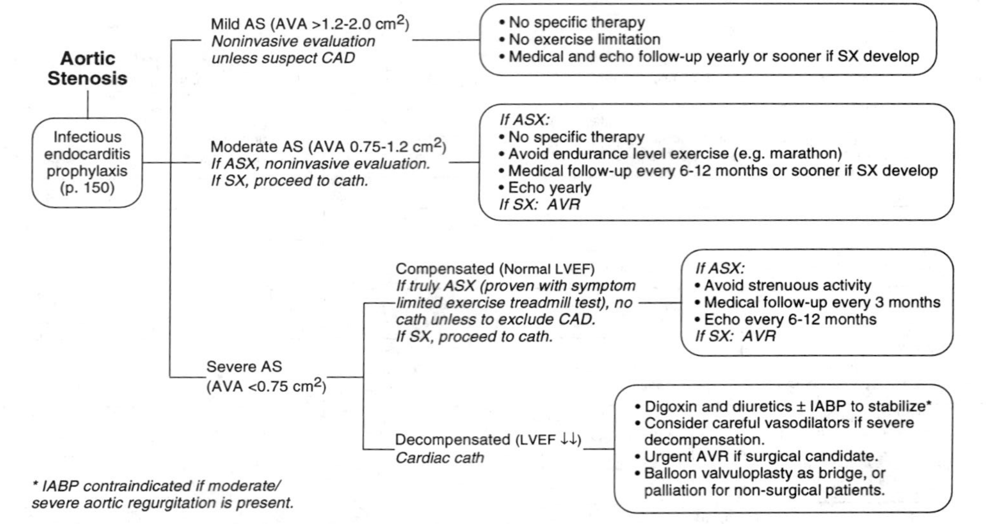


** IABP contraindicated if moderate/ severe aortic regurgitation is present.*

*AS = aortic stenosis; AVA = aortic valve area; CAD = coronary artery disease; ASX = asymptomatic; SX = symptomatic; ETT = exercise treadmill test; AVR = aortic valve replacement; IABP = intra-aortic balloon pump (counterpulsation); LVEF = left ventricular ejection fraction; NL = normal*

| II. AORTIC REGURGITATION (AR) | |
|---|---|
| Etiology | Valve disorders: Congenital bicuspid valve, rheumatic disease (mixed AS/AR), infective endocarditis (mitral valve involvement common), myxomatous valve (prolapse), valvulitis, trauma. Aortic root disorders: Connective tissue disease, systemic hypertension, syphilis, aortic dissection, supracristalar VSD. |
| Presentation<br>*Chronic AR* | Regurgitant volume induces slowly progressive LV dilatation and hypertrophy. **LV function ultimately declines, often while the patient remains asymptomatic.** Initial symptoms are typically those of pulmonary congestion (dyspnea). Angina may occur in the absence of CAD. Once symptoms develop, average survival is 2-5 years. |
| *Acute AR* | Presents as **acute pulmonary edema ± hypotension**. Severe diastolic dysfunction occurs despite intact systolic function as the normal LV and pericardium are unable to accommodate abrupt severe volume overload. Mortality is very high without acute surgical intervention. |
| Diagnosis | Echocardiography, cardiac catheterization. |

*See p. 1 for abbreviations and p. 199 for drug information.*

## SUMMARY: PHYSICAL EXAM IN AORTIC REGURGITATION

| | CHRONIC AR | | | | ACUTE AR |
|---|---|---|---|---|---|
| | | | Severe | | |
| | **Mild** | **Moderate** | *Intact LVEF* | *↓ LVEF* | |
| Vital signs | N | Normal or widened pulse pressure | ↑ Systolic BP, ↓↓ Diastolic BP | ↑ Systolic BP, ↓↓↓ Diastolic BP, ↑↑ HR, ↑ RR | ↑ Systolic BP, ↓ Diastolic BP, ↑↑↑ HR, ↑↑ RR |
| Lungs | N | N | N | Rales | Rales |
| Cardiovascular | | | | | |
| *JVP* | N | N | N | May be ↑ | N |
| *Carotid* | N | Mild ↑ | ↑↑ upstroke, ↑ volume, collapse | ↑↑ upstroke, ↑ volume, collapse | ↑ upstroke, lesser volume and collapse |
| *Precordium* | N | Mild LV heave | ↑↑ LV heave, Systolic + diastolic thrills | ↑↑↑ LV heave, thrill | Mild LV heave, thrill |
| *Auscultation* | Soft AR murmur | ↑↑ AR murmur | ↑↑ AR murmur | ↓ AR murmur, soft $S_1$, (+) $S_3$, Austin Flint rumble | Murmur loud or soft, $S_1$ very soft, (+) $S_3$ |

N = normal; ↑(↓) = increased (decreased); AOSP = aortic systolic pressure; AODP = aortic diastolic pressure; JVP = jugular venous pressure; HR = heart rate; RR = respiratory rate; LV = left ventricular; LVEF = LV ejection fraction; BP = blood pressure; (+) = present

*See p. 1 for abbreviations and p. 199 for drug information.*

## FIGURE 2. MANAGEMENT OF AORTIC REGURGITATION

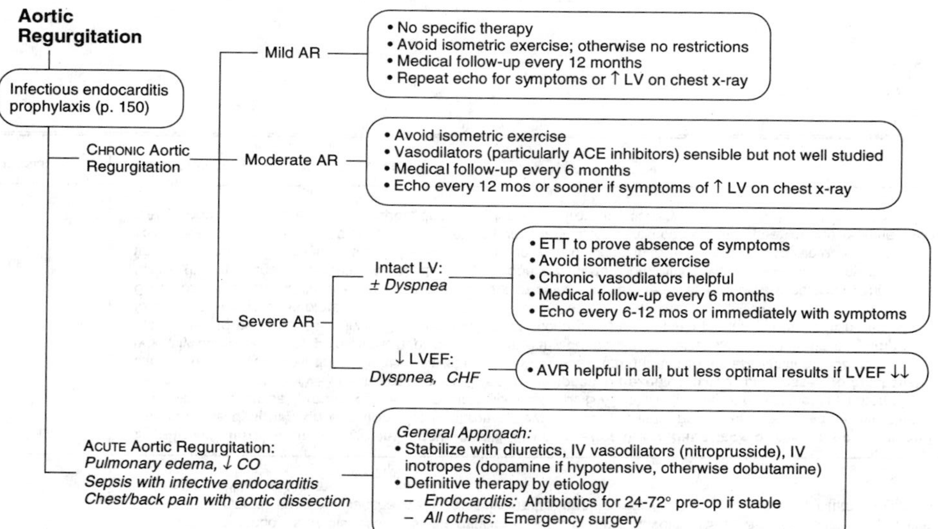


*ASX = asymptomatic; AVR = aortic valve replacement; ETT = exercise treadmill test; CO = cardiac output; LVEF = left ventricle ejection fraction; CHF = congestive heart failure; LV = left ventricle.*

## III. MITRAL STENOSIS (MS)

| | |
|---|---|
| Etiology | Acquired: Rheumatic heart disease (vast majority of cases), chronic valvulitis (SLE, amyloid, carcinoid), valve infiltration (carcinoid, mucopolysaccharides), massive mitral annular calcification, obstruction by tumors (atrial myxoma) of ball-valve thrombi. |
| Presentation | • **Significant mitral stenosis typically develops 5-20 years after the initial attack of rheumatic fever and presents as dyspnea on exertion** due to chronic elevations of left atrial pressure. Tachycardia—whether physiologic (exercise, pregnancy, fever) or pathologic (AFIB, SVT, etc.)—greatly exacerbates symptoms. As mitral valve area (MVA) decreases to 1.0-1.5 $cm^2$, dyspnea on exertion (DOE) progresses to functional class II-III exercise limitation. Tight mitral stenosis (MVA $< 1.0$ $cm^2$) leads to severe limiting DOE and is typically complicated by pulmonary hypertension. In early pulmonary hypertension, symptoms may improve but proves to be but a short lived "honeymoon" as pulmonary hypertension eventually results in profound fatigue and exercise intolerance.<br>• Other presentations include AFIB (occurs in 80% with severe mitral stenosis; emboli are common), right heart failure (hepatomegaly, ascites, edema due to pulmonary hypertension), infective endocarditis (may cause further obstruction or regurgitation), hemoptysis (usually mild; occasionally severe due to ruptured bronchial vein), hoarseness (compression of left atrium or pulmonary artery on recurrent laryngeal nerve), angina (from CAD, coronary artery embolism, subendocardial ischemia from pulmonary hypertension). |
| Diagnosis | Echocardiography, cardiac catheterization. |

*See p. 1 for abbreviations and p. 199 for drug information.*

| SUMMARY: PHYSICAL EXAM IN MITRAL STENOSIS (MS) | | | |
|---|---|---|---|
| | **Mild to Moderate MS (MVA > 2.0 cm$^2$)** | **Moderate to Severe MS (MVA 1.0-2.0 cm$^2$)** | **Critical MS (MVA < 1.0 cm$^2$)** |
| Vital signs | N | N or ↑ RR, ↑ HR | N or ↑ RR, ↑ HR |
| Chest | Clear | Clear; CHF if decompensated | Clear or CHF |
| Cardiovascular *JVP* | N | N; ↑ if pulmonary HTN | ↑ if RVH; ↑ V-wave if TR |
| *Carotid* | N | N upstroke, ↓ volume | N upstroke, ↓ volume |
| *Precordium* | N | Palpable pulmonary artery if PHTN; ↑ RV | Palpable pulmonary artery; ↑↑ RV; diastolic thrill |
| *Auscultation* | $S_1$↑, $P_2$ normal, (+) O.S. | $S_1$ ↑ if valve pliable and ↓ if nonpliable, $P_2$ ↑ if PHTN, ↓ $A_2$-O.S. interval | $S_1$ ↑ or ↓, $P_2$ ↑↑ = PHTN, ↓↓ $A_2$-O.S. interval |
| *Murmur* | Mid-diastolic rumble | Pandiastolic rumble | Diastolic rumble may ↓ with low cardiac output |

N = normal; JVP = jugular venous pressure; RV = right ventricle; RVH = right ventricular hypertrophy; RR = respiratory rate; HR = heart rate; TR = tricuspid regurgitation; CHF = congestive heart failure; PHTN = pulmonary hypertension; O.S. = opening snap; ↑(↓) = increased (decreased)

*See p. 1 for abbreviations and p. 199 for drug information.*

## Figure 3. Management of Mitral Stenosis (MS)

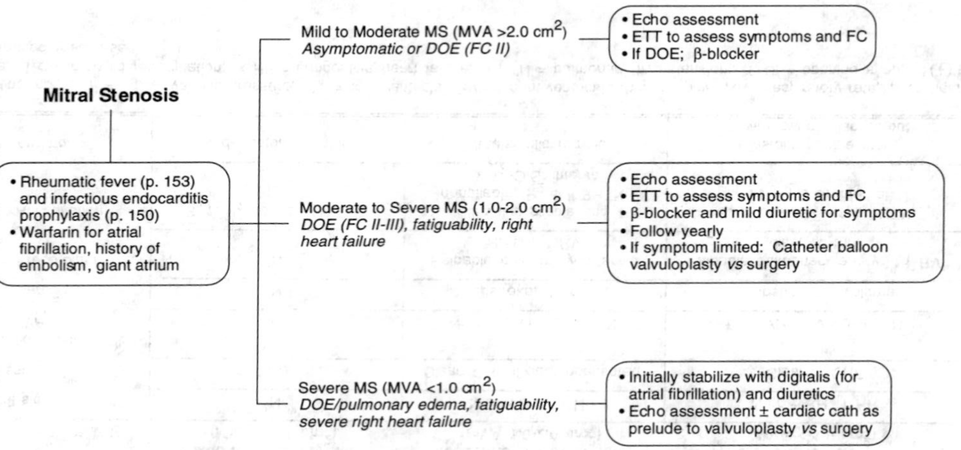


*DOE = dyspnea on exertion; FC = functional class; ETT = exercise treadmill test*

## IV. MITRAL REGURGITATION (MR)

| | |
|---|---|
| Etiology | Congenital (cleft valve, floppy valve), inflammatory (rheumatic heart disease, SLE, scleroderma, Takayasu's arteritis), degenerative (myxomatous), Marfan's, Ehler's Danlos, annular calcification, infective endocarditis, structural (ruptured chordae, ruptured or dysfunctional papillary muscle, dilatation of mitral annulus and/or LV cavity, hypertrophic cardiomyopathy, perivalvular prosthetic leak), post-valvuloplasty. |
| Presentation<br>*Chronic MR* | • Patients **may remain asymptomatic for many years**, during which time LV systolic dysfunction may develop insidiously. Course may be complicated by acute deterioration (ruptured chordae, endocarditis, etc). Five and 10-year survivals > 80% and 60%, respectively; prognosis is worse if MR is due to ischemia (5 yr. survival 30%).<br>• Symptoms include dyspnea (common; reflects either moderate-severe chronic MR or acute MR), fatigue (usually indicates severe MR with LV systolic dysfunction), hemoptysis (usually scanty; may be massive if due to a ruptured bronchial vein), and hoarseness (compression of recurrent laryngeal nerve by enlarged left atrium; more common in mitral stenosis). |
| *Acute severe MR* | Normal LV unable to acutely compensate for or accommodate diastolic volume overload. Increased wall stress may lead to **acute LV dysfunction, pulmonary edema, and hypotension**. Requires prompt intervention to reduce high mortality rates. |
| Diagnosis | Echocardiography, cardiac catheterization. |

*See p. 1 for abbreviations and p. 199 for drug information.*

## SUMMARY: Physical Exam in Mitral Regurgitation

| | CHRONIC MR | | | ACUTE SEVERE MR |
|---|---|---|---|---|
| | | Severe | | |
| | Mild-Moderate | *Compensated* | *Decompensated* | |
| Vitals | N | N | ↑ HR, ↑ RR | ↑↑ HR, ↑↑ RR |
| Chest | N | N | Rales | Rales |
| Pulses | N or ↑ upstroke | ↑ Upstroke | ↑ Upstroke, ↓ if EF ↓↓ | ↑ Upstroke, ↓ volume |
| JVP | N | N | ↑ with right heart failure (from pulmonary HTN) | ↑ with right heart failure (from pulmonary HTN) |
| Precordium | N or mild ↑ LV | ↑↑ LV ± thrill | ↑↑↑ LV, systolic thrill, palpable $P_2$ | ↑ V-wave, systolic thrill, palpable $P_2$ |
| Auscultation $S_1$ | N | N or ↓ | ↓↓ | ↓↓↓ |
| $S_2$ | N | N or slight ↑ with pulmonary HTN | ↑↑ $P_2$ | ↑↑ |
| $S_3$ | – | – | + | + |
| *Murmur* | Holosystolic murmur | Holosystolic murmur, ± diastolic flow rumble | Holosystolic murmur, diastolic flow rumble | Holosystolic murmur, diastolic flow rumble |

JVP = jugular venous pressure; N = normal; HR = heart rate; RR = respiratory rate; EF = ejection fraction; HTN = hypertension; LV = left ventricle; LVED(S)V = LV end-diastolic (systolic) volume; LVEF = LV ejection fraction; LA = left atrium; (–) = absent; (+) = present.

*See p. 1 for abbreviations and p. 199 for drug information.*

## FIGURE 4. MANAGEMENT OF MITRAL REGURGITATION (MR)

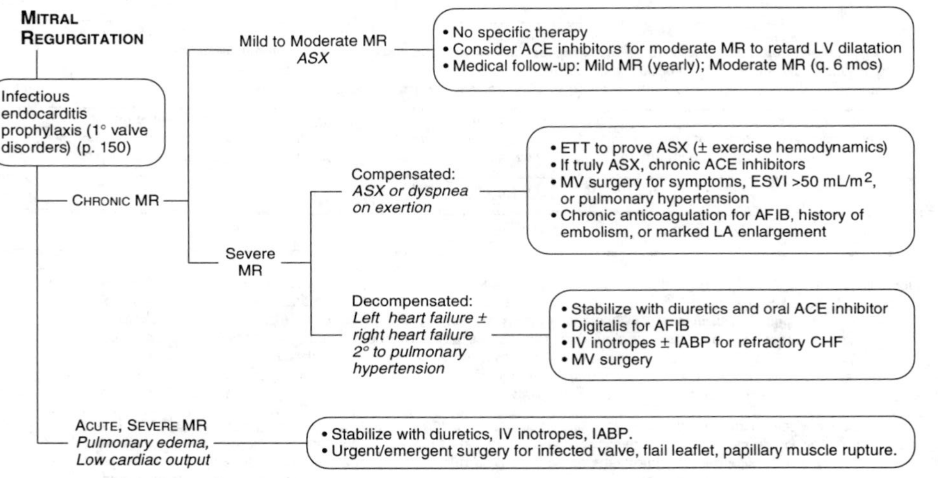


*ASX = asymptomatic; ACE = angiotensin converting enzyme; ETT = exercise treadmill test; LV = left ventricle; AFIB = atrial fibrillation; ESVI = end systolic volume index; CHF = congestive heart failure; IABP = intra-aortic balloon pump (counterpulsation)*

## V. MITRAL VALVE PROLAPSE

| | |
|---|---|
| Overview | Asymptomatic click/murmur is found in 10-15% of general population (much more common in females). **In most cases, mitral valve prolapse (MVP) is clinically silent, innocent, and benign**. Clinical associations include Marfan's, Ehlers-Danlos, atrial septal defect, hypertrophic cardiomyopathy, and congenitally corrected transposition; complications occur more often in these conditions. Auscultation: Early systolic click ± murmur of MR; maneuvers that ↓ LV volume (valsalva, supine → standing) make click-murmur occur earlier in systole. |
| Complications | • Chronic significant MR: Typically in those with myxomatous floppy valves related to Marfan's.<br>• Acute MR: Flail leaflet from ruptured chordae; classically in myxomatous or infected prolapsing valves.<br>• Infective endocarditis: Overall risk low but antibiotic prophylaxis is warranted for appropriate situations, p. 150.<br>• Non-ischemic atypical chest pain: Negative exercise thallium test; may improve with **β**-blockers.<br>• Increased incidence of SVT (AV nodal and AV reentry [Wolff-Parkinson-White syndrome]) and VT.<br>• Possible increased incidence of systemic emboli. When an embolism occurs and other causes have been excluded (e.g., AFIB, LV thrombus), aspirin is usually prescribed; warfarin (INR 2.0-3.0) may be considered for recurrences, although benefits are unknown. |

## VI. TRICUSPID REGURGITATION (TR)

| | |
|---|---|
| Etiology | Organic tricuspid valve disease: Rheumatic, infective endocarditis, RV infarction, trauma, right atrial myxoma, tricuspid valve prolapse, carcinoid, Ebstein's anomaly. Functional TR (annular dilatation and subvalvular dysfunction): Cardiomyopathies, pulmonary hypertension. |
| Presentation | Clinical picture **dominated by the underlying cause and right heart failure** (ascites, peripheral edema and GI symptoms [abdominal pain, anorexia, early satiety from bowel congestion, right upper quadrant pain from congestive hepatomegaly]). Other complaints include dyspnea, fatigue, and uncomfortable neck pulsations. |
| Diagnosis | Echocardiogram, cardiac catheterization. |

*See p. 1 for abbreviations and p. 199 for drug information.*

## VI. TRICUSPID REGURGITATION (TR)

| | |
|---|---|
| Management<br>*Medical therapy* | **Treat the underlying condition** (rheumatic aortic or mitral valve disease, infective endocarditis, cardiomyopathy, pulmonary hypertension, etc.).<br>• In the *absence of pulmonary hypertension*, even severe TR usually responds well to medical therapy with diuretics and venodilators (non-parenteral nitrates, ACE inhibitors added for severe refractory TR); dosages should be titrated to JVP height, weight loss, and extent of edema. Dobutamine may be helpful in refractory TR with severe RV failure.<br>• In the *presence of pulmonary hypertension*, in which the development of TR is devastating, interventions designed to lower pulmonary pressures are most likely to benefit (pp. 184-185). Diuretics and vasodilators may be helpful, but must be used with caution (may induce severe hypotension).<br>• Infectious endocarditis prophylaxis for organic tricuspid valve disease (p. 150); it is probably not necessary for TR secondary to pulmonary hypertension or RV dilatation with an otherwise normal valve. |
| *Surgical therapy* | Indications for TV repair or replacement: Severe refractory TR of any primary etiology (e.g., intractable infective endocarditis, trauma, carcinoid). Bioprosthetic valves preferred over mechanical valves in the tricuspid position (more durable, less thrombogenic). Annuloplasty is usually effective for secondary TR. |

## VII. TRICUSPID STENOSIS (TS)

| | |
|---|---|
| Etiology | Rheumatic heart disease (often "silent"; clinical picture dominated by mitral/aortic valve involvement), obstruction by right atrial myxoma or other tumors (renal, melanoma, testes, thyroid, liver). |
| Presentation | Chronic right heart failure with signs of systemic venous congestion: hepatomegaly, ascites, and pedal edema. If TS is very severe, low output symptoms (i.e., easy fatiguability) may also be present. Clinical picture is dominated by left heart valve involvement in rheumatic TS, or other tumor manifestations and complications in those with masses obstructing the tricuspid orifice. |
| Diagnosis | Echocardiography, cardiac catheterization. |

*See p. 1 for abbreviations and p. 199 for drug information.*

## VII. TRICUSPID STENOSIS (TS)

| | |
|---|---|
| Management | • Infective endocarditis prophylaxis: p. 150.<br>• Right heart failure: Diuretics and venodilators; overuse may ↓ cardiac output and BP.<br>• Rheumatic TS: If present at the time of mitral valve repair or replacement, the stenotic mitral valve may be improved via open valvotomy. On occasion, tricuspid valve replacement is required (bioprosthesis).<br>• Catheter balloon valvuloplasty can provide good results and may be considered an alternative to surgery.<br>• Surgical intervention should be considered for tumor involvement, which is usually definitive for myxomas and palliative ("debulking") for patients with metastatic obstruction. |

## VIII. PULMONARY VALVE REGURGITATION (PR)

| | |
|---|---|
| Etiology | Severe pulmonary hypertension (most common cause of chronic pulmonic regurgitation), infective endocarditis (most common cause of acute severe PR; usually drug abusers; often with gonococcus). Others: Congenital valve deformities, Marfan's, rheumatic heart disease, carcinoid, syphilis, and idiopathic pulmonary artery dilatation. |
| Presentation<br>*Chronic severe PR* | In *absence of pulmonary hypertension:* Usually asymptomatic and benign. In *setting of pulmonary hypertension:* Natural history dictated by severity of pulmonary hypertension and right heart failure. |
| *Acute severe PR* | Often presents as acute right heart failure. Infected pulmonary valve: In addition to acute PR, complications include pulmonary emboli and pulmonary artery abscesses. Natural history related to number of infected valves and associated complications; PR itself is rarely problematic. |
| Diagnosis | Echocardiography, cardiac catheterization. |
| Management | • Infective endocarditis prophylaxis (p. 150): Indicated for organic valve disease. Probably unnecessary if secondary to pulmonary hypertension.<br>• Right heart failure (diuretics, nitrates ± digoxin); infective endocarditis (Ch. 11); pulmonary hypertension (p. 184). |

*See p. 1 for abbreviations and p. 199 for drug information.*

## IX. PULMONARY VALVE STENOSIS (PS)

| | |
|---|---|
| Etiology | Most commonly congenital (associated with other complex congenital anomalies). Acquired PS is rare (carcinoid, massive vegetations). Pseudo-PS: External pulmonary artery compression from mediastinal tumors and rarely from Sinus of Valsalva aneurysm can simulate PS. Likewise, internal pulmonary artery luminal obstruction from a saddle embolus can simulate pulmonic valve obstruction, but is typically more acute. |
| Presentation | Fatigue, syncope, and right heart failure. |
| Diagnosis | Echocardiography, cardiac catheterization. |
| Management | • Isolated congenital PS: Often amenable to catheter balloon valvuloplasty (CBV).<br>• Acquired valvular PS: Rarely requires intervention but responds favorably to CBV.<br>• Others: External pulmonary artery compression from Sinus of Valsalva aneurysm requires surgical management of aortic root problem. Proximal pulmonary artery clots may improve with thrombolysis ± surgical embolectomy. External compression from tumors may respond to radiation or surgical debulking. |

## X. PROSTHETIC CARDIAC VALVES

| | |
|---|---|
| Valve selection<br>*Bioprosthetic valves (BPV)* | • **Patients with contraindications to chronic anticoagulation** (bleeding dyscrasias, recurrent GI bleeds, alcoholics, noncompliance). Note: Patients still require 3 months of anticoagulation post-op to allow for re-endothelialization of valve.<br>• **Patients over 65-70 years of age**, particularly in those requiring aortic valve replacement in whom the likelihood of primary valve failure in their expected life span is low.<br>• **Prosthetic replacement of the tricuspid valve**, even in patients undergoing concomitant mechanical valve implantation in the mitral or aortic position.<br>• **Women of child-bearing age planning pregnancy**. Although the risks of warfarin to mother and fetus can be avoided with BPV, the increased risk of accelerated primary valve failure is daunting. In such patients with mitral or aortic stenosis, catheter balloon valvuloplasty may be an attractive alternative. |

*See p. 1 for abbreviations and p. 199 for drug information.*

## X. PROSTHETIC CARDIAC VALVES

| | |
|---|---|
| *Mechanical valves* | The prosthesis of choice (especially in mitral position) in patients < 65 years of age who are reasonable candidates for chronic anticoagulation. |
| Management<br>*General* | • Infectious endocarditis prophylaxis for appropriate indications (p. 150); avoidance of bacteremia (indwelling IV lines, especially central catheters); physician follow-up every 6 months; echocardiogram yearly.<br>• Medical therapy: Careful anticoagulation with **warfarin** (INR 3.0-4.5). **Low-dose aspirin**: Patients with mechanical valves and high-risk patients with bioprosthetic valves may benefit from the addition of low-dose aspirin (100 mg/d) to warfarin (NEJM 1993;329:524).<br>• Management of anticoagulation prior to major noncardiac surgery: see p. 139. |
| *Embolization* | • **Non-infectious source, normal prosthetic valve function**: Heparinize acutely if INR is less than 3.0. If INR is 3.0-4.5, consider intensification of warfarin regimen (INR of 4.0-5.0) and/or the addition of aspirin (100-325 mg/qd). Recurrent emboli "umpired" as in baseball: "Three strikes and you're out." Role of acute lytic therapy for recurrent emboli is unknown.<br>• **Emboli with prosthetic valve infection**: One significant embolic episode will in many cases warrant surgery. However, must consider other factors: vegetation size, organism, presence of other mechanical complications (ring infection, regurgitation), stroke, risk of bleed with surgery, and candidacy for reoperation. |
| *Valve thrombosis* | May be managed initially with thrombolytic therapy in selected cases (exact role unknown); monitored by echo-doppler and/or fluoroscopy; re-thrombosis may occur and require surgery. Patients at risk for bleeding, with significant hemodynamic compromise, or with thrombus superimposed on pannus may be better managed with surgery (thrombectomy or valve replacement). |
| *Infective endocarditis* | Prosthetic valve endocarditis is associated with a high risk of complications (valve regurgitation, local extension of infection, emboli) and is exceedingly difficult to cure by antibiotics alone. Although patients with less virulent organisms (e.g., staph epidermidis) without mechanical complications can initially be treated medically, surgery should be considered early in the course. For specific antibiotic regimens, see pp. 145, 147. |
| *Bleeding from anticoagulation* | Very common in the lifetimes of patients with prosthetic valves; most can tolerate diminution or reversal of anticoagulation for several days (IV vitamin K, 5-10 mg ± fresh frozen plasma, 1-2 units). Persue measures to aggressively and quickly resolve primary hemorrhagic defects (radiologic or surgical interventions). |

## SUMMARY: PROSTHETIC CARDIAC VALVES

| | MECHANICAL | BIOPROSTHETIC |
|---|---|---|
| Hemodynamics | • Bileaflet central flow orifice designs (e.g., St. Jude) are the least obstructive, especially in smaller sizes.<br>• Tilting discs (Björk-Shiley) have good hemodynamic profiles.<br>• Caged-ball devices (Starr) have higher profiles and are intrinsically more stenotic. | • Hemodynamics of modified porcine designs (Hancock, Carpentier-Edwards) are similar to bileaflet central orifice mechanical types.<br>• Homograft hemodynamics are excellent, but the implant procedure may induce aortic regurgitation. |
| Durability | Excellent out past 20 years. | Major functional limitation by 5 years; replacement likely by 10-15 years. |
| Anticoagulants | Absolute in all valves in all positions. | All require 2-3 months post-implant. Some advocate long-term anticoagulation for valves in the mitral and tricuspid positions. |
| Thromboemboli | Valve thrombosis with thromboembolization is a major problem. | Uncommon in the aortic position; still problematic for mitral and tricuspid sites. |
| Infective endocarditis | Increased risk. Usually perivalvular in location. Results in regurgitation ± hemolysis. Bulky vegetations occasionally obstruct. Embolization from vegetations is always a risk. | Increased risk. Valvular or perivalvular in location. Infection commonly involves the valve leaflets to result in valvular regurgitation more often than stenosis; perivalvular abscess formation and regurgitation may also occur. |
| Mechanisms of valve failure | Obstruction is secondary to thrombosis, pannus, or bulky vegetations. Regurgitation is usually perivalvular and due to infective endocarditis. | Regurgitation is a major problem, which may be valvular from leaflet tears (usually caused by a degenerative or infectious process) or perivalvular from infective endocarditis. |

# 10. NONCARDIAC SURGERY FOR THE CARDIAC PATIENT

Thomas H. Lee, M.D.

| I. APPROACH TO PREOPERATIVE RISK ASSESSMENT | |
|---|---|
| Overview | **Although *"clearance"* is frequently requested, this term should be avoided since it implies a guarantee that complications will not occur,** and every surgical intervention entails some risk.<br>The highest rates of cardiovascular complications (~4%) occur in patients undergoing major aortic (e.g., AAA repair), intrathoracic (e.g., lung resection), and intra-abdominal operations (e.g., colon resection). Lower rates of complications are seen following major orthopedic procedures (~1%), whereas ophthalmological surgery and transurethral prostatic resection are almost always safe. The **risk of post-op MI or cardiac death is 4-fold higher when surgery is performed emergently** rather than electively. The preoperative assessment is an attempt to identify "needles in haystacks". |
| Physical exam | If the physical exam suggests aortic stenosis, LV dysfunction, peripheral/cerebrovascular disease, pulmonary disease, or infection, further evaluation is required to establish a diagnosis and assess the severity of the condition. |
| Labs | Minimum requirements include a complete blood count, platelet count, PT/PTT, glucose, serum electrolytes, renal and liver function tests. |
| ECG & Echo | • ECG: If the preoperative ECG is abnormal, it should be compared to a prior ECG to exclude a recent ischemic event. In patients with no old tracing and evidence of possible infarction on the preoperative ECG, an echocardiogram ± exercise test should be performed to confirm or undermine the diagnosis of CAD.<br>• Echo: Indicated for those with known or suspected congenital, valvular or ischemic heart disease, and when the physical exam suggests LV dysfunction. |
| Noninvasive cardiac testing | **Indicated for those with known or suspected coronary disease prior to high risk procedures, and for patients in whom the stability of ischemic symptoms and functional status are difficult to assess** (e.g., poor historian; sedentary lifestyle). |

*See p. 1 for abbreviations and p. 199 for drug information.*

| I. APPROACH TO PREOPERATIVE RISK ASSESSMENT | |
|---|---|
| Noninvasive cardiac testing (cont.) | If noninvasive testing is negative for ischemia, the likelihood of a perioperative complication is extremely low. However, the converse is not true: if noninvasive testing is positive for ischemia, only 10-40% will develop an ischemic complication. Therefore, **an abnormal test does not mean that coronary angiography is automatically warranted.** This decision should be individualized and based on the workload at which ischemia occurs, the amount of myocardium at risk, LV function, symptomatic status, and surgical risk. |
| *Exercise stress test* | Best direct measure of functional capacity for those able to perform graded exercise. The **ability to reach the third or fourth Bruce Protocol stage is associated with a very low perioperative cardiac complication rate, even if evidence of ischemia develops.** On the other hand, patients who cannot raise their heart rate to 85% of their predicted maximum due to fatigue or dyspnea should be considered at increased risk *even if no evidence of ischemia is detected.* |
| *Pharmacologic stress test* | Indicated for those who require noninvasive testing but cannot exercise (e.g., severe claudication, arthritis). |
| Coronary angiography | Indications:<br>• Class III or IV angina prior to high-risk surgery<br>• Known/suspected CAD and inability to reach 85% of predicted maximal heart rate or severe ischemia on provocative testing |

## Figure 1. Estimating Preoperative Coronary Risk

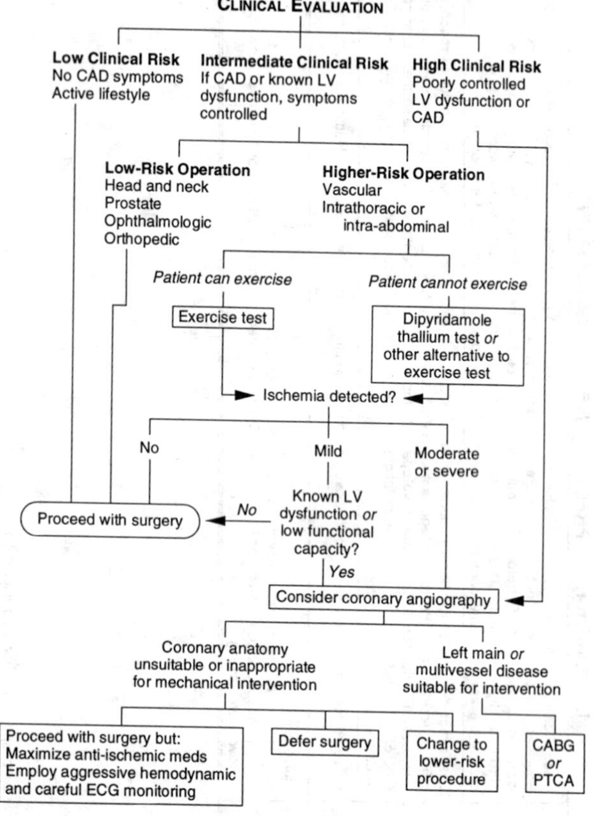


In assessing patients for surgery consider clinical risk profile, type of surgery, and results of noninvasive testing or coronary angiography. Urgent surgery may preempt risk stratification.

CAD = coronary artery disease; LV = left ventricular; ECG = electrocardiogram; CABG = coronary artery bypass graft; PTCA = percutaneous transluminal coronary angioplasty.

*Modified from Eagle KA, Boucher CA: Cardiac Risk of Noncardiac Surgery. N Eng J Med 1989;321:1330.*

## II. PREOPERATIVE RISK REDUCTION

| | |
|---|---|
| Prophylactic measures | • Deep venous thrombosis/pulmonary embolism: See p. 183.<br>• Infectious endocarditis: See p. 150.<br>• Adrenal insufficiency: Err on side of overreplacement. One protocol includes hydrocortisone 100 mg IM or IV on-call to the operating room followed by 50 mg IM or IV in the recovery room and every 6 hrs for 24 hrs. If progress is satisfactory, the dose can then be reduced to 25 mg every 6 hrs for 24 hrs, and then tapered to maintenance doses over 3-5 days. Fludrocortisol (Florinef, 0.05-0.2 mg po qd) is restarted when the patient is able to take oral medications.<br>• Anticoagulation: Discontinue warfarin 5-7 days prior to surgery when anticoagulation is being prescribed for prophylaxis against DVT or systemic emboli from atrial fibrillation. For mechanical valves, see p. 139. |

## III. PREOPERATIVE MANAGEMENT OF COMMON MEDICAL CONDITIONS

| Pre-Op Condition | Therapy |
|---|---|
| Arrhythmias<br>*AFIB/flutter* | Ventricular response must be controlled before surgery, but there is **no need to attempt cardioversion specifically for pre-op purposes if the patient is hemodynamically stable**. Discontinue warfarin 3-5 days prior to surgery and reinstitute 1-3 days post-op. |
| *Premature atrial contractions (>5/hr)* | Associated with an increased risk of SVT post-op, but usually does not warrant pre-op intervention. Some advocate prophylactic digitalis for patients with frequent PACs and subcritical valvular disease, a prior history of SVT, or for elderly patients undergoing pulmonary surgery. |
| *Supraventricular tachycardia* | Sustained arrhythmias should be controlled before patient enters operating room with an AV nodal blocker ± Class IA or IC antiarrhythmic (pp. 63-64). High likelihood of recurrence postoperatively. |
| *Wolff-Parkinson-White syndrome* | Risk of intra- and postoperative SVT is increased, but preoperative intervention (drug therapy, catheter ablation) is not necessary if the patient is asymptomatic. |

*See p. 1 for abbreviations and p. 199 for drug information.*

## III. PREOPERATIVE MANAGEMENT OF COMMON MEDICAL CONDITIONS

| | |
|---|---|
| Arrhythmias (cont.)<br>*PVCs, nonsustained VT* | Exclude ischemia, LV dysfunction, hypoxemia, and electrolyte disorders. **Antiarrhythmic therapy should not be started unless the patient meets the usual criteria for long-term treatment**. Some advocate prophylactic lidocaine for patients with a history of symptomatic ventricular arrhythmias or cardiac arrest, and for those with very high grades of asymptomatic ventricular arrhythmias. |
| Conduction system disturbances<br>*$1^o$ or $2^o$ (Type I) AV block* | If possible, discontinue drugs that slow AV conduction including $\beta$-blockers, verapamil, diltiazem, and digoxin. **If the patient is asymptomatic (no syncope or presyncope), noncardiac surgery may proceed without prophylactic placement of a temporary pacemaker**. |
| *$2^o$ (Type II) or $3^o$ AV block* | Temporary followed by permanent pacing (possible exception: congenital heart block). |
| *Fascicular block* | No intervention needed for isolated left anterior or posterior fascicular block. |
| *Left or right bundle branch block* | • LBBB: No intervention is needed if the patient is asymptomatic and lacks evidence of other cardiovascular disease. **A temporary pacemaker should be immediately available when a pulmonary artery catheter is placed** due to an ↑ risk of complete heart block.<br>• RBBB: No intervention needed. |
| *Bifascicular block ± ↑ PR interval* | Preoperative pacemaker placement is indicated for patients with symptomatic bradyarrhythmias, unexplained syncope, or a history of either Type II second-degree AV block or complete heart block. Permanent pacing may be indicated for these patients as well. |
| Carotid artery disease | • Severe carotid artery stenosis (> 70% luminal narrowing): If the patient is asymptomatic or symptoms are remote, proceed with noncardiac surgery. **If the patient has a history of recurrent TIAs or a nondisabling stroke, consider carotid endarterectomy prior to high-risk elective surgery**.<br>• Slight or moderate carotid stenosis (< 70% narrowing): Platelet inhibitors, proceed with surgery. |

*See p. 1 for abbreviations and p. 199 for drug information.*

## III. PREOPERATIVE MANAGEMENT OF COMMON MEDICAL CONDITIONS

| Condition | Management |
|---|---|
| Coronary disease<br>*Stable angina* | • Active patients with normal or new normal functional capacity should be able to tolerate surgery without further testing or intervention. **Prophylactic revascularization is of no added benefit to medical therapy alone unless symptoms would otherwise warrant revascularization**. Possible exception: Pre-op PTCA should be considered prior to high-risk surgery for patients with no or minimal symptoms but a high-grade coronary stenosis that supplies a large area of viable myocardium.<br>• For patients with peripheral vascular disease, functional class is not a reliable gauge of functional capacity. Therefore, pharmacological stress testing (e.g. dipyridamole or adenosine thallium scintigraphy) ± ambulatory ischemia monitoring is advised. |
| *Unstable angina* | **Coronary angiography and revascularization should be performed preoperatively if possible**. Elective procedures should be postponed until coronary disease and symptoms are treated. If urgent surgery is required, options include emergency angioplasty, combined noncardiac and cardiac surgery, or full hemodynamic monitoring and anti-ischemic pharmacotherapy (± intraaortic balloon counterpulsation) with emergency PTCA reserved for the development of acute MI. |
| *Myocardial infarction* | **Risk of reinfarction ~ 6% and 2% if surgery is performed < 3 months and 3-6 months post-MI.**<br>- MI within 6 months: Elective procedures should be delayed. If surgery must be performed and post-infarct angina is present, coronary angiography and PTCA should be performed preoperatively when feasible. All others require stress testing. Hemodynamic monitoring is recommended, especially if LV ejection fraction < 40%.<br>- MI > 6 months: Elective procedures need not be delayed. Preoperative coronary angiography should be performed for patients with recurrent ischemic pain despite medical therapy. Noninvasive testing should be performed for asymptomatic patients undergoing high-risk procedures and for symptomatic patients undergoing low-risk procedures. |
| LV dysfunction<br>*No $S_3$, JVD, pulmonary edema* | Check orthostatic signs to identify hypovolemic patients. Consider intraoperative hemodynamic monitoring. Check hemodynamic status frequently post-op. Not an indication for prophylactic digitalis. Risk of post-op pulmonary edema is 6%. |

*See p. 1 for abbreviations and p. 199 for drug information.*

## III. PREOPERATIVE MANAGEMENT OF COMMON MEDICAL CONDITIONS

| | |
|---|---|
| LV dysfunction (cont.) +$S_3$ *gallop* ± *JVD* | Postpone surgery if further medical therapy can lead to improved hemodynamic status. If surgery must be performed, strongly consider **hemodynamic monitoring** (continue for 24-72 hours after high-risk procedures). Risk of post-op pulmonary edema is 16%. |
| *Pulmonary edema* | **Postpone all but emergent surgery**. If possible, stabilize for 5-7 days prior to surgery. Avoid overdiuresis and hypokalemia. Full hemodynamic monitoring prior to and for 24-72 hrs post-op. |
| Hypertension | Patients with preoperative hypertension, even if controlled, **may have labile BP during anesthesia/surgery**. Proceed with surgery unless the diastolic BP exceeds 110 mmHg. Patients on chronic diuretics may need fluids to restore intravascular volume and prevent intraoperative hypotension. |
| Hypertrophic obstructive cardiomyopathy | Avoid volume depletion, preload or afterload reduction, and the use of inotropes (may ↑ outflow tract obstruction). Consider use of a pulmonary artery catheter, especially for high-risk procedures. **General anesthesia may be less likely to cause hypotension than spinal or epidural** anesthesia. Intraoperative hypotension unresponsive to fluids should be treated with a pure *α*-agonist (phenylephrine). |
| Pulmonary disease | • Avoid preload reduction; urge patient to stop smoking days-weeks prior to surgery; consider preoperative respiratory therapy and hemodynamic monitoring. Early mobilization, incentive spirometry, ECG and cardiac enzymes postoperatively.<br>• Acute exacerbation: Treat infection, maximize bronchodilators and steroids (inhaled ± oral), and postpone all but emergent surgery. If steroid dependent, the daily dose of oral steroids should be doubled and given as an equipotent dose of IV methylprednisolone.<br>• Pulmonary hypertension: Optimize lung function with $O_2$, bronchodilators, antibiotics, and steroids as needed. **Patients with Class IV symptoms due to pulmonary hypertension are at increased risk of sudden death** during general anesthesia/surgery; a pulmonologist should be consulted to optimize care and pulmonary pressures should be monitored during and after surgery. |

*See p. 1 for abbreviations and p. 199 for drug information.*

## III. PREOPERATIVE MANAGEMENT OF COMMON MEDICAL CONDITIONS

| Condition | Management |
|---|---|
| Valve disease | |
| *Aortic stenosis (AS)* | Patients with severe AS are **prone to perioperative pulmonary edema and sudden cardiac death**. Valve replacement before noncardiac surgery is indicated for patients with symptomatic critical aortic stenosis and probably for asymptomatic patients with severe stenosis. Balloon valvuloplasty can be used as a "bridge" for patients who require urgent noncardiac surgery or are seriously ill; valve replacement can then be performed on a semi-elective basis after noncardiac surgery. Hemodynamic monitoring is indicated for moderate-severe AS. |
| *Aortic insufficiency* | Hemodynamic monitoring for patients with moderate-severe LV enlargement. |
| *Mitral stenosis (MS)* | Patients with severe MS are **prone to perioperative pulmonary edema and sudden cardiac death**. Valvuloplasty or valve replacement is recommended before high-risk noncardiac surgery for patients with severe symptoms. Acute or chronic tachyarrhythmias should be treated with drugs that slow sinus node activity or ventricular response (e.g., ***β***-blockers, verapamil). Hemodynamic monitoring should be considered for symptomatic patients. |
| *Mitral regurgitation* | Hemodynamic monitoring for patients with moderate-severe LV enlargement. |
| Prosthetic valve | |
| *Tissue valves* | Antibiotic prophylaxis for high and intermediate risk procedures (see p. 150). |
| *Mechanical valves* | • **Anticoagulation**: (1) Switch from warfarin to heparin 2-3 days prior to surgery (esp. mitral valve); (2) discontinue heparin ~ 6 hours prior to surgery; (3) restart heparin and warfarin 36-48 hours later; and (4) discontinue heparin once INR is in therapeutic range.<br>• **Antibiotic prophylaxis** for high and intermediate risk procedures (see p. 150). |

*See p. 1 for abbreviations and p. 199 for drug information.*

## IV. PERIOPERATIVE MANAGEMENT OF ORAL MEDICATIONS

| Drug | Recommendations |
|---|---|
| Antiarrhythmics<br>*Quinidine* | If patient cannot take oral medications after surgery, consider switching to IV procainamide. Alternatively, quinidine can be given IV if infused slowly and levels are followed. |
| *Procainamide* | Can be given IV while NPO. |
| *Disopyramide* | Consider switching to IV procainamide while NPO. |
| *Mexilitine* | Consider switching to IV lidocaine while NPO. |
| Antithrombotics<br>*Aspirin* | Surgeon should decide whether the increased risk of bleeding should lead to cessation of aspirin. |
| *Heparin* | Can be stopped about 6 hours before the operation and restarted 36-48 hours later. |
| *Warfarin* | Should be stopped 2-3 days before surgery. Patients with mechanical prosthetic valves should receive IV heparin as warfarin effects diminish (see p. 139). |
| Antidepressants | Tricyclic antidepressants may precipitate arrhythmias and slow AV conduction via quinidine-like effects. MAO inhibitors may exaggerate the hypertensive response to indirect sympathomimetics (e.g. ephedrine), and interact with meperidine to produce agitation, hyperpyrexia, hypertension, rigidity, and convulsions. Therefore, some experts recommend that MAO inhibitors be discontinued 2-3 weeks before surgery. There is no reason to discontinue lithium before elective surgery. |
| Antihypertensives<br>*ACE inhibitors* | Should be continued up to and including the morning of surgery. |
| *Antiadrenergics* | Centrally-acting agents: Transdermal clonidine can be substituted for the oral drug to ensure maintenance of drug levels during perioperative period. Withdrawal can cause severe rebound hypertension (p. 9). |

*See p. 1 for abbreviations and p. 199 for drug information.*

## IV. PERIOPERATIVE MANAGEMENT OF ORAL MEDICATIONS

| Drug | Recommendations |
|---|---|
| *Antiadrenergics (cont.)* | Peripheral agents: Reserpine and guanethidine may reduce sensitivity to indirect vasopressors such as ephedrine. Hypotension can be treated with direct vasopressors, such as phenylephrine. |
| ***β**-blockers* | Older teaching that **β**-blockers should be discontinued before surgery is now in disfavor. **β**-blockers should be continued up to and including the morning of surgery. IV **β**-blockers can be substituted for oral preparations while NPO. Intraoperative effects may be overcome by isoproterenol (2-10 mcg/min IV infusion) or glucagon (5-10 mg IV bolus; maintenance infusion 2-5 mg/hr). |
| *Calcium channel blockers* | Should be continued up to the morning of surgery. Negative inotropic effects may lead to hemodynamic deterioration with general anesthesia. |
| *Diuretics* | May cause hypovolemia; pre-op evaluation should include orthostatic vital signs. Correct hypokalemia. |
| *Vasodilators* | Hydralazine and minoxidil may reduce the sensitivity to vasopressor agents. |

## V. MANAGEMENT OF POSTOPERATIVE COMPLICATIONS

| Complication | Therapy | Comments |
|---|---|---|
| Arrhythmias | Indications for treatment: tachy- or bradyarrhythmias that cause hypotension, heart failure, or myocardial ischemia. Long-term therapy is often unnecessary. | Usual causes include stress, electrolyte shifts, hypoxemia, acid-base disturbances, myocardial ischemia, heart failure, infection, and pulmonary embolism. **If ventricular arrhythmias develop for the first time in the post-op setting, rule out MI**. |
| Fever | Workup should include blood cultures, chest x-ray, and inspection of wound. | Common causes include infection (pulmonary, wound, urinary tract, endocarditis), atelectasis, and PE. |

*See p. 1 for abbreviations and p. 199 for drug information.*

## V. MANAGEMENT OF POSTOPERATIVE COMPLICATIONS

| Complication | Therapy | Comments |
|---|---|---|
| Heart failure | Consider inotropic therapy to improve oxygen delivery after major surgery. Hemodynamic monitoring is indicated if patient has pulmonary congestion and low blood pressure. Diuretic therapy alone is often sufficient. | **May occur immediately postoperatively or at post-op day 3-5** (intravascular volume expansion from resorption of extracellular fluid). **Rule-out MI**. Usually no adjustment in long-term medical therapy is needed. |
| Hypertension | Determine whether oxygenation, pain control, and fluid balance are adequate. If not, hypertension may be effectively treated with supplemental $0_2$, morphine, and diuretics. Otherwise, use antihypertensive agents as needed (Ch. 1). | Post-op systolic BP > 210 mmHg or an increase > 50 mmHg above baseline occurs in 25% of patients with, and 5% of patients without a history of hypertension. **If large doses of antihypertensives are administered, blood pressure may fall when pain is relieved**. |
| Hypotension | First treatment should be volume infusion, followed by inotropic/vasopressor therapy if patient does not respond quickly. | Causes include hypovolemia (volume depletion, hemorrhage), cardiogenic (ischemic, valvular), pulmonary embolism, sepsis, drug effect, and adrenal insufficiency. |
| Myocardial infarction | Urgent cath/PTCA if large MI or clinically unstable. For small MI, patient should be monitored in an intensive care unit and undergo coronary angiography/PTCA if ischemia recurs. Lytics contraindicated. Treat in conventional manner with long-term $\beta$-blocker and/or ACE inhibitor. | Most present with hypotension, heart failure, arrhythmias or a change in mental status. **Diagnosis may be complicated by lack of chest pain** (due to analgesia, sedation, post-op pain) **and high false-positive rate of cardiac enzymes**. Consider clonidine or $\beta$-blocker withdrawal as the etiology. |
| Pulmonary embolism | Therapeutic heparin. If risk of bleeding is excessive, an inferior vena caval filter should be placed. If PE is massive, consider surgical embolectomy. | This diagnosis should be suspected in any postoperative patient with unexplained dyspnea or chest pain. Lytics are contraindicated. |

*See p. 1 for abbreviations and p. 199 for drug information.*

# 11. INFECTIOUS AND INFLAMMATORY CARDIAC DISEASES

Jeffrey D. Band, M.D.

## I. INFECTIOUS ENDOCARDITIS (IE)

| | |
|---|---|
| Diagnosis | IE remains a clinical diagnosis and should be suspected in any patient with an unexplained fever and a heart murmur (Caveat: murmur may be absent with right-sided or mural infection and the classic "changing murmur" or new murmur is found in only 15%). **Single most important diagnostic test is the blood culture,** which is (+) in over 95% of patients, but may be negative if antibiotics had been given within the previous 2 weeks or if fungal endocarditis is present. Obtain ≥ 3 sets of blood cultures (10-15 cc of blood per culture tube) at least 15 minutes apart (one set per venipuncture site). **If initial cultures are positive, they should be repeated every other day until they turn negative**. Blood cultures obtained 2-6 wks after antibiotic therapy can detect the majority of relapses. |
| Principles of therapy | • **Need for hospitalization**: All patients with suspected or proven endocarditis should initially be managed in the hospital setting. If clinically stable after ≥ 10-14 days of observation, patients at low risk for complications (i.e., prompt defervescence, negative repeat blood culture, stable ECG without conduction defects, no emboli, hemodynamically stable) can be considered for treatment and close monitoring in the ambulatory setting<br>• **Timing of therapy**: Antimicrobial therapy should be administered *after* blood cultures have been obtained. IV antibiotics are preferred to oral antibiotics. For acutely ill patients, empiric treatment should be initiated within 2 hrs. of presentation and based on the type of valve (native, prosthetic) and patient characteristics (p. 145).<br>• **Susceptibility testing**: If the minimum bactericidal concentration (MBC) exceeds the minimum inhibitory concentration (MIC) by at least 4-fold, tolerance may be present (antimicrobial inhibits but does not kill infecting organism) and cure rates lower: the addition of a second antibiotic may improve outcome. This is especially important for infections due to enterococci and relatively penicillin-resistant streptococci.<br>• **Serum cidal levels:** Once treatment has been initiated, the efficacy of the patient's serum in killing the infecting organism can be monitored. Peak bactericidal levels ≥ 1:8 dilution and trough levels > 1:2 dilution usually indicate adequate therapy.<br>• **Antibiotic levels:** Whenever potentially toxic antibiotics are used, antibiotic levels should be obtained to ensure that the circulating concentration is within therapeutic--but not toxic--range. For this purpose, *peak* levels (30-60 min after dose #4) and *trough* levels (immediately prior to dose #4) levels are commonly obtained, particularly when vancomycin or gentamicin is prescribed. |

## A. ANTIBIOTIC DOSAGE AND DOSING INTERVALS BASED ON GFR (cc/min)†

| Antibiotic | > 90 cc/min | 50-90 | 10-50 | <10 |
|---|---|---|---|---|
| Amphotericin B | 0.3-0.7 mg/kg/day IV piggy back (IVPB) infused over 4-6 hrs | q24h | q24h | q24h |
| Ampicillin | 2 gm IVPB q 4 hrs up to 200 mg/kg/day | q6 | q6-12h | q12-24h |
| Ampicillin-sulbactam | 3 gm IVPB q 4-6 hrs | | | |
| Cefazolin | 2 gm IVPB q 6-8 hrs | q8h | q12h | q24-48h |
| Fluconazole | 200-600 mg po qd | q24h | q24-48h | q48-72h |
| 5-Flucytosine | Up to 100-150 mg/kg/day po in 3-4 divided doses | q6-8h | q8-12h | q24-48h |
| Gentamicin 1 | 1 mg/kg IVPB q 8-12 hrs: peak of 3-4 mcg/mL & trough < 1 mcg/mL | q8-12h | q12h | q24-48h |
| Gentamicin 2 | 1.7 mg/kg IVPB q 8 hrs or 2.5 mg/kg q 12 hrs: peak 7-11 mcg/mL & trough < 1 mcg/mL | q8-12h | q12h | q24-48h |
| Nafcillin | 200 mg/kg/day IVPB divided into 6 doses | q4h | q4h | q4h |
| Penicillin G | 200-250 x $10^3$ U/kg/day IVPB in 6 divided doses | q6h | q8h | q12h |
| Piperacillin | Up to 3 gm IVPB q 4 hrs | q4-6h | q6-8h | q8h |
| Rifampin | 300 mg po q 8 hrs | q24h | q24h | q24h |
| Tobramycin | 1.7 mg/kg q 8 hrs or 2.5 mg/kg q 12 hrs: peak 7-11 & trough < 1 mcg/mL | q8-12h | q12h | q24-48 |
| Vancomycin | 15 mg/kg IVPB q 12 hrs: peak of 25-40 mcg/mL & trough of 5-10 mcg/mL | q1-3d | q3-10d | q10d |

† GFR (estimated): Males = [(140 — age) x (ideal body wt, kg)] / [72 x (serum creatinine, mg/dL)]. For females, multiply x 0.85

References: Inf Dis N Amer 1989;3:517; West J Med 1992;156:633; Drug Prescribing in Renal Failure (Eds: Bennett et al) 1991; Guide to Antimicrobial Therapy (Ed: J.P. Sanford) 1993.

### B. NATIVE VALVE ENDOCARDITIS: EMPIRIC THERAPY (AWAITING CULTURES)

| Subgroup | Common Pathogens | Therapy* | Comments |
|---|---|---|---|
| Non-toxic patient | Viridans strep., enterococci, strep bovis, microaerophilic strep. | Pen G (or amp) + gent[1]<br>Alternate: Vanco + gent[2] | Perform serum bactericidal test to confirm peak cidal levels ≥ 1:8 dilution. |
| Toxic patient | Staph. aureus, enterococcus, group B strep | Vanco + gent[1] | Observe in monitored setting for complications (CHF, emboli, arrhythmias). |
| IV drug abuse | S. aureus (60%), group B strep., pseudomonas, serratia, yeast, polymicrobial, bacillus cereus | Vanco + gent[2] ± extended spectrum penicillin (piperacillin) | Right-sided involvement is common and often presents with septic pulmonary emboli. |
| Hemodialysis or indwelling central venous catheter | S. aureus, pseudomonas, serratia; yeast | Vanco + gent[2] ± extended spectrum pen (piperacillin); Amphotericin B for yeast | **Hold blood cultures at least 4 weeks** to exclude fungi and other fastidious organisms. Remove & culture device. |
| Colon CA/polyp | S. bovis, viridans strep. | Pen G + gent[1] | Polyp may be malignant. |

### C. PROSTHETIC VALVE ENDOCARDITIS (PVE): EMPIRIC THERAPY (AWAITING CULTURES)

| Subgroup | Common Pathogens | Therapy* | Comments |
|---|---|---|---|
| Early PVE: < 2 months post-op | Coagulase ⊖ Staph. > *Staph. aureus* > Gram ⊖ bacilli. Yeast (candida, aspergillus) ~ 10% | Vanco + gent[2] + extended spectrum penicillin (piperacillin). Empiric ampho B rarely warranted | High mortality. If coagulase ⊖ staph, triple therapy x 5-14 d; vanco + rifampin to complete 6 wks |
| Late PVE | Viridans strep enterococci, staph | Vanco + gent[1] | Indolent or fulminant course. |

* *See p. 144 for antibiotic dosages*

## D. NATIVE VALVE ENDOCARDITIS: THERAPY BASED ON INFECTING ORGANISM

| Pathogen | Therapy* | Comments |
|---|---|---|
| "Penicillin-sensitive" streptococci (MIC ≤ 0.1 mcg/mL)<br>• Viridans strep.<br>• Group B Strep | Pen G + gent[1] x 2 weeks (Rev Inf Dis 1986;8:54) *or* Pen G x 4 wks.<br>Alternate: Cefazolin or vanco x 4 wks. | Separate gent dose from pen dose by at least 2 hrs. **If *S. bovis* is isolated, look for GI pathology such as colon cancer or polyps.** |
| "Penicillin-intermediate" streptococci (MIC 0.1-0.5 mcg/ml)<br>• Viridans Strep. (esp. *S. mutans*)<br>• Nutritionally dependent Strep. | Pen G + gent[1] x 2 wks, followed by Pen G alone x 2 wks. | |
| "Penicillin-resistant" streptococci (MIC ≥0.5 mcg/ml)<br>• Enterococci<br>• Some viridans<br>• Nutritionally deficient Strep. | Pen G (or amp.) + gent[1] x 4-6 wks. | Test enterococcus for high level (≥2000 mcg/ml) resistance to gent and streptomycin. Occasional strains may be resistant to gent but susceptible to streptomycin, although gent is preferred if both are active. |
| Staph. aureus<br>*β-lactam sensitive*<br><br>*β-lactam resistant* | Nafcillin x 4-6 wks.<br>------<br>Vancomycin x 4-6 wks. | Gent[1] may be added for the first 3-5 days if pt. appears "toxic" (Ann Intern Med 1982; 97:496). Rifampin (300 mg po q 8 hrs.) should be considered if the response is slow or there is a high likelihood of abscess. Obtain MIC and MBC to **exclude the presence of a "tolerant" strain** (p. 143). If tolerance is present, add a second agent for synergy (gent or rifampin). |

* *See p. 144 for antibiotic dosages*

## D. NATIVE VALVE ENDOCARDITIS: THERAPY BASED ON INFECTING ORGANISM

| Pathogen | Therapy* | Comments |
|---|---|---|
| HACEK group: *H. parainfluenza, H. aphrophilus, Actinobacillus, Cardiobacterium, Eikenella, Kingella* | Ampicillin-sulbactam + gent[1] x 4-6 wks. pending ID and specific susceptibilities. | Common cause of "culture-negative" endocarditis. **Difficult to cure medically**. *H. aphrophilus* with propensity for large vessel embolization. |
| Pseudomonas | Tobramycin plus antipseudomonal pen. (ticarcillin or piperacillin) x 6 wks. | Treat aggressively; **often requires surgical removal** of infected valve for cure. |
| Culture-negative | Ampicillin-sulbactam plus gent.[1] If IV drug abuse suspected or recent indwelling central venous catheter, add vanco initially. | Less than 5% of IE is culture-negative. Recovery rate is improved if an adequate volume of blood is cultured (10-15 cc). The use of special media ($B_6$ supplements), neutralization of antibiotic (if currently receiving), and serologic studies to exclude organisms such as chlamydia, rickettsia, and fungi also improve recovery rates. |

## E. PROSTHETIC VALVE ENDOCARDITIS (PVE): THERAPY BASED ON INFECTING ORGANISM

| Pathogen | Therapy* | Comments |
|---|---|---|
| Coagulase-negative staphylococci | Vanco + gent[1] + rifampin x 2 wks, followed by vanco + rifampin x 4 wks. | More than 70% of coag ⊖ staph are resistant to nafcillin and all other beta-lactams (including cephalosporins) despite *in-vitro* susceptibility. |
| Staph aureus ***β-lactam susceptible*** | Nafcillin + gent[1] x 2 wks, followed by nafcillin x 4 wks. | Monitor with telemetry until clinically stable. |

* *See p. 144 for antibiotic dosages*

## E. PROSTHETIC VALVE ENDOCARDITIS (PVE): THERAPY BASED ON INFECTING ORGANISM

| Pathogen | Therapy* | Comments |
|---|---|---|
| Staph aureus (cont.)<br>*β-lactam resistant* | Vanco + gent[1] x 2 wks, followed by vanco x 4 wks. | Besides clinical monitoring, follow CBC with differential (weekly) and renal function (3 x per week) to exclude toxicity. |
| Diphtheroids | Pen G+ gent[1] x 6 wks *or* vanco x 6 wks. | Have lab speciate and perform MIC & MBC; variable susceptibilities have been reported. |
| Aerobic gram ⊖ bacilli | Tobramycin + piperacillin x 6 wks. | Two bactericidal agents are required for cure. |
| Fungi<br>*Candida* | Amphotericin B (minimum 1 gm) ± 5 flucytosine | If organism is *C. albicans*, high dose fluconazole may be used instead of ampho B if susceptible. Surgical intervention usually required. |
| *Aspergillus* | Amphotericin B (minimum 1 gm) | Surgical intervention usually required. |

## F. INFECTIOUS ENDOCARDITIS: MANAGEMENT OF COMPLICATIONS

| Complication | Comments |
|---|---|
| Cardiac abscess | **Surgical intervention** required; drainage, debridement and valve replacement as indicated. New onset of first degree AV block may presage complete heart block; consider temporary pacing. |
| Coronary emboli | Small emboli may result in ischemia, infarction, ventricular dysfunction, and arrhythmias. |
| Metastatic infection | Most common in staph. endocarditis. High-dose antibiotics required; abscesses may require drainage. Search for metastatic abscess in patients who re-develop fever or fail to respond to therapy. If history and physical do not point to source, order chest x-ray, abdominal CT scan and urinalysis. |

* *See p. 144 for antibiotic dosages*

## F. INFECTIOUS ENDOCARDITIS: MANAGEMENT OF COMPLICATIONS

| Complication | Comments |
|---|---|
| Mycotic aneurysm | Search for cerebral mycotic aneurysm (e.g., MRI) in patients with headaches or neurologic findings. Other common sites of involvement include the abdominal aorta, Sinus of Valsalva, and mesenteric artery. Usually persists despite microbiologic cure; **may require resection** to prevent rupture months-years later. |
| Organ infarction | Large emboli may result in "bland" organ infarction with or without abscess formation. |
| Purulent pericarditis | **Surgical drainage** (subxyphoid pericardiotomy) is required. |
| Persistent fevers | Differential diagnosis: Unremitting infection, abscess formation, embolization, new foci of infection (IV device), and drug-hypersensitivity reaction (eosinophilia with normal WBC count). |

## G. INFECTIOUS ENDOCARDITIS: SURGICAL INTERVENTION

| Indication | Comments |
|---|---|
| Refractory heart failure due to destruction of valve or chordae | Most frequent cause of death in patients with IE. Heart failure in absence of valve destruction may be managed medically. |
| Outflow tract obstruction | Caused by large vegetation; may result in heart failure and/or shock. |
| Recurrent major emboli | First episode not an indication for surgery in native valves but possibly for prosthetic valves. Avoid anticoagulants (↑ risk of bleeding into cerebral infarct and from mycotic aneurysm). |
| Persistent bacteremia despite antibiotics x 10 d | Must exclude metastatic abscess formation at another site. |
| Ineffective therapy (fungal endocarditis) | Operate early since medical cure rate is low. |

## G. INFECTIOUS ENDOCARDITIS: SURGICAL INTERVENTION

| Indication | Comments |
|---|---|
| Suppurative extension into myocardium or pericardium | Septal abscess usually manifests as progressive heart block. Suppurative pericarditis requires immediate drainage. |
| Recurrent relapses | Timing controversial; consider valve replacement for 2 or more relapses. |
| Early prosthetic-valve endocarditis | Surgical indications include prosthetic valve dehiscence or obstruction and those listed above. |

## H. PROPHYLAXIS AGAINST INFECTIOUS ENDOCARDITIS

**Prophylaxis is indicated for high-risk and intermediate-risk patients** (see below) **undergoing procedures commonly associated with significant bacteremias** (pp. 151-152). Note: Episodes of infectious endocarditis commonly occur in patients without predisposing factors or recent exposure to high-risk procedures. Therefore, prophylaxis may only prevent a minority of episodes from occurring.

### 1. PATIENT SUBGROUPS REQUIRING PROPHYLAXIS

| High Risk | Intermediate Risk | Low Risk |
|---|---|---|
| Prosthetic valves<br>Previous infectious endocarditis<br>Patent ductus arteriosus (PDA)<br>Ventricular septal defect (VSD)<br>Tetralogy of Fallot<br>Coarctation of aorta<br>Aortic/mitral stenosis or regurgitation<br>Marfan's syndrome<br>AV fistula | Mitral valve prolapse with insufficiency<br>Tricuspid or pulmonary valve disease<br>Asymmetric septal hypertrophy | MVP without insufficiency<br>Isolated secundum atrial septal defect (ASD)<br>Cardiac pacemakers and internal cardioverter/defibrillators<br>Six or more months after surgical repair of secundum ASD, VSD, or PDA *and* no evidence of residual disease<br>Previous coronary artery bypass surgery |

## 2. PROPHYLACTIC REGIMENS BASED ON TYPE OF PROCEDURE

For high-risk and intermediate-risk groups as defined on p. 150. Modified from JAMA 1990;264:2919.

| Category | Procedure | Regimen |
|---|---|---|
| Dental | • Prophylaxis for procedures likely to cause bleeding, such as cleaning, scaling, extractions, oral surgery.<br>• No prophylaxis is required for simple fillings above the gum line. | • **Amoxicillin 3 gm po 1 hr before procedure followed by 1.5 gm po 6 hrs later**. If pen allergic, consider erythromycin 1 gm po 2 hrs before procedure, then 500 mg 6 hrs later. If unable to take oral medications, then ampicillin 2 gm IV 30 min before procedure, followed by 1 gm IV 6 hrs later.<br>• If at very high risk, some recommend ampicillin 2 gm IV plus gentamicin 1.5 mg/kg IV 30 min before procedure, followed by same doses 8 hrs later.<br>• If allergic to penicillin and IV prophylaxis is required, give vancomycin 1 gm IV 1 hr before procedure (no repeat dose is necessary). |
| Upper respiratory | • Prophylaxis for tonsillectomy & adenoidectomy, operations involving infected tissue, and bronchoscopy using a rigid scope.<br>• No prophylaxis is required for flexible bronchoscopy or endotracheal intubation. | Same as above for dental. |
| Gastrointestinal | • Prophylaxis for endoscopy with biopsy, operations involving infected tissue or drainage of abscess, sclerotherapy for esophageal varices, esophageal dilatation, and gall bladder surgery.<br>• No prophylaxis is required for endoscopy without biopsy, barium enema, liver biopsy. | **Ampicillin 2 gm IV plus gentamicin 1.5 mg/kg 30 min before procedure, followed by amoxicillin 1.5 gm po 6 hrs later.** If allergic to penicillin, give vancomycin 1 gm IV plus gentamicin 1.5 mg/kg IV 1 hr before procedure and repeat 8 hrs later. |

## 2. PROPHYLACTIC REGIMENS BASED ON TYPE OF PROCEDURE

For high-risk and intermediate-risk groups as defined on p. 150. Modified from JAMA 1990;264:2919.

| Category | Procedure | Regimen |
|---|---|---|
| Genitourinary | • Prophylaxis for delivery other than spontaneous, abortion, D & C in the presence of cervicitis, urethral dilatation, urethral catheter or urinary tract surgery in the presence of infection, cystoscopy, and prostatectomy. | Same as above for GI. |
| Cutaneous and soft tissue | • Prophylaxis for incision and drainage of infected tissue. | Author preference: **Dicloxacillin 1.5 gm po 1 hr before the procedure, followed by 750 mg po 6 hrs later**. Treatment—not prophylaxis—is needed whenever operating on infected tissue or draining abscess. Duration of treatment is ~ 7-10 d post-procedure. |
| Others | **Not at significant risk:** Cardiac catheterization and angioplasty, caesarean section, uncomplicated vaginal delivery, intrauterine device, D & C in absence of cervicitis, urethral catheterization in absence of infection. | |

## II. MYOCARDITIS

| | |
|---|---|
| Presentation | Suspect diagnosis in patients with **unexplained tachycardia, arrhythmias and/or heart failure.** |
| Diagnostic studies | Endomyocardial biopsy limited by poor sensitivity and problems with interpretation. Viral etiology may be established by body fluid culture or a 4-fold rise in antibody titers between acute and convalescent periods. |
| Prognosis | Majority of patients have subclinical myocarditis and recover completely. Among those with symptoms, 50% recover while 50% progress at variable rates to a dilated cardiomyopathy. **Sudden death may occur**. |

## II. MYOCARDITIS

| | |
|---|---|
| Principles of therapy | • Treatment should be initiated in the hospital setting and include **modified bed rest, oxygen and antipyretics**.<br>• *Cause-specific therapy:* Enterovirus (no specific therapy; avoid strenuous exercise and steroids); influenza (rimantidine 100 mg po bid x 7 days beginning within 48 hrs from symptom onset); varicella zoster or herpes simplex (acyclovir 5-10 mg/kg IVPB q 8 hrs); cytomegalovirus (gancyclovir 5 mg/kg IVBP q 12 hrs); HIV (retrovir 200 mg po tid); mycoplasma (erythromycin 0.5-1.0 gm IVPB q 6 hrs); chlamydia or rickettsia (doxycycline 100 mg IVPB q 12 hrs); borrelia burgdorferi (Lyme disease; ceftriaxone 2 gm IVPB daily or pen G 18-21 million units IVPB in 6 divided doses/d); S. aureus (vancomycin pending susceptibility); C. diphtheria (antibiotic + urgent antitoxin); trypanosomiasis (Chagas disease; none); trichinella spiralis (corticosteroids if severely ill); toxoplasma gondii; (pyrimethamine + sulfadiazine + folinic acid); rheumatic fever (salicylates; steroids if severe); heart transplant rejection (high-dose steroids; antithymocyte globulin and/or OKT3 monoclonal antibody for severe cases); and others. **Immunosuppressive therapy is usually not helpful.**<br>• *Control of complications:* (1) Heart failure: $Na^+$ restriction, diuretics, digitalis, and dobutamine. May be sensitive to digitalis and develop toxicity at routine dose; (2) Shock: IABP, ventricular assist device, cardiac transplantation; (3) Arrhythmias/heart block: Pharmacologic therapy, pacemaker; (4) Thromboembolism: Anticoagulation (except when complicated by pericarditis or endocarditis). |

## III. PROPHYLAXIS AGAINST RECURRENCE OF RHEUMATIC FEVER (CIRCULATION 1988;78:1082)

| Patient groups | Regimens | Comments |
|---|---|---|
| • Acute RF in all age groups<br>• Rheumatic carditis<br>• Frequent recurrences<br>• Rheumatic heart disease (RHD) | Benzathine penicillin 1.2 million units IM q month | Lifetime prophylaxis is required. |
| • Adult more than 5 yrs. from initial episode without evidence of carditis or rheumatic heart disease<br>• Adults free of recurrences for ≥ 5 yrs. | Sulfadiazine 1 gm po daily or Pen V 250 mg po BID | Oral agents are not as good as IM pen but more convenient. All patients with residual rheumatic heart disease must also receive endocarditis prophylaxis before "at risk" procedures. |

# 12. PERICARDIAL DISEASE

Mark Freed, M.D.
Jeffrey D. Band, M.D.

| I. PERICARDITIS | |
|---|---|
| Presentation | **Chest pain, a pericardial friction rub, and serial ECG changes** dominate the acute presentation. Pericardial chest pain is typically sharp, retrosternal, and may radiate to the shoulders, trapezius ridge and neck. The pain may be aggravated by deep breathing (and therefore easily mistaken for pleuritis), lying supine, coughing and swallowing; it is often improved or relieved by sitting up and lying forward. On occasion, the **pain may mimic an acute abdominal process, aortic dissection or myocardial infarction**. Pericarditis may also initially present as supraventricular tachycardia or cardiac tamponade. A **pericardial friction rub** is diagnostic of pericarditis, but **may be missed on auscultation** due to its often intermittent nature. **ECG abnormalities occur in 90%** of cases. Early changes include PR segment depression and diffuse concave upward ST segment elevation without reciprocal ST segment depression or pathological Q waves. **Pulsus paradoxus** (inspiratory fall in systolic BP) > 12-15 mmHg indicates impending hemodynamic compromise and should be considered a cardiac emergency! |
| Prognosis | **The majority of episodes are self-limited** and resolve within 2-6 wks. Complications: Cardiac tamponade (15%, p. 157), constrictive pericarditis (< 10%, p. 158), recurrent chest pain (25%, p. 158), and arrhythmias (PACs/SVT). |
| Principles of therapy | • **Hospitalization and bed rest** are recommended for all patients who present with pericarditis to exclude acute MI, rule-out a pyogenic process, and observe for tamponade.<br>• For pericardial chest pain: **Aspirin** (650 mg PO q 3-4 hrs) or **indomethacin** (25-50 mg PO q 6 hrs) results in dramatic relief of symptoms in most patients. Supplemental therapy with meperidine (25-150 mg PO/IM/IV q 3-4 hrs) or morphine (2-15 mg IM/IV q 4-6 hrs) may also be required. If pain persists beyond 48-72 hrs or is extremely severe, **steroids** should be considered (e.g., prednisone 60-80 mg/d in divided doses). In general, high-dose therapy is required for 5-7 days followed by tapering doses of anti-inflammatory agents.<br>• **Anticoagulation is not recommended** (↑ risk of cardiac tamponade). If necessary (e.g., prosthetic valve), use IV heparin (protamine sulfate for abrupt clinical deterioration in association with an increasing effusion). |

*See p. 1 for abbreviations and p. 144 for antibiotic dosages.*

## A. TREATMENT OF PERICARDITIS BASED ON ETIOLOGY

| Etiology | Therapy | Comments |
|---|---|---|
| Aortic dissection | See p. 172. | Bloody effusion (also seen in neoplasm, uremia and TB). |
| Collagen vascular *Lupus, rheumatoid arthritis* | Nonsteroidal anti-inflammatory drugs. Corticosteroids for severe disease. Immunosuppressive therapy for steroid-resistant cases. | Must exclude drug-induced lupus states (procainamide, hydralazine, isoniazid [INH]). |
| Drug-induced | Eliminate inciting agent. Steroids may hasten recovery. | Primary agents: procainamide, hydralazine and INH. Others: minoxidil, methysergide, anthracycline neoplastic agents, and hypersensitivity to penicillin or cromolyn. |
| Idiopathic | Rest and nonsteroidal anti-inflammatory drugs. Steroids should be avoided. | Majority of cases due to undiagnosed viral infection. |
| Infectious *Strep. pneumococcus* | Penicillin G (200-250 x $10^3$ units/kg/d IV divided into 6 doses) for at least 10-14 d. Pericardial and blood isolates must be sent for susceptibility testing. | Acute dramatic presentation with fever, chills, and dyspnea. **Diagnosis is often missed**; chest pain and friction rub may be absent. Drainage is usually required. Mortality rates are high. |
| *Staph. aureus* | Vancomycin (15 mg/kg IV to produce peak of 25-40 mcg/mL and trough of 5-10 mcg/mL ) or nafcillin (200 mg/kg/d IV divided into 6 doses if susceptible) for at least 14-21 d. | |
| *Fungal* | Amphotericin B (0.3-0.7 mg/kg/d IV over 4-6 hrs. up to minimum of 1 gm) ± 5-flucytosine (up to 100-150 mg/kg/d in 3-4 divided doses). | Pericarditis is an uncommon complication of fungal infections. Histoplasmosis pericarditis is usually self-limited, whereas other etiologies are associated with high mortality rates. |

*See p. 1 for abbreviations and p. 144 for antibiotic dosages.*

## A. TREATMENT OF PERICARDITIS BASED ON ETIOLOGY

| Etiology | Therapy | Comments |
|---|---|---|
| *TB* | Combination therapy with isoniazid (300 mg/day), rifampin (600 mg/day), pyrazinamide (PZA, 25 mg/kg/day), and corticosteroids (prednisone 1 mg/kg/day). | Many develop chronic constrictive pericarditis and extensive pericardial calcification ("concretio cordis") despite therapy. |
| *Viral* | Rest, nonsteroidal anti-inflammatory drugs, and close observation. Corticosteroids should be avoided. | Patients usually highly symptomatic. Vast majority of cases are self-limited and uncomplicated. Recurrences in 15%. |
| Malignant | • Terminally ill patient: Pericardiocentesis as needed. Secondary interventions include balloon pericardiostomy, sclerotherapy, or surgery through subxyphoid route for palliative "partial window".<br>• Recurrent, symptomatic effusions when longterm prognosis is good: Radiation therapy for sensitive tumor types; otherwise, complete pericardiectomy. Intrapericardial sclerotherapy falling out of favor. | Malignant pericarditis frequently manifests as hemopericardium with tamponade. Common etiologies include cancer of the lung and breast, melanoma, leukemia, and lymphoma. **50% of pericardial effusions in cancer patients are due to non-malignant causes** including radiation, idiopathic, infection (TB, fungal), and impaired lympathic drainage. |
| Post-MI | Symptomatic therapy including rest, aspirin, analgesics, and close monitoring. | NSAIDs sparingly (may impair infarct healing and increase the risk of rupture). |
| Post-pericardiotomy | Routine therapy with aspirin, nonsteroidal anti-inflammatory drugs. If no response within 48 hrs, steroids are given. | Usually self-limited. Disabling recurrences and constriction may develop months-years later. |
| Radiation | None recommended if asymptomatic. Steroids for severe intractable pain. Extensive pericardiectomy for large recurrent effusions, severe effusive-constrictive or constrictive pericarditis in those with good prognoses. | Exclude radiation-induced hypothyroidism as a cause. Restrictive cardiomyopathy may coexist. |

*See p. 1 for abbreviations and p. 144 for antibiotic dosages.*

## A. TREATMENT OF PERICARDITIS BASED ON ETIOLOGY

| Etiology | Therapy | Comments |
|---|---|---|
| Uremic | Dialysis (intensify regimen if already on). Surgical drainage for nonresponders or recurrences. | Occurs in 20% of those with end-stage renal disease. Pain is uncommon: **may first manifest as hypotension during dialysis**, acute or chronic tamponade, or constriction. Pericardiocentesis may induce hemorrhage. |

## B. COMPLICATIONS OF PERICARDITIS

### 1. CARDIAC TAMPONADE

| | |
|---|---|
| Diagnosis | **Combined clinical & hemodynamic assessment** (cath and/or echo) **are essential for the diagnosis.**<br>• Physical exam: Increased jugular venous pressure with prominent X-descent and absent Y-descent; pulsus paradoxus (inspiratory fall in systolic BP) > 12-15 mmHg is usually present.<br>• ECG: Low voltage QRS complex; QRS alternans or total alternans (P, QRS, T; virtually pathognomonic).<br>• Echocardiogram: Pericardial effusion with diastolic compression of the inferior vena cava, right atrium and right ventricle (unless RV hypertrophy is present). Findings may occur prior to hemodynamic compromise and are *not* by themselves an indication for pericardiocentesis.<br>• Cardiac cath: Equalization of intrapericardial, mean RA, RV diastolic, LV diastolic, and pulmonary capillary wedge pressures; pronounced pulsus paradoxus; decreased or absent Y-descent. |
| Treatment *Acute episode* | **Urgent or emergent pericardiocentesis.** Intravascular volume expansion (300-500 cc of normal saline over 30-60 minutes) and parenteral inotropes (isoproterenol 2-20 mcg/min or dobutamine 5-20 mcg/kg/min) may be used to temporarily support hemodynamics while preparing for pericardiocentesis. |

*See p. 1 for abbreviations and p. 144 for antibiotic dosages.*

## 1. CARDIAC TAMPONADE

| | |
|---|---|
| Rx (cont.) *Recurrences* | • Subxyphoid pericardiotomy as a palliative procedure for pts with poor prognoses; reaccumulations are common.<br>• Complete pericardiectomy when long-term survival can be expected, especially for patients with effusive-constrictive pericarditis or loculated effusions. Operative mortality 10-15%. |

## 2. CONSTRICTIVE PERICARDITIS

| | |
|---|---|
| Presentation | Insidious but progressive symptoms of low cardiac output (fatigue, tachycardia, relative hypotension) and right-sided heart failure (jugular venous distension, hepatomegaly, ascites, peripheral edema). |
| Diagnosis | • Physical exam: Increased jugular venous pulse with **prominent X and Y descents,** pericardial knock. A normal appearing pericardium on CT or MRI speaks strongly against the diagnosis.<br>• Cardiac cath: Less than 5 mmHg difference between the mean right atrial pressure, RV diastolic pressure, LV diastolic pressure, and pulmonary capillary wedge pressure; "dip and plateau" in ventricular waveform. |
| Treatment | Mild symptoms may respond to long-term diuretic therapy. However, **many patients develop progressive disability and require complete pericardiectomy.** |

## 3. OTHER COMPLICATIONS OF PERICARDITIS

| Complication | Therapy |
|---|---|
| Effusive-constrictive pericarditis | Definitive treatment requires pericardiectomy. Presents with cardiac tamponade; after pericardiocentesis, right atrial pressure remains elevated and typical features of constriction appear. |
| Recurrent, relapsing pericarditis | Chronic nonsteroidal anti-inflammatory agents. Long-term steroid use may be required (alternate day therapy preferred to avoid adverse effects). |

*See p. 1 for abbreviations and p. 144 for antibiotic dosages.*

# 13. CARDIAC DISEASE AND PREGNANCY

Pamela S. Douglas, M.D.

| I. MATERNAL CARDIAC DISEASE: OVERVIEW OF THERAPY | |
|---|---|
| Antepartum | **Most pregnant females with cardiac disease will deteriorate by at least 1 functional class** due to the increase in cardiac work required to maintain the uteroplacental circulation (especially weeks 28-32). **Moderate-to-severe maternal cardiac disease is associated with preterm labor, fetal growth retardation, and fetal wastage**. Therapeutic recommendations include:<br>• Bedrest to decrease cardiac work and increase diuresis.<br>• Salt restriction (4-6 gm/d).<br>• Diuretics: Used only for heart failure not responding to above measures. Overdiuresis results in contracted intravascular volume, which is associated with increased fetal morbidity.<br>• Digoxin: Often administered empirically for prophylaxis against CHF for patients with severe LV dysfunction.<br>• Tocolysis: **β**-mimetics ↑ cardiac work and should be avoided in patients with moderate-to-severe disease.<br>• Therapeutic abortion for high-risk pregnancy (see below).<br>• Genetic counseling. |
| Intrapartum | **Many maternal deaths occur during this period** as cardiac reserve is exhausted from a 15-20% increase in cardiac output consequent to pain, relief of inferior vena caval (IVC) obstruction, and autoperfusion from the uteroplacental circulation during contractions. Therapeutic measures include:<br>• Lateral supine position to relieve IVC obstruction and increase preload.<br>• Hemodynamic monitoring and pulse oximetry.<br>• Anesthesia: Should be local, if possible. Avoid general anesthesia.<br>• Antibiotic prophylaxis: See p. 166.<br>• IV fluids: Minimize in volume overload states.<br>• Oxytocin: Avoid if possible.<br>• Method of delivery: Vaginal unless obstetrical indications for Caesarean are present. |

*See p. 1 for abbreviations and p. 199 for drug information.*

## I. MATERNAL CARDIAC DISEASE: OVERVIEW OF THERAPY

| | |
|---|---|
| Postpartum | **Maternal death may occur in this period**. Cardiac demands remain high and right-to-left shunting may occur or worsen if pulmonary hypertension is present, resulting in progressive hypoxemia.<br>• Anticoagulants (subcutaneous heparin 5,000 units every 12 hrs) to prevent DVT in patients at high risk of thromboembolic events. |

## II. USE OF CARDIAC DRUGS DURING PREGNANCY

| | |
|---|---|
| Probably safe (but no adequate studies) | • Aldomet • Hydralazine • Nifedipine • Verapamil • **β**-blockers<br>• Digoxin • Lasix • Quinidine • Procainamide • Heparin<br>• Atropine • Epinephrine • Diphenhydramine HCl • Aspirin (until term) |
| Evidence of fetal risk | • Warfarin • ACE inhibitors • Thiazide diuretics • Spironolactone • Reserpine • Diazoxide<br>• Indomethacin |

## III. HYPERTENSION

| Presentation | Therapy |
|---|---|
| Pre-existing hypertension | Bed rest, low-salt diet. Drug therapy: May continue previous antihypertensive regimen during gestation except for ACE inhibitors (associated with fetal toxicity). |
| Pregnancy-induced (gestational) | Primary prevention: Rest periods, low salt diet. Medical therapy for diastolic BP >100 mmHg: **Aldomet** is considered by many the drug of choice. Useful alternatives include hydralazine, **β**-blockers, prazosin, and labetalol. |

*See p. 1 for abbreviations and p. 199 for drug information.*

## III. HYPERTENSION

| Presentation | Therapy |
|---|---|
| Pre-eclampsia, eclampsia | • **Hospitalization** and bedrest for moderate and severe cases.<br>• **Control BP**: Lower diastolic BPs > 105-110 mmHg to < 95 mmHg. May require IV therapy with **hydralazine or labetalol**. Hydralazine dose: 5-20 mg IV bolus q 20-30 min as needed. Alternatively, infuse 0.5-1.0 mg/min IV to a mean arterial pressure of 100-110 mmHg; the total dose (mg) is then given as an hourly maintenance infusion. Aggressive lowering of BP (≤ 120/80 mmHg) may cause acute renal shutdown and should be avoided.<br>• **Seizure prophylaxis**: **Magnesium sulfate** 4-6 gm IV bolus over 15-30 min followed by a continuous infusion of 1-2 gm/hr to maintain serum $Mg^+$ at 4.8-9.6 mg/dL. Magnesium toxicity is suggested by increased lethargy or decreased patellar tendon reflexes.<br>• **Immediate delivery** for uncontrolled hypertension, progressive renal insufficiency or hepatic dysfunction, and signs of impending eclampsia (severe headache, visual disturbances, hyperreflexia).<br>• Prevention: Low-dose aspirin (JAMA 1991;226:261) and dietary calcium (2 gm/d) appear promising. |

## IV. MATERNAL CONGENITAL HEART DISEASE

| Category | Comments |
|---|---|
| ***High-Risk Lesions:***<br>• Symptomatic prior to conception<br>• Moderate-severe valvular stenosis<br>• Moderate-severe hypertrophic cardiomyopathy<br>• Severe valvular regurgitation<br>• Cyanotic congenital heart disease<br>• Right-to-left shunt<br>• Eisenmenger's syndrome<br>• Severe symptoms during gestation (NYHA Class III-IV) | • Preconception counseling.<br>• Sterilization or therapeutic abortion should be considered.<br>• Fetal monitoring including echocardiography.<br>• If carried to term: Hospitalization, bed rest, anticoagulation, non-induced labor with pulmonary artery pressure monitoring, vaginal delivery with forceps, and epidural anesthesia. Forceps are used to shorten the second stage of labor and to avoid maternal Valsalva.<br>• Caesarean section for obstetrical indications only.<br>• Endocarditis prophylaxis during delivery (see p. 166). |

## IV. MATERNAL CONGENITAL HEART DISEASE

| Category | Comments |
| --- | --- |
| ***Low-Risk Lesions:***<br>• Asymptomatic patients<br>• ASD, VSD, PDA with normal PA pressure<br>• Mild-to-moderate valve regurgitation<br>• Mild-to-moderate pulmonic stenosis<br>• Mild-to-moderate hypertrophic cardiomyopathy | • Preconception counseling.<br>• Fetal monitoring including echocardiography.<br>• Non-induced labor, epidural anesthesia, vaginal delivery.<br>• Caesarean section for obstetrical indications only.<br>• Endocarditis prophylaxis as outlined on p. 166. |

## V. ACQUIRED VALVULAR HEART DISEASE

| Presentation | Therapy |
| --- | --- |
| Rheumatic heart disease | • **High-risk lesions**: Symptomatic prior to conception, moderate-severe mitral or aortic stenosis, severe valvular regurgitation, pulmonary hypertension, AFIB:<br>- As above for high-risk congenital heart disease.<br>- Digoxin or ***β***-blockers to control heart rate in AFIB.<br>- Cardioversion for uncontrolled tachycardia.<br>- Reduce PCWP to ≤14 mmHg prior to delivery in anticipation of average 10 mmHg rise postpartum.<br>- Balloon mitral and aortic valvuloplasty for severe symptoms.<br>- Endocarditis prophylaxis during delivery (p. 166).<br>• **Low-risk lesions**: Mild-moderate valvular regurgitation, mild mitral stenosis with normal PA pressure, asymptomatic or mild symptoms in third trimester:<br>- Routine antepartum, intrapartum, and postpartum considerations.<br>- See p. 166 for indications for endocarditis prophylaxis during pregnancy. |

*See p. 1 for abbreviations and p. 199 for drug information.*

## V. ACQUIRED VALVULAR HEART DISEASE

| Presentation | Therapy |
|---|---|
| Mitral valve prolapse | *β*-blockers for severe chest pain and/or arrhythmias. Endocarditis prophylaxis is controversial for patients undergoing normal vaginal delivery without mitral regurgitation and/or a thickened valve. |
| Prosthetic valves | • Mechanical valves/bioprosthetic mitral valves: Endocarditis prophylaxis (p. 166), anticoagulation (p. 165).<br>• Bioprosthetic aortic valves: Routine care and endocarditis prophylaxis.<br>• There is an **increased risk of valve thrombosis and systemic bleeding** from fluctuating anticoagulation status during pregnancy. |
| Infectious endocarditis | Antibiotic choice dictated by microbiology (Ch. 11). **Probably "safe"**: Penicillin, cephalosporin, erythromycin, clindamycin; **Use with caution**: Metronidazole, bactrim, aminoglycosides, vancomycin; **Unsafe**: Tetracycline. |

## VI. MYOCARDIAL DISEASE

| Presentation | Therapy |
|---|---|
| Myocarditis | Bed rest and oxygenation. Heart failure: Digoxin, diuretics, and vasodilators (hydralazine, prazosin). Arrhythmias: p. 165. Use of steroids/immunosuppressives is controversial but should probably be avoided. |
| Hypertrophic obstructive cardiomyopathy | Preconception counseling. Medical therapy: see pp. 112-113. Avoid *β*-mimetic tocolytic therapy, hypovolemia, inotropes, and most vasodilators. If tocolysis is needed, consider magnesium sulfate. Spinal and epidural anesthesia should be avoided; consider inhalation agents and/or paracervical/pudendal blocks. Vaginal delivery with endocarditis prophylaxis (p. 166); hemodynamic monitoring during labor and delivery for symptomatic patients and those with an LV outflow tract gradient. |

*See p. 1 for abbreviations and p. 199 for drug information.*

## VI. MYOCARDIAL DISEASE

| Presentation | Therapy |
| --- | --- |
| Peripartum cardiomyopathy (PPCM) | • Bed rest and oxygenation. Consider anticoagulation during 3rd trimester with heparin (5,000 units subcutaneous bid) and postpartum with warfarin (INR 2.0-3.0) due to an ↑ risk of thromboembolic events.<br>• For systolic ventricular failure: Digitalis, diuretics, vasodilators ± dobutamine. Nonresponders: Consider IABP or ventricular assist device as a temporizing measure (until recovery occurs) or a bridge to cardiac transplantation (severe unremitting cases).<br>• Use of immunosuppressives and steroids is controversial but should probably be avoided.<br>• Nitroprusside should be used prior to delivery *only if* CHF is unresponsive to other vasodilators (may cause fetal toxicity). Avoid ACE inhibitors during pregnancy (↑ fetal toxicity). |

## VII. VASCULAR AND EMBOLIC DISEASE

| Presentation | Therapy |
| --- | --- |
| Primary pulmonary hypertension | • Preconception counseling; therapeutic abortion.<br>• If carried to term: Oxygen and management as in high-risk congenital heart disease (p. 161). |
| DVT, pulmonary embolism | Anticoagulation (p. 165), even for calf phlebitis. If anticoagulation is contraindicated or PE recurs despite anticoagulation, inferior vena caval interruption or umbrella is indicated. |
| The Marfan Syndrome | • Pre-pregnancy counseling (50% of offspring develop Marfan's, ↑ risk of aortic dissection).<br>• Baseline cardiac and aortic assessment prior to conception, frequent echocardiograms during gestation.<br>• Consider prophylactic bedrest and $\beta$-blockers to possibly ↓ the rate of aortic dilatation.<br>• **Therapeutic abortion for significant aortic dilation (> 40-45 mm)**.<br>• Delivery: Vaginal with forceps, endocarditis prophylaxis if valvular regurgitation is present (p. 166). |
| Aortic dissection | See p. 172. Caesarean section with epidural anesthesia, depending on fetal viability. |

*See p. 1 for abbreviations and p. 199 for drug information.*

## VIII. CORONARY ARTERY DISEASE AND ARRHYTHMIAS

| Presentation | Therapy |
|---|---|
| Coronary artery disease | For atherosclerotic disease: Exercise restriction, nitrates, $\beta$-blockers; hemodynamic monitoring during labor and delivery; adequate anesthesia and analgesia; and caesarean section only for obstetrical indications. **Avoid oxytocin and ergot derivatives** to suppress lactation (may provoke coronary spasm). |
| Arrhythmias | • Evaluate and treat underlying heart disease; exclude other contributing causes such as pulmonary embolism thyroid disease, caffeine, drug abuse, electrolyte disturbances, etc.<br>• Teach vagal maneuvers for SVT.<br>• **Cardioversion is considered safe**: Indications include AFIB/flutter, SVTs that cause hypotension, heart failure or angina, and ventricular tachycardia/fibrillation (see Ch. 5,6).<br>• Avoid drug therapy in absence of organic heart disease or potentially life-threatening arrhythmias. If treatment is required, use "safe" agent at lowest dose possible: **"Safe":** Lidocaine, digoxin, $\beta$-blockers; **"Probably safe":** Quinidine, procainamide, IV calcium channel blockers, adenosine; **Unknown:** Mexiletine, disopyramide; **Unsafe:** Phenytoin, amiodarone, oral (chronic) calcium channel blockers. |

## IX. OTHER TOPICS

| Topic | Comments |
|---|---|
| Anticoagulation<br>*Pre-pregnancy* | Counseling, discontinue warfarin, begin subcutaneous heparin; dose adjusted to PTT of 1.5-2.0 x control (usually 10-15,000 U bid). |
| *Pregnancy* | Continue heparin at least through the 1st trimester; warfarin is contraindicated at this time. May switch back to warfarin in 2nd and 3rd trimesters, but will need to overlap heparin and warfarin for 3-5 days until a therapeutic INR is achieved. If warfarin is used, switch to heparin from 35-37 weeks until delivery. |

*See p. 1 for abbreviations and p. 199 for drug information.*

## IX. OTHER TOPICS

| | |
|---|---|
| Anticoagulation (cont.) *Delivery* | Discontinue heparin at start of labor. If the patient is on warfarin at the time of delivery, reverse anticoagulation with fresh frozen plasma (2 units). Warfarin's effects may persist in the fetus for 7-10 days after drug discontinuation. |
| *Postpartum* | Restart heparin at 2-4 hours postpartum. Restart warfarin at 24 hours (does not enter breast milk). |
| *Complications* | All drugs increase the risk of maternal and fetal hemorrhage. Heparin may cause maternal thrombocytopenia, osteoporosis, and hypoaldosteronism; does not cross the placenta. Warfarin with high incidence of fetal wastage, stillbirths, blindness, and mental retardation. If used in the 1st trimester, up to 25% develop *coumarin embryopathy* (nasal hypoplasia, epiphyseal stippling, CNS abnormalities). Antiplatelet agents may cause fetal cardiac abnormalities and early ductal closure. |
| Tocolysis | Tocolytic therapy may precipitate heart failure and arrhythmias in patients with underlying heart disease. If tocolysis is needed, consider adjunctive use of steroids to accelerate fetal maturity. |
| *Specific agents* | **$\beta_2$-selective sympathetic amines** (ritodrine, terbutaline, orciprenaline, salbutamol) may precipitate heart failure, arrhythmias, hypokalemia, hyperglycemia, and hypotension; these agents are **contraindicated in patients with moderate-to-severe symptoms or "high-risk" heart disease** (pp. 161-162). |
| *Recommendations* | • Bed rest, hydration, and treatment of underlying disorders (e.g., infection) prior to tocolytic therapy.<br>• Mild-moderate cardiac disease: Magnesium sulfate for tocolysis; avoid $\beta$-agonists.<br>• Severe or high-risk cardiac disease: Avoid all tocolytics. |
| Endocarditis prophylaxis | Indications: (1) Complicated delivery in patients with prosthetic heart valves, congenital or rheumatic heart disease, hypertrophic obstructive cardiomyopathy, and mitral valve prolapse with thickened leaflets and regurgitation; (2) Uncomplicated vaginal delivery in patients with prosthetic heart valves; (3) Antibiotic prophylaxis is controversial for uncomplicated vaginal delivery in pts with acquired valvular heart disease. |
| *Antibiotic regimen* | Ampicillin 2 gm (IM or IV) plus gentamicin 1.5 mg/kg (IM or IV: max 80 mg) 30-60 minutes prior to delivery and 8 hours later. If allergic to penicillin, substitute vancomycin 1 gm (IV over 60 minutes). |

# 14. ADULT CONGENITAL HEART DISEASE

James Boatman, M.D.

## I. PATENT DUCTUS ARTERIOSUS (PDA)

| | |
|---|---|
| Natural history | The ductus arteriosus exists in the fetus as a functional vessel that connects the pulmonary artery to the descending aorta, typically just distal to the origin of the left subclavian artery. PDAs may remain patent after birth and result in chronic volume overload of the pulmonary vasculature and left heart from left-to-right shunting (i.e., aorta → pulmonary artery).<br>• Small PDA: Usually does not affect life expectancy, although the risk of infectious endocarditis is increased.<br>• **Moderate or large PDA**: Congestive heart failure, pulmonary hypertension and/or infectious endocarditis may occur, **reducing life expectancy**. Infective endocarditis is almost exclusively seen with left-to-right shunts; a "jet lesion" in the pulmonary artery serves as the nidus for infection and multiple pulmonary emboli. As pulmonary hypertension progresses, there may be reversal in the direction of the shunt to result in isolated lower extremity cyanosis, exercise-induced leg fatigue, and paradoxical embolization. |
| Management<br>*Medical* | Antibiotic prophylaxis against infectious endocarditis prior to and 6 months following repair (p. 150). Routine measures to treat congestive heart failure may be needed (Ch. 8). |
| *Surgical* | **Elective surgical closure** via simple ligation is safe (mortality < 0.5%) and is recommended **for all patients more than 1 year of age**. If an aneurysmal or calcified PDA is found, surgical resection with cardiopulmonary bypass may be required. Once severe pulmonary hypertension and irreversible pulmonary vascular obstructive disease develop, surgery is of no benefit. Following surgery, abnormalities on physical examination usually disappear and regression of LV hypertrophy is common. Unfortunately, pulmonary hypertension may persist or even progress. Transcatheter closure (double umbrella technique) has shown early promise but is currently considered investigational. |

*See p. 1 for abbreviations and p. 199 for drug information.*

## II. VENTRICULAR SEPTAL DEFECT (VSD)

| | |
|---|---|
| Overview | VSD is the most common congenital cardiac abnormality in infants and children, and occurs equally among males and females. 25-40% of VSDs spontaneously close, 90% by age eight. In large VSDs (shunt > 2:1), both pulmonary blood flow and pulmonary vascular resistance (PVR) are markedly increased; as PVR continues to rise, the left-to-right shunt may reverse direction and result in cyanosis, clubbing, and an increased risk of paradoxical embolization. Untreated, RV ± LV failure and irreversible pulmonary vascular obstruction (Eisenmenger's Syndrome) ensue. |
| Natural history | • Small VSD: Little impact on longevity, although the risk of infective endocarditis is increased.<br>• Moderate-sized VSD: CHF usually occurs during infancy; symptoms may improve with spontaneous narrowing or closure. Severe pulmonary hypertension is rare.<br>• Large (nonrestrictive) VSD: Most are diagnosed early, 10% lead to Eisenmenger's Syndrome, and most patients die in early childhood or adolescence.<br>• **Maternal mortality in Eisenmenger's syndrome exceeds 50% during pregnancy/delivery**; 3% of first degree relatives of VSD patients will also have a VSD. |
| Management<br>*Medical* | • Asymptomatic children with normal pulmonary pressures (even with a large VSD) can be managed medically. If spontaneous closure does not occur by 3-5 years of age, elective surgical repair should be performed.<br>• For CHF, hydralazine (or nitroprusside acutely) may reduce systemic vascular resistance relative to pulmonary vascular resistance. This results in a reduction in left-to-right shunting and improved symptomatic status. Diuretics may be useful for right heart failure.<br>• Antibiotic prophylaxis against infective endocarditis before, and for 6 mos. after uncomplicated repair (p. 150). |
| *Surgical* | **Surgical repair** is recommended for asymptomatic infants without spontaneous closure by 3-5 years of age, infants with symptoms of CHF or pulmonary hypertension, and **all adults with a left-to-right shunt > 1.5:1**. Surgery is of no benefit once the ratio of pulmonary-to-systemic vascular resistance exceeds > 0.9. Direct surgical closure, usually with a patch, results in perioperative mortality in 3% and complete heart block in less than 2%. Following surgery, most patients improve symptomatically and ECG signs of RV hypertrophy frequently reverse. Unfortunately, pulmonary hypertension usually persists. |

*See p. 1 for abbreviations and p. 199 for drug information.*

## III. ATRIAL SEPTAL DEFECT (ASD)

| | |
|---|---|
| Overview | ASDs constitute 30% of congenital heart defects found in adults. In small shunts, there is a mild increase in right heart blood volume, although pulmonary pressures remain normal. Even when the shunt is large, pulmonary hypertension may only be mild. Rarely, severe pulmonary hypertension develops and results in right heart failure (hepatomegaly, ascites) and R → L shunting (cyanosis, clubbing, paradoxical embolus). |
| Natural history | Young patients with isolated ASDs generally tolerate even large volume shunts well. When complicated by mitral regurgitation, the incidence of atrial arrhythmias and pulmonary hypertension is increased. **Patients with untreated moderated-sized ASDs frequently die in the 4th or 5th decade**; however, prolonged survival to an elderly age is not uncommon, especially for those without manifest pulmonary hypertension. Pulmonary and systemic (paradoxical) emboli are relatively common in older patients with ASDs complicated by AFIB and right heart failure. Eisenmenger's physiology (irreversible severe pulmonary arteriolar disease) is rare; when present, it usually manifests in young adulthood and carries a high mortality from embolic events, arrhythmias, and progressive RV failure. Infective endocarditis is rare in ASDs without valve abnormalities or other congenital heart disease. **Pregnancy is usually well-tolerated**. |
| Management<br>*Medical* | **Antibiotic prophylaxis is unnecessary for uncomplicated secundum ASDs**, although patients with primum ASDs and prominent sinus venosus ASDs should receive coverage before, and for 6 months after surgical repair (see p. 150). Diuretics may be useful in treating right heart failure. |
| *Surgical closure* | Surgical closure, using a single suture or patch, is **indicated if the pulmonary-to-systemic flow ratio (shunt ratio) is ≥ 1.5:1**, even in asymptomatic patients. This prevents the development of pulmonary hypertension and right-heart failure, and decreases the risk of infectious endocarditis. In contrast, surgery is of no benefit once severe pulmonary vascular disease has developed (ratio of pulmonary-to-systemic vascular resistance ≥ 0.9). Operative mortality for uncomplicated secundum ASD repair is less than 1% but slightly higher for primum ASDs that also require mitral valve repair. Postoperative complications include sinus node dysfunction (after repair of sinus venosis defect) and complete heart block (after primum repairs). If mitral regurgitation is present preoperatively, symptoms may worsen following ASD closure as regurgitant volume "run-off" across the ASD is blocked. If AFIB or SVT is present prior to surgical repair, they most likely will persist postoperatively. |

# 15. PERIPHERAL VASCULAR DISEASE

John A. Spittell, Jr., M.D.
Peter C. Spittell, M.D.

## I. AORTIC ANEURYSM

| | THORACIC AORTIC ANEURYSM | ABDOMINAL AORTIC ANEURYSM (AAA) |
|---|---|---|
| Clinical presentation | Most are first discovered on chest x-ray. When symptomatic, the most common complaint is **pain in the upper chest or back.** Pressure on surrounding mediastinal structures may also cause hoarseness, cough, dyspnea, and dysphagia. | **50% are asymptomatic.** The most common complaint is **awareness of a pulsating abdominal mass.** Other complaints include pain in the abdomen, back, flank or groin, and abdominal tenderness. With atheroembolism, a lacy, irregular, bluish discoloration of the skin of the lower extremities (livedo reticularis) and/or blueness of one or more toes may be present. |
| Natural history | Average life expectancy is reduced, with **untreated 5 year survival of 25-50%.** Principal causes of premature death include rupture and atherosclerotic coronary/cerebral artery disease. The risk of rupture increases with aneurysms > 6.0 cm in diameter, especially if the patient is hypertensive. | The most frequent complication and cause of death is rupture. The **risk of rupture becomes significant when the aneurysm reaches 5.0 cm in diameter** (30-40% at 1-year) and increases with increasing size. Aneurysms enlarge at variable rates but average 0.5 cm per year. |
| Medical therapy | For **asymptomatic aneurysms < 5.0 cm in diameter**, recommendations include careful control of hypertension and ultrasound observation twice yearly (to detect changes that would warrant surgical intervention). Screen for coronary artery and cerebrovascular disease. | For **asymptomatic aneurysms < 4.5 cm in diameter,** serial observation with ultrasound twice yearly--or sooner if symptoms develop--is recommended. Screen for coronary artery and cerebrovascular disease. |

*See p. 1 for abbreviations and p. 199 for drug information.*

## I. AORTIC ANEURYSM

| | THORACIC AORTIC ANEURYSM | ABDOMINAL AORTIC ANEURYSM (AAA) |
|---|---|---|
| Surgical therapy, indications | • Atherosclerotic aneurysms: ≥ 6.0 cm in diameter, those causing symptoms, those enlarging under observation (particularly in hypertensives), and for post-traumatic aneurysms.<br>• Marfan syndrome: ≥ 6.0 cm even if asymptomatic. | Elective surgical treatment is indicated for aneurysms that produce symptoms or are larger than 4.5 cm in diameter. |

## II. AORTIC DISSECTION

Acute aortic dissection is the most frequent acute aortic lesion encountered in clinical practice. The variable and protean manifestations account for the diagnostic difficulty. **A correct diagnosis is made in only about 50%** of most reported series. Thus, a high index of suspicion in likely settings and prompt application of appropriate screening imaging techniques are essential requisites to an improved management strategy and clinical outcome (Mayo Clin Proc 1993;68:642).

| | PROXIMAL AORTIC DISSECTION (Types I, II: Type A) | DISTAL AORTIC DISSECTION (Type III: Type B) |
|---|---|---|
| Clinical presentation | Acute onset of **severe anterior chest pain** which usually migrates distally. The patient appears acutely ill, often shock-like but with an elevated blood pressure. **Aortic valve regurgitation** occurs in ~ 50%; manifestations of **ischemia to various organ systems** (e.g., brain, spinal cord, kidneys, extremities, heart) and cardiac tamponade may also be evident. | Acute onset of **severe interscapular or epigastric pain.** The pain may migrate to chest, neck, back and/or lower extremities. Hemopericardium and aortic regurgitation are not part of the clinical picture. |

| | PROXIMAL AORTIC DISSECTION (Types I, II: Type A) | DISTAL AORTIC DISSECTION (Type III: Type B) |
|---|---|---|
| Diagnosis | Transesophageal echocardiography, CT scan and MRI can be used to demonstrate the intimal flap, true and false lumens, pericardial fluid, and aortic valve regurgitation (NEJM 1993;328:1). Transesophageal echo (TEE) has the advantage of being portable, requires no contrast media, provides an accurate diagnosis with a sensitivity and specificity >90%, and allows rapid triage to surgery to decrease early mortality. If noninvasive imaging does not provide adequate information, urgent angiography is indicated prior to surgical repair. If the patient is stable and CAD is suspected, consider cardiac cath prior to surgery. | |
| Natural history | **Without treatment, 70% die within 2 weeks** and > 50% of survivors die within the ensuing 12 months. The most common cause of death is external rupture, even if re-entry has occurred. | |
| Medical therapy | When acute aortic dissection is suspected, drug therapy is started while the definitive diagnosis is pursued:<br>• **Elevated BP: β-blockade** (e.g. metoprolol: 5 mg IV bolus every 2-5 minutes x 3, then 50 mg po q 6 hours starting 15 min after the last IV dose) **followed by sodium nitroprusside,** or monotherapy with labetalol to decrease BP, contractility, and shear force.<br>• Normotensive: β-blocker alone.<br>• **Aspirin, heparin, thrombolytics are contraindicated**. | • **Acute pharmacotherapy as for proximal aortic dissection.** For those whose pain and BP are controlled on medical therapy, either a β-blocker (e.g. propranolol, metoprolol, atenolol) or labetalol may be continued long term.<br>• Follow-up imaging (CT scan) at least annually. **Aspirin, heparin, and thrombolytics are contraindicated**. |
| Surgical therapy | • **Prompt surgical resection** (aortic valve repair when necessary) **is the treatment of choice** to prevent the serious and unpredictable complications of external rupture and proximal extension.<br>• **Following successful surgery, chronic β-blocker therapy** and annual imaging (CT scan) are indicated. | • **Surgery is indicated if symptoms of aortic dissection recur, and for patients on medical therapy who develop enlargement of the aorta, aneurysm formation, or deterioration in distal organ function**. β-blockers should be continued indefinitely after successful surgical therapy along with annual imaging (CT scan). Continued... |

*See p. 1 for abbreviations and p. 199 for drug information.*

| | PROXIMAL AORTIC DISSECTION (Types I, II: Type A) | DISTAL AORTIC DISSECTION (Type III: Type B) |
|---|---|---|
| Surgical therapy (cont.) | See previous page. | • For patients with stable dissections < 70 years old without serious comorbid conditions, some recommend surgical repair after stabilization on drug therapy for several months, while others advocate medical therapy alone. |

## III. ACUTE ARTERIAL OCCLUSION

| | THROMBOTIC OCCLUSION | EMBOLIC OCCLUSION |
|---|---|---|
| Presentation | One or more of the "5 P's:" Pain, parasthesia, paralysis, pallor, pulselessness. In general, **restoration of flow within 8 hours is necessary to ensure limb survival.** Co-morbid conditions determine life expectancy. | Same as for thrombotic occlusion. |
| Medical therapy | **IV heparin** should be instituted at time of diagnosis to protect the collateral circulation. **The ischemic limb should be protected from trauma and should not be elevated, heated, or cooled**. | **Same as for thrombotic occlusion** plus stabilization of cardiac problems. Long-term oral anticoagulant therapy is indicated for persistent cardiac source of emboli (e.g., chronic AFIB). **Thrombolytic therapy may be of value** (agents, dosages, adjuncts identical to those used for acute MI, p. 49). The role of lytic therapy vs. acute surgical intervention is under investigation. |

*See p. 1 for abbreviations and p. 199 for drug information.*

## III. ACUTE ARTERIAL OCCLUSION

| | THROMBOTIC OCCLUSION | EMBOLIC OCCLUSION |
|---|---|---|
| Surgical therapy | **Surgical thrombectomy** should be performed acutely if the limb is threatened and the condition of the patient permits. Arterial surgery or angioplasty is indicated for the relief of ischemic rest pain and disabling claudication. The prognosis for limb salvage is good if pulsatile flow is restored before irreversible changes occur (muscle necrosis or gangrene). Life expectancy depends on co-morbid conditions. | **Embolectomy by Fogarty catheter** (or surgery if necessary) should be performed as soon as cardiac status has stabilized. The prognosis for limb salvage is good if embolectomy is successful before irreversible changes occur. Life expectancy depends on co-morbid conditions. |

## IV. CHRONIC ATHEROSCLEROTIC OCCLUSIVE DISEASE

When symptomatic, the hallmark of chronic occlusive peripheral arterial disease is **intermittent claudication**--distress in the affected extremity that occurs with walking and is relieved by standing still. As atherosclerotic narrowing progresses and ischemia becomes more severe, the patient may have pain in the foot or toes at rest, which is typically worse at night and better when placed in a dependent position. Even trivial injury may result in ulceration or gangrene. Fifty percent of patients have significant coronary artery disease, which may be symptomatic and is the principal cause for their shortened life expectancy.

*See p. 1 for abbreviations and p. 199 for drug information.*

## A. CHRONIC ATHEROSCLEROTIC OCCLUSIVE DISEASE

| Presentation | TRIAGE Medical Therapy | TRIAGE Angioplasty or Surgery | Comments |
|---|---|---|---|
| Claudication *Non-diabetic* | General measures,[1] walking program[2] and Trental 300 mg tid during meals | Elective. Goal is to increase walking distance | Risk of limb loss without treatment is 4-5% in 5 years. Walking distance over 5 years is stable in 50% |
| *Diabetic* | Same as above plus control of diabetes | Indicated due to the increased risk of limb loss | Risk of limb loss is 4 times greater than in the nondiabetic with claudication |
| Foot ulcer *Non-infected* | Rest,[3] general measures[1] | Indicated due to the increased risk of limb loss | Risk of limb loss with ischemic ulceration ~ 12% in 5 years |
| *Infected* | Rest,[3] systemic antibiotics based on culture, general measures[1] | Indicated after control of infection | |
| Rest pain | Rest, general measures[1] | Indicated due to the increased risk of limb loss | Risk of limb loss ~ 12% in 5 years |

1. General measures are essential for all patients with occlusive disease regardless of any other therapy planned or instituted. These include interdiction of tobacco, properly fitted and protective footwear, regular foot hygiene, protection of the ischemic limb from all types of trauma, control of hyperlipidemia and diabetes, and the avoidance of medications known to cause a worsening of symptoms (e.g., $\beta$-blockers).
2. 30-minute walk, stopping as needed to relieve discomfort, 5 times/week.
3. Avoid weight bearing on affected limb until healed.

*See p. 1 for abbreviations and p. 199 for drug information.*

## B. NON-MEDICAL THERAPY OF PERIPHERAL VASCULAR DISEASE

| Modality | Indications |
|---|---|
| Percutaneous revascularization | Selection of the optimal technique (balloon angioplasty, atherectomy, laser) is based on lesion morphology and location (Curr Opin Cardiol 1990;5:666, JACC 1990;15:1551). Ideal lesions include iliac stenosis ≤ 5 cm in length and femoropopliteal occlusion or stenosis ≤ 10 cm in length. When thrombus is present, thrombolysis is used in conjunction with the mechanical procedures. |
| Surgery<br>*Indications* | Surgical treatment of symptomatic occlusive peripheral arterial disease is "elective" for the nondiabetic person whose only symptom is intermittent claudication; the goal of surgery is to allow the patient to walk further. For patients with **ischemic pain at rest, ischemic ulceration, and for diabetics with symptomatic disease,** restoration of pulsatile flow is indicated to decrease the incidence of limb loss. |
| *Preoperative assessment* | Coronary artery disease is present in 50%, may be asymptomatic, and is responsible for the shortened life expectancy among patients with peripheral vascular disease. It also is the most common cause of morbidity and mortality associated with vascular surgical procedures. Accordingly, **the first objective when considering surgery is to determine the risk of perioperative cardiac complications** and institute medical and surgical measures to minimize the level of risk (see Ch. 10). |

## V. DEEP VENOUS THROMBOSIS (DVT)

| | PROXIMAL DVT | DISTAL DVT |
|---|---|---|
| Presentation | Soft pitting edema of the lower extremity, pain and tenderness over the superficial femoral, common femoral and/or popliteal veins. **Proximal DVT may be "silent" and first present as pulmonary embolism.** | Calf pain or tenderness, which may be minimally symptomatic, is the most common presentation. May also be asymptomatic. **Edema is not a feature of calf DVT.** |

*See p. 1 for abbreviations and p. 199 for drug information.*

## V. DEEP VENOUS THROMBOSIS (DVT)

| | PROXIMAL DVT | DISTAL DVT |
|---|---|---|
| Natural history | **Pulmonary embolism occurs in 40-50%,** the majority of which are clinically silent. Venous flow returns to normal by recanalization and/or collateral formation in 2/3 of cases within 3 months. Valvular damage is common. | **Spontaneous lysis is the rule,** although in 20% of patients, extension occurs into the proximal leg veins. Pulmonary embolism occurs in 1-5% of isolated calf vein thromboses; if extension into the proximal leg vein occurs, this risk increases to 40-50%. The majority of these PEs are clinically silent. |
| Diagnostic tests | • **Duplex ultrasound:** Procedure of choice for the diagnosis of **femoral and popliteal DVT**. A negative test does not exclude calf vein or iliac vein DVT, which require contrast venography for definite diagnosis.<br>• Impedance plethysmography (IPG): Noninvasive, reproducible, reliable. Can be used if ultrasound is not available. | • **Contrast venography** is the definitive diagnostic procedure for **calf vein DVT**, but is usually not necessary when the clinical presentation is classic.<br>• Duplex ultrasound and IPG lack sensitivity for calf vein DVT. |
| Medical therapy<br>*Anticoagulation* | Indicated for all patients without a contraindication:<br>• Obtain baseline PT, PTT, platelet count.<br>• **IV heparin followed by warfarin:** Follow recommendations for pulmonary embolism, p. 181.<br>• Monitor platelet count daily; if platelets fall to < 100,000/mcl, stop heparin.<br>• Warfarin dosage is regulated to keep INR at 2.0-3.0 for 3 months, or for at least 6 months if risk factors persist. | Controversial. Some prefer to withhold treatment unless there is an extension into proximal deep veins on serial evaluation and IPG, while others (the authors included) treat as described for acute proximal DVT. |

*See p. 1 for abbreviations and p. 199 for drug information.*

## V. DEEP VENOUS THROMBOSIS (DVT)

| | |
|---|---|
| Medical Rx (cont.)<br>*Thrombolysis* | • Indications: **Massive proximal DVT or recent extensive axillary/subclavian DVT**, particularly in younger persons. Lytic therapy has been associated with a decreased incidence of valvular damage and postphlebitic venous insufficiency; **its impact on the development of PE is unknown**. Not indicated for isolated calf vein DVT.<br>• Regimens (see p. 181):<br>- Streptokinase: Often necessary to continue the infusion for 48-72 hours. Best results are seen when the process is < 7 days duration, preferably < 36 hours. Thrombolysis is achieved in 70-80%.<br>- Urokinase: Continue infusion for 24-48 hours. Clot lysis is more rapid than with streptokinase and is achieved in about 80%. |
| Complications | Chronic deep venous insufficiency (CVI) occurs in as many as 80% of patients with acute proximal DVT. When not properly managed, complications of venous stasis may occur in the distal medial leg (pigmentation, dermatitis, chronic induration, and **venous stasis ulceration**). CVI is best managed with regular use of good elastic support up to knee level (i.e., elastic stockings with 30-40 mm compression at the ankle). |
| Prophylaxis | See p. 183. |

## VI. RAYNAUDS

Raynaud's phenomenon is a **vasospastic disorder**, the hallmark of which is paroxysmal color change of acral parts (fingers, toes, ears, nose) on exposure to cold or with emotional stress. The typical sequence of color change is pallor to cyanosis; with rewarming, rubor is followed by return to normal color. The digits appear normal in color between episodes of vasospasm.

## VI. RAYNAUDS

| | RAYNAUD'S DISEASE | RAYNAUD'S PHENOMENON |
|---|---|---|
| Etiology | Idiopathic. | Secondary to a local or systemic process (e.g., disorders of connective tissue, arterial occlusive disease, neurologic disease, myxedema, repetitive trauma to hands). |
| Natural history | A **benign** disorder, but vasospasm may occur at progressively warmer temperatures. Minor digital ulcerations, chronic paronychia, and sclerodactyly occur in a minority of patients. | The course is variable and depends on the underlying cause. With connective tissue disease, particularly scleroderma, **digital ischemia and ulceration** are often problematic. |
| Treatment<br>*Primary* | • Protection from cold exposure, stop tobacco.<br>• Prazosin (1 mg po bid-tid) or doxazosin (1-2 mg po qd).<br>• Biofeedback benefits many patients. | • Protection from the cold, avoidance of tobacco, and treatment of underlying disorder.<br>• Prazosin (1 mg po bid-tid) or doxazosin (1-2 mg po qd). |
| *Surgical* | **Regional sympathectomy** produces symptomatic relief in 50-60% of cases, especially in Raynaud's of lower extremities. | Response to regional sympathectomy is less predictable and more persistent than for Raynaud's disease, but may be useful for refractory ischemic ulceration. |

*See p. 1 for abbreviations and p. 199 for drug information.*

# 16. PULMONARY VASCULAR DISEASE

Stuart Rich, M.D.

## I. PULMONARY EMBOLISM

| | |
|---|---|
| Presentation | Pulmonary embolism usually presents as one of the following syndromes: **Pulmonary infarction** (pleuritic pain, dyspnea ± hemoptysis); **acute cor pulmonale** (acute dyspnea, cyanosis, RV failure, hypotension; may result in syncope or cardiac arrest); **acute unexplained dyspnea**; or **chronic pulmonary hypertension** (dyspnea, jugular venous distension, hepatomegaly, ascites, lower extremity edema). There is often a discrepancy between the size of PE and severity of symptoms; small PEs may result in pulmonary infarction and severe pleuritic chest pain, while mod-large PEs may only result in mild dyspnea. Symptoms and signs may occur in many other conditions including MI, CHF, COPD, pericarditis, pneumothorax, sepsis and others. |
| Natural history | If diagnosed and treated early, **most PEs are well tolerated**; recovery is usually complete without long-term sequelae; mortality is < 10%. Once therapy is initiated, mortality is more closely related to underlying cardiopulmonary status than the PE itself. **Progression to chronic pulmonary hypertension is rare (< 1%).** |
| Diagnostic strategy | 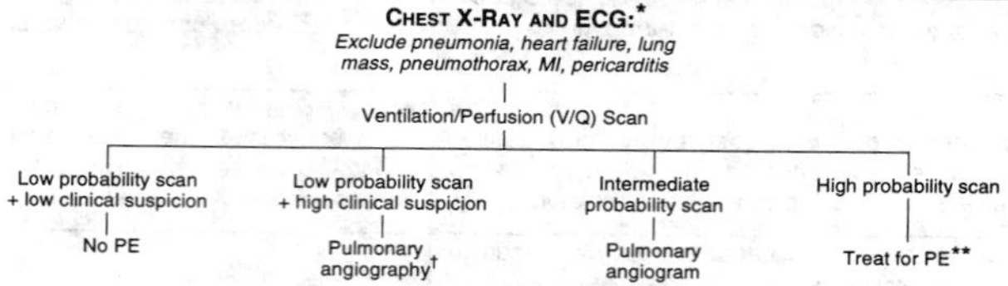 **CHEST X-RAY AND ECG:*** *Exclude pneumonia, heart failure, lung mass, pneumothorax, MI, pericarditis* → Ventilation/Perfusion (V/Q) Scan →<br>• Low probability scan + low clinical suspicion → No PE<br>• Low probability scan + high clinical suspicion → Pulmonary angiography†<br>• Intermediate probability scan → Pulmonary angiogram<br>• High probability scan → Treat for PE**<br><br>* *Echocardiogram may be of value when acute cor pulmonale is suspected and lytic therapy is being considered.*<br>† *Some advocate serial non-invasive leg scan: If negative for proximal DVT, may not require pulmonary angiogram or treatment for PE.*<br>** *Patients with lung cancer or previous PE may require pulmonary angiogram to confirm diagnosis.*<br><br>*DVT = deep venous thrombosis; MI = myocardial infarction; PE = pulmonary embolism* |

## A. PULMONARY EMBOLISM: PRINCIPLES OF DRUG THERAPY

| Drug | Comments |
|---|---|
| Heparin | **Initial therapy:** IV bolus (5-10,000 units) followed by continuous IV infusion (10-15 units/kg/min). May need higher-than-usual dose (increased heparin clearance in early PE). Ensure adequate anticoagulation: Monitor PTT every 4 hours until at least 2 consecutive recordings demonstrate PTT levels 1.5-2.5 x control; thereafter, follow daily PTT levels. If PTT < 1.5 x control, administer a mini re-bolus (2,000-5,000 units) and increase the infusion rate by 25%. If PTT > 2.5-3.0 x control, decrease the infusion rate by 25%. |
| Warfarin | **Initiate therapy on day 1-2:** 10 mg po daily x 2-4 days, then adjust the daily dose until the INR is 2.0-3.0. **It is essential to *overlap* warfarin with heparin** for at least 5 days. Even if risk factors for development of DVT and PE are no longer present, anticoagulation should be **continued for a minimum of 3-6 months** (some anticoagulate for one year). If risk factors persist or recurrent PE develops after warfarin is discontinued, lifelong therapy is required. |
| Thrombolysis<br>*Regimens* | • Streptokinase: 250,000 IU load over 30 minutes, followed by 100,000 IU/hr x 24 hours.<br>• Urokinase: 4,400 IU/kg load over 10 minutes, followed by 4400 IU/kg/hr x 12-24 hours.<br>• tPA: 100 mg infusion over 2 hours. |
| *Administration* | Administer through **peripheral IV**. Obtain PT/PTT, fibrinogen, fibrin split products and thrombin time at baseline and 4 hours post-lytic: **if labs fail to show evidence of a lytic state, consider doubling the infusion dose**. Following discontinuation of lytic therapy, an IV heparin infusion should be started when the PTT < 2 x control, followed by warfarin (see above). Unlike acute MI, **heparin should *not* be given at the same time as the lytic infusion.** |

*See p. 1 for abbreviations and p. 199 for drug information.*

## B. MANAGEMENT OF PULMONARY EMBOLISM

| Presentation | Therapy |
|---|---|
| Stable BP | |
| *Small-moderate PE* | Heparin followed by warfarin. |
| *Large PE* | Initial therapy is controversial: heparin vs. thrombolytic therapy. |
| *Acute RV failure* | Heparin vs. lytic therapy. Lytic therapy should probably be used; several reports show early improvement in RV function due to rapid clot lysis. |
| *Pulmonary infarct* | Heparin followed by warfarin. Hemoptysis is not a contraindication to anticoagulation. |
| *Anticoagulation contraindicated* | Inferior vena cava filter or interruption (clipping/ligation). |
| Hypotension<br>*Anticoagulation O.K.* | • Neck veins low: Fluid challenge and re-evaluate.<br>• Neck veins elevated or hypotension persists despite fluids: Thrombolysis. (To date, no study has demonstrated a survival benefit for thrombolytic therapy. However, rapid improvement in RV function following massive PE may confer a survival benefit for select patients.)<br>• Parental inotropes (dobutamine, amrinone) and vasopressors (dopamine, norepinephrine) are often required for BP support. |
| *Anticoagulation contraindicated* | • Neck veins low: Fluid challenge and re-evaluate.<br>• Neck veins elevated or hypotensive persists despite fluids: Emergency pulmonary angiography and embolectomy (mortality 20-30%). Parental inotropes and vasopressors for BP support. |
| Recurrent PE<br>*On anticoagulants* | Options include (1) addition of aspirin, (2) intensification of INR to 3.0-4.5, (3) IVC filter/interruption plus warfarin (to decrease insertion-site DVT, propagation of clot, and recurrent DVT). |
| *Off anticoagulants* | Life-long warfarin. Evaluate for underlying cor pulmonale. |

*See p. 1 for abbreviations and p. 199 for drug information.*

## C. PREVENTION OF PULMONARY EMBOLISM

| Condition | Preventive Measures | Comments |
|---|---|---|
| High-risk surgery | • Orthopedic surgery on lower extremity (esp. total hip or knee replacement, hip fracture) or gyne cancer surgery: Intermittent pneumatic compression device (IPC) + low-dose warfarin. Low molecular weight heparin (30 mg subcutaneous q12 hours) approved for prophylaxis of total hip repair. Dextran 40 advocated by some.<br>• General or urologic surgery: Either IPC alone or subcutaneous heparin ± gradient compression stockings.<br>• Neurosurgery and other surgeries with contraindication to pharmacologic prophylaxis: Graded compression stockings ± IPC. | • **Low-dose heparin: 5,000 units subcutaneous every 8-12 hours,** with the first dose 2 hrs prior to surgery. Continue therapy at least 7 days postoperatively or until ambulatory (may require continued prophylaxis at home). Inadequate for hip/knee reconstruction.<br>• **Low-dose warfarin: INR 2.0-3.0.** 5-10 mg the night prior to surgery, 5 mg the day of surgery, followed by a daily dose adjusted to maintain INR 2.0-3.0 for at least one month. |
| Low-risk surgery | None. | Low risk patients: Age < 40 years, surgery < 1 hour, no history of cancer or prior PE/DVT, and early ambulation after surgery. |
| Medical patients | IPC alone or graded compression stockings ± low dose subcutaneous heparin. | Prophylactic measures are especially important for patients with a history of DVT/PE and for medical conditions associated with venous stasis, prolonged immobilization, or a hypercoagulable state. |
| Where recurrence may be fatal | Anticoagulation + IVC filter + compression stockings. | Combined preventive measures are recommended for patients with refractory hypercoagulable states or severe cardiopulmonary compromise. |

*See p. 1 for abbreviations and p. 199 for drug information.*

## II. PULMONARY HYPERTENSION

| | PRIMARY PULMONARY HTN | SECONDARY PULMONARY HTN |
|---|---|---|
| Presentation | Dyspnea on exertion, weakness, precordial chest pain, palpitations, syncope and/or RV failure. Cyanosis occurs late. | Same as primary. |
| Natural history | **Progressive RV failure** is the rule. **Sudden death may occur**, usually in Class IV patients, especially during general anesthesia, surgery, cardiac cath, PTCA, and pulmonary angiography. Mean survival 2.8 years. | **Progressive RV failure**. Survival relates to both the severity of underlying disease and hemodynamics. |

## A. MEDICAL THERAPY OF PULMONARY HYPERTENSION

| Etiology | Therapy |
|---|---|
| Primary pulmonary hypertension | General measures: Instruct patient to avoid isometric activity, administer annual influenza and pneumonia vaccines, treat pulmonary infections aggressively, and appropriate use of drug therapy:<br>• **Anticoagulation:** Warfarin (INR 2.0-3.0) **may improve survival** (NEJM 1992;327:76), although symptoms are not usually improved.<br>• **Digoxin:** Given empirically; animal data suggests improvement in RV function. Clinical trial in progress.<br>• **Diuretics:** Given to those with markedly elevated right atrial pressures or clinical manifestations of right-sided venous hypertension (ascites, edema). May require high-dose therapy. Dyspnea may or may not improve.<br>• **Oxygen:** Given for marked hypoxemia at rest or during exercise testing (benefit unproven).<br>• **Testing for reversibility (*performed at experienced centers only*):** Responsiveness to vasodilators (adenosine, acetylcholine, $PGI_2$, nitric oxide) is tested during right heart catheterization. For patients who respond favorably to the acute challenge, oral calcium channel blockers are prescribed on a chronic basis.<br>• **Dobutamine** for acute right heart failure and dopamine if accompanied by hypotension. |

*See p. 1 for abbreviations and p. 199 for drug information.*

## A. MEDICAL THERAPY OF PULMONARY HYPERTENSION

| Etiology | Therapy |
|---|---|
| Hypoxic lung disease (e.g., COPD) | General measures: Influenza and pneumonia vaccines, aggressive treatment of infections, and appropriate use of drug therapy:<br>• **Oxygen and diuretics** (for right heart failure) **are the mainstays of therapy**. Bronchodilators with or without corticosteroids if bronchospasm is evident.<br>• Anticoagulation untested.<br>• Digoxin may be more likely to induce arrhythmias when used in this setting and is not routinely prescribed unless overt right heart failure supervenes.<br>• Empiric use of vasodilators should be avoided. Agents such as calcium channel blockers may antagonize hypoxic pulmonary vasoconstriction, exaggerate V/Q mismatch, and worsen hypoxemia. |
| Others | For pulmonary hypertension due to collagen vascular disease, congenital shunt, peripheral PE not amenable to thromboendarterectomy, and interstitial lung disease without hypoxemia:<br>• General measures: Same as for COPD, above.<br>• **Primary therapy directed at underlying disease** (e.g., immunosuppressive for collagen vascular disease, valvuloplasty or valve replacement for mitral stenosis, thromboendarterectomy for proximal chronic PE, repair of congenital shunt).<br>• Drug therapy:<br>- Anticoagulation, digoxin, diuretics, and oxygen as for primary pulmonary hypertension. Oxygen is of no help in congenital heart disease with right-to-left shunts.<br>- Less than 5% of patients respond to reversibility testing (see primary pulmonary hypertension). |

*See p. 1 for abbreviations and p. 199 for drug information.*

## B. SURGICAL THERAPY OF PULMONARY HYPERTENSION

| Modality | Indications | Comments |
|---|---|---|
| Thrombo-endarterectomy | Symptomatic patients with chronic pulmonary hypertension. | Location of pulmonary thromboembolism should be proximal to lobar bifurcations. Anticoagulants and thrombolytics of no value. **High risk surgery**; requires referral to specialized center. |
| Transplant<br>*Lung* | Symptomatic patients despite medical therapy. | Single-lung adequate to reduce pulmonary artery pressures in most cases of pulmonary hypertension. Double-lung transplant provides greater functional reserve in the event of acute rejection, but is a more difficult operation. Prognosis: **2-year survival 60%.** One-half of pts develop obliterative bronchiolitis (chronic rejection) by the 4th year. |
| *Heart-lung* | Symptomatic patients with congenital heart disease or underlying coexistent LV dysfunction. | Poor organ supply and very long wait times limit utility. |

*See p. 1 for abbreviations and p. 199 for drug information.*

# 17. CEREBROVASCULAR DISEASE

Louis R. Caplan, M.D.

## I. OVERVIEW

Stroke is the third most common cause of death in the United States. Each year, approximately 500,000 Americans have a stroke and about 150,000 people die from a stroke or its immediate complications. At any one time, 2 million people in the United States have had strokes. The American Heart Association estimates the annual cost of stroke-related healthcare to be $13.5 billion.

## II. CLASSIFICATION

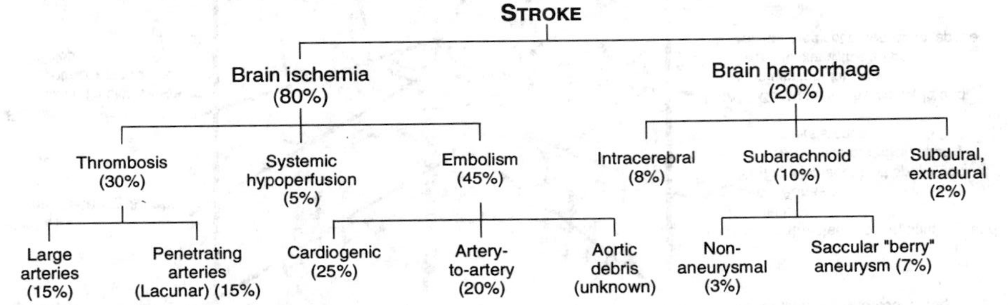


*See p. 1 for abbreviations and p. 199 for drug information.*

## Figure 1. Clinical Presentation of Common Stroke Syndromes

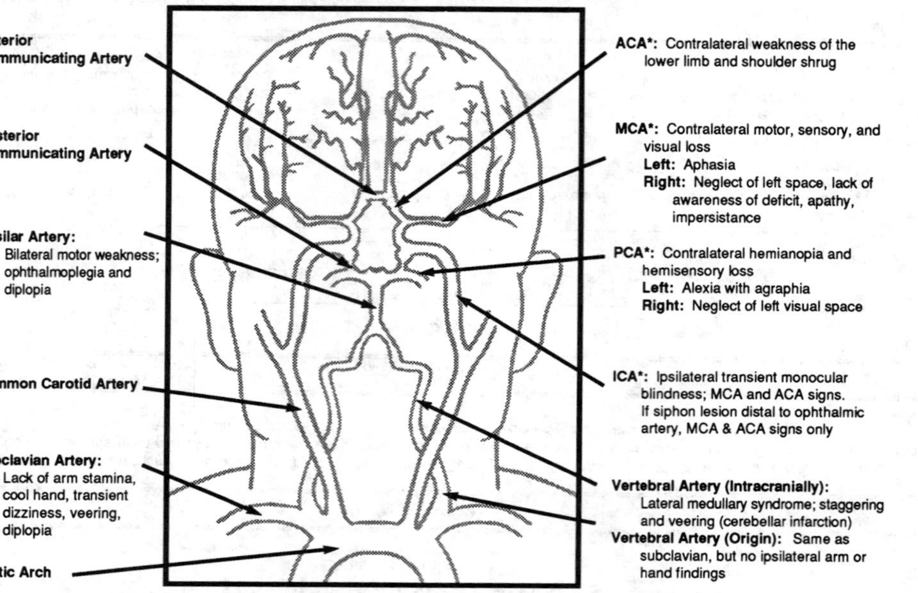


*ACA = Anterior Cerebral Artery; MCA = Middle Cerebral Artery; PCA = Posterior Cerebral Artery; ICA = Internal Carotid Artery

## Figure 2. Initial Evaluation and Management of Stroke

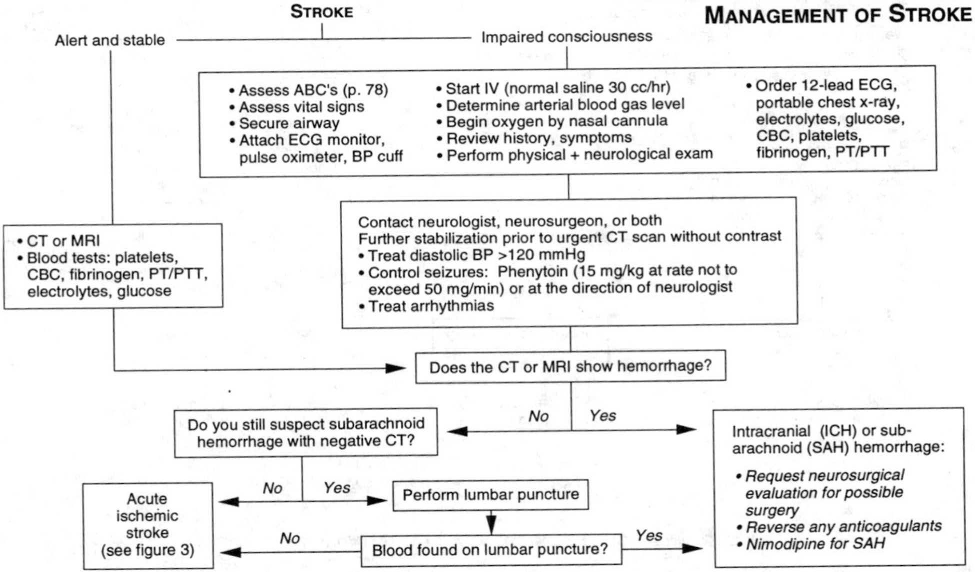

**Stroke**

Alert and stable

- CT or MRI
- Blood tests: platelets, CBC, fibrinogen, PT/PTT, electrolytes, glucose

→ Does the CT or MRI show hemorrhage?

Impaired consciousness

- Assess ABC's (p. 78)
- Assess vital signs
- Secure airway
- Attach ECG monitor, pulse oximeter, BP cuff
- Start IV (normal saline 30 cc/hr)
- Determine arterial blood gas level
- Begin oxygen by nasal cannula
- Review history, symptoms
- Perform physical + neurological exam
- Order 12-lead ECG, portable chest x-ray, electrolytes, glucose, CBC, platelets, fibrinogen, PT/PTT

Contact neurologist, neurosurgeon, or both
Further stabilization prior to urgent CT scan without contrast
- Treat diastolic BP >120 mmHg
- Control seizures: Phenytoin (15 mg/kg at rate not to exceed 50 mg/min) or at the direction of neurologist
- Treat arrhythmias

Does the CT or MRI show hemorrhage?

*No* → Do you still suspect subarachnoid hemorrhage with negative CT?

- *No* → Acute ischemic stroke (see figure 3)
- *Yes* → Perform lumbar puncture → Blood found on lumbar puncture?
  - *No* → Acute ischemic stroke (see figure 3)
  - *Yes* → Intracranial (ICH) or subarachnoid (SAH) hemorrhage

*Yes* → Intracranial (ICH) or sub-arachnoid (SAH) hemorrhage:

- *Request neurosurgical evaluation for possible surgery*
- *Reverse any anticoagulants*
- *Nimodipine for SAH*

*See p.194 for SAH & p.195 for ICH. CT = computerized tomography; MRI = magnetic resonance imaging; CBC = complete blood cell count*

## Figure 3. Evaluation and Management of Ischemic Stroke

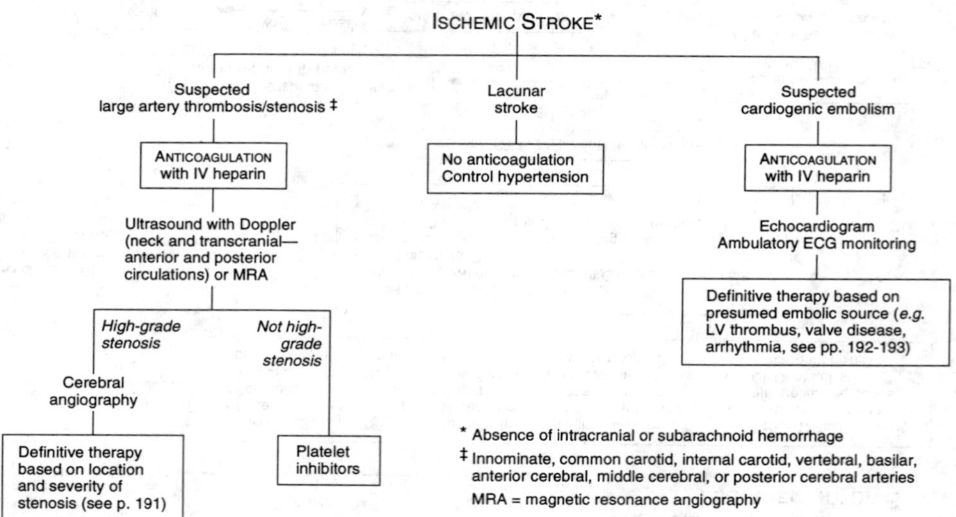

# III. CEREBRAL ISCHEMIA

The characterization of ischemia by tempo alone (transient ischemic attack, progressing stroke), is *not* a useful guideline for treatment. Specific treatment depends primarily on the cause of stroke and the functional status of the patient.

## A. LARGE ARTERY STENOSIS

| Etiology | Therapy |
|---|---|
| Internal carotid | |
| *Total occlusion (100%)* | Short-term heparin (PTT 1.5-2.0 x control) followed by warfarin (INR 2.0-3.0) x 6 weeks. Empiric anticoagulation may prevent embolization of fresh clot and clot propagation. |
| *Severe stenosis (70-99%)* | Carotid endarterectomy (CEN); urgent for progressing neurologic deficit, at 3-6 wks for stable deficit. CEN shown to reduce stroke rate and improve survival (NEJM 1991;325:445). If not a surgical candidate, options include long-term warfarin or balloon angioplasty. |
| *Plaque disease (< 70%)* | Aspirin (≥ 325 mg/day). Ticlopidine (250 mg bid) for aspirin allergy, side effects or failure (neutropenia occurs in 1%). Others: Indomethacin, omega-3 oils. |
| Vertebral artery | |
| *Total occlusion (100%)* | Short-term heparin (PTT 1.5-2.0 x control) followed by warfarin (INR 2.0-3.0) for 3-6 weeks. Empiric anticoagulation may prevent embolization of fresh clot and clot propagation. |
| *Severe stenosis (70-99%)* | Long-term warfarin (INR 2.0-3.0). Surgery and balloon angioplasty have also been successfully performed. Monitor stenosis non-invasively every 6 months. If total occlusion develops, continue anticoagulant therapy for an additional 3-6 weeks (to prevent propagation of clot in-situ). |
| *Plaque disease (< 70%)* | Aspirin (≥ 325 mg/day). Ticlopidine (250 mg po bid) for aspirin allergy, side-effects, or failure. |

*See p. 1 for abbreviations and p. 199 for drug information.*

## A. LARGE ARTERY STENOSIS

| Etiology | Therapy |
|---|---|
| Intracranial disease<br>*Total occlusion (100%)* | Short-term anticoagulation (3-6 weeks). Investigational: Acute fibrinolysis with tPA or kinases. |
| *Severe stenosis (70-99%)* | Long-term warfarin (INR 2.0-3.0) while monitoring stenosis with ultrasound/MRA. If total occlusion develops, continue anticoagulation for an additional 3 weeks (to prevent propagation of clot in-situ). |
| *Plaque disease (<70%)* | Aspirin (≥325 mg/day). Ticlopidine (250 mg po bid) for aspirin allergy, side-effects, or failure. |

## B. BRAIN EMBOLISM

| Embolic Source | Therapy |
|---|---|
| Atrial fibrillation (AFIB) | **Heparin** (PTT 1.5-2.0) **followed by warfarin** (INR 2.0-3.0) as long as AFIB persists. Some neurologists initiate anticoagulation only if a CT scan or MRI at day 3-5 is negative for hemorrhage (especially if a large area of infarction is present). For acute embolism with occlusion of an intracranial artery, consider **acute thrombolysis** with tPA or kinases. |
| Valve disease | As for AFIB, above. If embolization occurs on warfarin, options include intensification of warfarin, addition of low-dose aspirin (80-160 mg/d), or surgery in selected patients. |
| Acute MI | Acute stroke during thrombolytic therapy is often hemorrhagic and may require drainage of hematoma. |
| Cardiomyopathy | As above for AFIB. |

*See p. 1 for abbreviations and p. 199 for drug information.*

## B. BRAIN EMBOLISM

| Embolic Source | Therapy |
|---|---|
| Paradoxical embolism | As above for AFIB followed by repair of the atrial septal defect. Contrast echo (with valsalva maneuver) is recommended for all young patients who present with unexplained stroke. |
| Atrial myxoma | As above for AFIB followed by surgical excision. |
| Other cardiac | • Embolic stroke from mitral valve prolapse, mitral annular calcification, calcified aortic valve, marantic endocarditis: Aspirin ($\geq$ 325 mg/day). Recurrences treated with warfarin.<br>• Infectious endocarditis: Control of infection. Anticoagulation does not prevent embolization and increases the risk of bleeding from a mycotic aneurysm or cerebral embolus. Single embolus is not an indication for valve surgery (see Ch. 9). |

## C. OTHER CAUSES OF CEREBRAL ISCHEMIA

| | |
|---|---|
| Lacunar stroke | Due to ruptured microaneurysms of small penetrating arteries. Prognosis is good for recovery of function, although other lacunes frequently develop. Therapy: Longterm control of hypertension ± platelet inhibitors empirically. Anticoagulation is not indicated. |
| Systemic hypoperfusion | Prognosis depends on the cause, degree, and duration of hypotension. Most who eventually recover awaken by 72 hrs. **Adverse prognostic factors include dilated non-reactive pupils > 12 hrs (in the absence of atropine), and absent corneal, oculocephalic (doll's eyes) and oculovestibular reflexes (cold water calorics)**. Therapy: Maintenance of blood pressure with fluids, vasopressors, pneumatic antishock garment and/or intra-aortic balloon pump until cause-specific therapy can be instituted (Ch. 7). |

*See p. 1 for abbreviations and p. 199 for drug information.*

# IV. BRAIN HEMORRHAGE

Separation into subarachnoid (SAH), intracerebral (ICH), and subdural/extradural hemorrhage is usually relatively simple. **SAH presents with sudden onset severe headache, cessation of activities, and vomiting without focal neurologic signs**. CT shows blood in the subarachnoid space and brain cisterns; spinal fluid is always bloody. In contrast, **ICH presents with focal neurologic symptoms**. In large hemorrhages, headache, vomiting, progressive neurologic focal signs, and decreased consciousness develop. CT and MRI show a hematoma within the brain. In subdural and extradural hemorrhage, the cause is usually head trauma and the lesions are outside the brain, either inside (subdural hemorrhage) or outside the dura mater (extradural hemorrhage).

## A. SUBARACHNOID HEMORRHAGE (SAH)

| Etiology | Therapy |
|---|---|
| Saccular ("Berry") aneurysm | • **Bedrest, gentle hydration, and prophylactic anticonvulsant** therapy (phenytoin; 300-400 mg/day in divided doses to maintain plasma levels at 10-20 mcg/mL).<br>• Angiography (4-vessel) and **surgical clipping/ligation** to reduce rebleeding and improve survival. Surgery should be performed as soon as possible (within 72 hrs) for patients who are alert, oriented, and without focal deficit (Hunt and Hess Class I or II, J Neurosurg 1968;28:14). For the remaining patients, surgical intervention is recommended at 10-14 days.<br>• **Nimodipine** to reduce vasospasm; 60 mg po q 4 hrs x 21 days starting within 4 days of event (Br Med J 1989;298:636). |
| AV malformation | • Delayed surgical excision for younger patients in good condition (early rebleed rare). Consider radiation therapy or embolization for the elderly and those with severe neurologic deficits.<br>• Seizures without SAH: Anticonvulsants without surgery. |
| Complications | • **Rebleeding**: Complicates 50% of untreated berry aneurysms; 20% of rebleeds occur within 2 weeks (mortality 40%). Uncommon following ruptured AV malformation. **Prevention is the key** to therapy and includes adequate analgesia, control of hypertension, sedation, laxatives, and early surgery. |

*See p. 1 for abbreviations and p. 199 for drug information.*

## A. SUBARACHNOID HEMORRHAGE (SAH)

| Etiology | Therapy |
|---|---|
| Complications (cont.) | • **Vasospasm**: Complicates 25-35% of ruptured berry aneurysms, usually between days 4-14. The majority of episodes go on to cerebral infarction. Uncommon after ruptured AV malformation. Treat with **hypervolemic hemodilution** (3 L of fluid/day) to decrease blood viscosity and maintain cerebral blood flow. **Nimodipine** may be of value in the prevention of vasospasm and secondary stroke (60 mg po every 4 hrs for 21 days starting within 4 days of bleed).<br>• Increased intracranial pressure: See p. 198.<br>• Hydrocephalus: Surgical (ventricular) drainage or repeat lumbar punctures.<br>• Intracerebral hematoma: Surgical evacuation for mass effect.<br>• Cardiac: **ECG** abnormalities occur in > 50%, may persist for days, and include long QT interval, ST segment elevation or depression, giant upright or inverted T-waves and prominent U waves. **May mimic acute myocardial ischemia/infarction**. Arrhythmias are common and include sinus tachycardia, sinus bradycardia, tachy-brady syndrome, wandering atrial pacemaker, and AV junctional rhythm. Ventricular tachycardia is infrequent (occurs most commonly in the setting of a long QT interval).<br>• Hyponatremia: May be due to the syndrome of inappropriate ADH. Associated with a poor prognosis. |

## B. INTRACEREBRAL HEMORRHAGE

| Etiology | Therapy |
|---|---|
| Hypertension | • Control hypertension (systolic BP ≤ 160 mmHg). If neurologic function deteriorates during antihypertensive therapy, reduce dosage or discontinue. Avoid hypotension.<br>• Reduce intracranial pressure (p. 198): papilledema may lag behind clinical improvement and is not necessarily a sign of worsening.<br>• **Surgical drainage for large putaminal, lobar, and cerebellar hematomas**. Rebleeding is uncommon. |

*See p. 1 for abbreviations and p. 199 for drug information.*

## B. INTRACEREBRAL HEMORRHAGE

| Etiology | Therapy |
|---|---|
| Others | • Treat bleeding diathesis when present (e.g., vitamin K, fresh frozen plasma, factor VIII, cryoprecipitate, platelets).<br>• Surgery for AV malformations.<br>• Anticoagulant-related: High morbidity and mortality. If anticoagulant therapy is essential, do not resume for at least 2 weeks following intracranial hemorrhage. |
| Cerebellar hemorrhage | • **Surgical drainage** if hemorrhage is ≥ 3 cm in diameter, especially if there is decreased consciousness. |

## V. TREATMENT OF STROKE-RELATED COMPLICATIONS

| Complication | Comments |
|---|---|
| ↑ intracranial pressure | See p. 198. |
| Seizures | May occur in 5-20% of stroke patients. Management is usually successful with **single-drug therapy**. |
| Deep venous thrombosis | High incidence during recovery. **Prevention is the key**: Early ambulation if possible, bedside physical therapy, and support hose or inflated stockings. Mini-heparin (5,000 units subcutaneous q 12 hrs) in the absence of brain hemorrhage or other contraindications. |
| Pulmonary embolus (PE) | Treat with **IV heparin** unless recent brain hemorrhage. If multiple or life-threatening PEs occur in the setting of recent brain hemorrhage, inferior vena caval umbrella or interruption is indicated. |
| Depression | Depressive syndromes may be difficult to recognize in the stroke patient. Suspect if there is slower than expected recovery, poor cooperation in therapy, emotional lability, or flattened affect. |

*See p. 1 for abbreviations and p. 199 for drug information.*

## V. TREATMENT OF STROKE-RELATED COMPLICATIONS

| Complication | Comments |
|---|---|
| Hypertension | **Hypertension should not be treated in the acute stages of stroke unless BP > 200/120 mmHg**; aggressive ↓ in BP increases the risk of further ischemia. Useful agents: nitroprusside, *β*-blockers, calcium blockers & labetalol. |
| Myocardial infarction (MI) | MI occurs in up to 20% of patients with acute stroke and is the **most common cause of death between 1-4 weeks**. High catecholamine levels, which accompany most strokes, may precipitate angina and infarction. |
| Arrhythmia | Sinus tachycardia, sinus bradycardia, and tachy-brady syndrome are not uncommon following stroke. Ventricular tachycardia has been reported, most often in association with long QT interval (Torsade de Pointes). Cardioversion, drugs, and pacemaker reserved for hemodynamic instability or symptoms. |
| Sepsis | **Most commonly due to urinary tract infections or pneumonia**. Prevention includes intermittent bladder catheterization (preferred over continuous drainage), physical therapy with feeding guidance (feeding tube may be necessary), coughing and deep breathing exercises. A high index of suspicion is essential; **fever, leukocytosis, and a fluctuating mental status often accompany stroke *without* infection**. |
| Upper GI bleed | **Cushing's ulcers** (stress-related gastric mucosal damage) can develop rapidly and may perforate or result in severe GI bleed. **Prevention is the key**: Maintain gastric pH >3.5 with $H_2$ blocker or sucralfate. |
| Hyponatremia | **Adverse prognostic factor**. May be due to the syndrome of inappropriate antidiuretic hormone release (SIADH). Ensure euvolemia and exclude renal, adrenal, and thyroid disease. |
| Undernutrition | Give supplemental multivitamins and thiamine. NG-tube supplements are recommended if intake is still poor by day 4-5. A gastric feeding tube may be required. |
| Contractures | Preventive therapy with early physical therapy. |
| Decubitus ulcers | Meticulous attention to skin care is essential: Keep skin clean and dry, turn the patient frequently, and use padded boots and mattress. Wound debridement and skin grafting may be required in severe cases. |

*See p. 1 for abbreviations and p. 199 for drug information.*

## VI. SELECTED TOPICS

| Category | Therapy |
|---|---|
| Asymptomatic carotid disease<br>*> 70% stenosis* | • General measures: Treat hypertension and hyperlipidemia. Carotid endarterectomy (CEN) vs. antiplatelet trials in progress.<br>• Prior to coronary artery bypass surgery (CABG): If the patient is asymptomatic or symptoms are remote, proceed to CABG without carotid surgery. **If the patient has recurrent TIAs or a nondisabling stroke, CEN should be performed simultaneous with CABG**.<br>• Prior to PTCA: If the patient is asymptomatic or symptoms are inactive, proceed with PTCA. If neurologic symptoms are active and the patient has stable coronary artery disease, perform CEN before PTCA. If the patient has both active neurologic symptoms and unstable angina, PTCA followed by CEN is recommended. |
| *< 70% stenosis* | **Aspirin** (≥ 325 mg/d). Ticlopidine (250 mg bid) for aspirin allergy, intolerance, or failure. Treat hypertension and hyperlipidemia. |
| Unruptured aneurysm | Surgical clipping or ligation for aneurysms that are greater than 5-7 mm in diameter or cause progressive neurological symptoms secondary to compression. |
| Increased intracranial pressure | • Head of bed elevated; decrease usual fluid intake by 1/3.<br>• **Hyperventilation** with hypocapnia ($pCO_2$ 20-35 mmHg).<br>• **Osmotic agents** (mannitol, glycerol) to achieve serum osmolality of 300-310 mOsm/L. Rebound may occur upon withdrawal. Osmotic agents may reduce extracellular edema but are of little value for intracellular edema.<br>• **High dose corticosteroids** if due to tumor, trauma, abscess. Not for anoxia or infarction.<br>• **Surgical removal or drainage** of hematomas, removal of infarcted temporal lobe/cerebellum. |

*See p. 1 for abbreviations and p. 199 for drug information.*

# 18. CARDIAC DRUGS

Richard L. Lucarotti, Pharm.D., Matthew H. Johnson, Pharm.D.,
Maureen A. Smythe, Pharm.D., Heidi A. Pillen, Pharm.D.,
Mary Beth Sancimino, Pharm.D.



This section provides information pertinent to the clinical use of common cardiovascular drugs. Each monograph includes dosing by indication, dose adjustment, adverse reactions, drug interactions, and contraindications. Hypersensitivity, common to all medications, is not listed in the contraindication or adverse reaction sections.

Dose adjustment based on creatinine clearance is indicated in many of the monographs. One method used to estimate creatinine clearance is [(weight, kg) x (140 - age)] *divided by* [72 x serum creatinine, mg/dL]. The calculated value is multiplied by 0.85 for females.

The information provided is not exhaustive and the reader is referred to other drug information references and the manufacturer's product literature for further information. Primary references used for the compilation of these monographs include *Drug Facts and Comparisons*, Facts and Comparisons, St. Louis, Missouri; *American Hospital Formulary Service Drug Information 1994*, American Society of Hospital Pharmacists, Bethesda, Maryland; and the *Physicians' Desk Reference 1994, 48th Edition,* Medical Economics Data Production Company, Montvale, New Jersey.

Clinical use of the information provided and any consequences that may arise from its use is the responsibility of the clinician. The authors, editors, and publisher cannot be responsible for errors or omitted information in these monographs or any consequences that may occur from such.

# TRADE NAME INDEX

# DRUG CLASS INDEX
## (Generic and Trade Names)

### ALPHA ADRENERGIC AGENTS
**Peripheral Alpha-Adrenergic Blockers**
Doxazocin (Cardura)
Terazocin (Hytrin)
Prazosin (Minipress)
**Central Alpha-Adrenergic Agonists**
Clonidine (Catapres, Catapres-TTS)
Guanfacine (Tenex)
Guanabenz (Wytensin)
Methyldopa (Aldomet)
**Peripheral Alpha-Adrenergic Agonists**
Guanadrel (Hylorel)
Guanethidine (Ismelin)
Reserpine

### ANGIOTENSIN CONVERTING ENZYME (ACE) INHIBITORS
Benazepril (Lotensin)
Captopril (Capoten)
Enalapril (Vasotec)
Enalaprilat (Vasotec I.V.)
Fosinopril (Monopril)
Lisinopril (Prinvil, Zestril)
Quinapril (Accupril)
Ramipril (Altace)

### ANTIARRHYTHMICS
Adenosine (Adenocard)
Amiodarone (Cordarone)
Bretylium (Bretylol)
Brevibloc (Esmolol)
Digoxin (Lanoxin)
Disopyramide (Norpace)
Flecainide (Tambocor)
Lidocaine (Xylocaine)
Moricizine (Ethmozine)
Mexilitine (Mexitil)
Phenytoin (Dilantin)
Procainamide (Pronestyl, Procan SR)
Propafenone (Rhythmol)
Quinidine (Quinidine Sulfate - Quinidex, Quinidine Gluconate - Quiniglute, Quinidine Polygalacturonate - Cardioquin)
Sotalol (Betapace)
Tocainide (Tonocard)
Verapamil (Isoptin)

### ANTIPLATELET AGENTS
Aspirin
Dipyridamole (Persantine)
Ticlopidine (Ticlid)

## ANTICOAGULANTS
Warfarin (Coumadin)
Enoxaparin (Lovenox)
Heparin

## HEPARIN ANTAGONIST
Protamine

## BETA ADRENERGIC BLOCKERS
Acebutolol (Sectral)
Atenolol (Tenormin)
Betaxolol (Kerlone)
Bisoprolol (Zebeta)
Carteolol (Cartrol)
Esmolol (Brevibloc)
Labetolol (Normodyne, Trandate)
Metoprolol (Lopressor)
Nadolol (Corgard)
Penbutolol (Levatol)
Pindolol (Visken)
Propranolol (Inderal)
Sotalol (Betapace)
Timolol (Blockadren)

## CALCIUM CHANNEL BLOCKERS
Amlodipine (Norvasc)
Bepridil (Vascor)
Diltiazem (Cardizem, Cardizem CD, Cardizem CR, Cardizem Inj., Cardene I.V., Dilacor XR)
Felodipine (Plendil)
Isradipine (DynaCirc)

## CALCIUM CHANNEL BLOCKERS *(cont.)*
Nicardipine (Cardene)
Nifedipine (Procardia, Procardia XL)
Verapamil (Calan, Calan SR, Isoptin, Isoptin SR, Isoptin Injection, Verelan)

## DIGITALIS GLYCOSIDES
Digoxin (Lanoxin)
Digitoxin (Crystodigin)

## DIURETICS
Bendroflumethiazide (Naturetin)
Benzthiazide (Exna)
Bumetanide (Bumex)
Chlorthalidone (Hygroton)
Chlorothiazide (Diuril)
Ethacrynic Acid (Edecrin)
Furosemide (Lasix)
Hydrochlorothiazide (Hydrodiuril)
Hydroflumethiazide (Diucardin, Saluron)
Indapamide (Lozol)
Methyclothiazide (Enduron)
Metolazone (Zaroxolyn)
Polythiazide (Renese)
Quinethiazone (Hydromox)
Trichlormethiazide (Metahydrin, Naqua)

## DIURETICS - POTASSIUM SPARING
Amiloride (Midamor)
Spironolactone (Aldactone)
Triamterene (Dyrenium)

## HYPOLIPIDEMICS

Cholestyramine (Questran, Questran Light, Cholybar)
Colestipol (Colestid)
Niacin
Clofibrate (Atromid-S)
Gemfibrozil (Lopid)
Probucol (Lorelco)
Lovastatin (Mevacor)
Pravastatin (Pravachol)
Simvastatin (Zocor)

## INOTROPES/VASOPRESSORS

Amrinone (Inocor)
Dobutamine (Dobutrex)
Dopamine (Intropin)
Ephedrine
Epinephrine (Adrenalin)
Isoproterenol (Isuprel)
Metaraminol (Aramine)
Methoxamine (Vasoxyl)
Milrinone (Primacor)
Norepinephrine (Levophed)
Phenylephrine (Neo-Synephrine)

## NITRATES

Isosorbide dinitrate sublingual (Isordil, Sorbitrate)
  tablet (Isordil Titradose, Sorbitrate)
  sustained release (Isordil Tembids, Sorbitrate SA, Dilatrate SR)
Isorbide mononitrate (IMDUR, ISMO, Monoket)
Nitroglycerin sublingual (Nitrostat)

## NITRATES (cont.)

  sustained release tablets and capsules (Nitrong)
  ointment (Nitrol, Nitro-Bid)
  patch (Deponit NTG, Minitran, Nitrodisc, Nitro-Dur, Transderm Nitro)
  injection (Nitrobid IV, Nitrostat IV, Tridil)
Pentaerythritol Tetranitrate (Peritrate)
Erythritol Tetranitrate (Cardilate)

## POTASSIUM SUPPLEMENTS

Potassium Chloride, Kaon CL, Kay Ciel, K-Dur, Klorvess, Klotrix, K-Lyte/CL

## MAGNESIUM

Magnesium Carbonate, Magnesium Glucontate (Magonate), Magnesium Sulfate, Magnesium Chloride

## THROMBOLYTICS

Alteplase (Activase)
Anistreplase (Eminase)
Streptokinase (Streptase, Kabikinase)
Urokinase (Abbokinase)

## VASODILATORS - DIRECT ACTING

Diazoxide (Hyperstat IV)
Hydralazine (Apresoline)
Nitroprusside (Nipride)
Minoxidil (Loniten)

## GANGLIONIC BLOCKER

Trimethaphan (Arfonad)

## Acebutolol (Sectral, *Wyeth-Ayerst*)

**CLASS** *β*-blocker; *β*-1 selective with ISA

**DOSE** **Hypertension**: 400 mg po given as single dose or in 2 divided doses with a maximum of 1200 mg/d; **Ventricular arrhythmia**: 200 mg BID, ↑ dose gradually to 600-1200 mg/d

**DOSAGE ADJUSTMENT** *Elderly*: Avoid doses > 800 mg/d. *Renal impairment*: reduce daily dose by 50% when CrCl is < 50 ml/min and by 75% when CrCl < 25 ml/min. *Hepatic impairment*: Use cautiously.

**DRUG INTERACTIONS** *Calcium Channel Blockers:* may ↑ *β*-blocker effects.

**ADVERSE EFFECTS** *CV*: bradycardia, heart failure, edema, pulmonary edema; *CNS*: dizziness, tiredness/fatigue, headache, peripheral neuropathy, nervousness; *GU*: sexual dysfunction, impotence, ↓ libido; *Endocrine*: hyperglycemia, hypoglycemia; Raynaud's phenomenon.

**DISCONTINUATION** When discontinuing chronically administered *β*-blockers, ↓ dosage gradually over 1-2 weeks.

**CONTRAINDICATIONS** Not recommended for patients with sinus bradycardia, greater than first degree heart block, overt heart failure, cardiogenic shock, congenital or acquired long QT syndromes. Caution in patients with bronchospasm, peripheral vascular disease, or diabetes mellitus.

## Adenosine (Adenocard, *Fujisawa*)

**CLASS** Antiarrhythmic

**DOSE** **Paroxysmal supraventricular tachycardia (PSVT) including that associated with accessory bypass tracts (Wolff-Parkinson-White Syndrome):** Initial dose 6 mg given as rapid IV bolus (over 1-2 seconds); if desired response not achieved within 1-2 minutes, 12 mg should be given as rapid IV bolus; (may be repeated a second time). Doses exceeding 12 mg are not recommended.

**DRUG INTERACTIONS** *Caffeine, Theophylline*: antagonize effects of adenosine; *Dipyridamole*: potentiate effects of adenosine; *Atropine*: adenosine effect not blocked by atropine

**ADVERSE EFFECTS** Facial flushing (18%), dyspnea (12%), chest pressure (7%).

**CONTRAINDICATIONS** Second or third degree AV block or sick sinus syndrome (unless functioning artificial pacemaker).

**OTHER COMMENTS** Inhaled adenosine induces bronchoconstriction in asthmatic patients.

## Alteplace tPA (Activase, *Genentech*)

**CLASS** Thrombolytic

**DOSE** **Coronary artery thrombosis/Acute MI**: 100 mg given IV as 60mg (over first hr) of which 6-10 mg is given as a bolus dose over 1-2 min, 20 mg (2nd hr), and 20 mg (3rd hr); patients < 65 kg give 1.25 mg/kg over 3 hrs; see p. 49 for accelerated dosing. **Pulmonary embolism**: 100 mg IV over 2 hrs; follow with heparin when PTT or thrombin time ≤ 2 x control.

**DOSAGE ADJUSTMENT** Dose > 150 mg not recommended (4-fold increase in intracranial hemorrhage).

**DRUG INTERACTIONS** *Heparin:* has been given with and after alteplace to ↓ risk of rethrombosis; both may cause bleeding; *Antiplatelet agents (aspirin, dipyridamole, indomethacin, phenylbutazone, sulfinpyrazone) and warfarin (Coumadin)*: may ↑ bleeding if given before, during or after alteplace.

## Alteplace tPA (cont.)

**ADVERSE EFFECTS** *Bleeding* (> 250 ml): GI (5%), GU (4%), intracranial (0.4%), other sites (≤ 1%); *Mild hypersensitivity* reactions (e.g. urticaria); *Arrhythmias:* (ventricular & atrial) associated with reperfusion.

**CONTRAINDICATIONS** Active internal bleeding, history of stroke, recent (< 2 mo) intracranial or intraspinal surgery or trauma, intracranial neoplasm, A-V malformation or aneurysm, bleeding diathesis, severe uncontrolled hypertension; avoid in patients with arterial emboli originating from left side of heart (mitral stenosis with atrial fibrillation, LV thrombi)

**OTHER COMMENTS** Start treatment as soon as possible after onset of symptoms of acute MI (within 6-12 hrs). Preferred thrombolytic in patients who have received streptokinase or anistreplace within 6 mo, have had a streptococcal infection, and in patients where potential hypotension from streptokinase should be avoided.

## Amiloride (Midamor, *Merck*)

**CLASS** Diuretic-potassium sparing

**DOSE Heart failure, Hypertension (in conjunction with potassium wasting diuretic or antihypertensive)**: 5 mg po and ↑ to 10 mg prn; 15-20 mg/d has been used for persistent ↓ $K^+$.

**DRUG INTERACTIONS** *Potassium preparation*: may cause severe hyperkalemia; *ACE Inhibitors*: ↑ serum potassium

**ADVERSE EFFECTS** *CNS:* headache (3-8%), dizziness, encephalopathy (1-3%); *GI:* nausea, anorexia, diarrhea, vomiting (3-8%), abdominal pain, appetite changes, constipation (1-3%); *CV:* orthostatic hypotension; *Hematologic:* aplastic anemia, neutropenia; *Other:* cough, dysuria, impotence (1-3%), polyuria, dyspnea, skin rash, itching, visual disturbances, tinnitus

**CONTRAINDICATIONS** Serum potassium > 5.5 mEq/L; potassium supplements; acute and chronic renal insufficiency

**OTHER COMMENTS** Use cautiously in patients with diabetes mellitus.

## Amlodipine (Norvasc, *Pfizer*)

**CLASS** Calcium channel blocker

**DOSE Hypertension:** Initial: 5 mg po QD; titrate dose over 7-14 days to maximum dose (10mg/d); **Angina (chronic stable or vasospastic)**: 5-10 mg/d; most patients require 10 mg/d

**DOSAGE ADJUSTMENT** In geriatric patients, small frail individuals, and patients with hepatic insufficiency, an initial dose of 2.5 mg daily is recommended for hypertension and 5 mg daily for angina.

**DRUG INTERACTIONS** *β-blockers:* may ↑ depressant effect on contractility and AV conduction.

**ADVERSE EFFECTS** *CNS*: dizziness/lightheadedness (1.1-3.4%), headache (7.3%), *CV*: peripheral edema (1.8-14.6%), palpitations (0.7-4.5%), tachycardia (1%), CHF (1%); *Other*: fatigue/lethargy (4.5%), flushing (0.7-4.5%)

**OTHER COMMENTS** Use with caution in CHF patients

## Amiodarone (Cordarone, *Wyeth-Ayerst*)

**CLASS** Antiarrhythmic; Class III

**DOSE Life-threatening recurrent ventricular fibrillation or recurrent hemodynamically unstable ventricular tachycardia not responsive to other antiarrhythmics or when alternative agents**

## Amiodarone (cont.)

**are not tolerated**: Loading dose of 800-1600 mg po QD for 1-3 wks (occasionally longer) until therapeutic response occurs. Administer in divided doses with meals for total daily doses of ≥ 1000 mg or when GI intolerance occurs. When adequate arrhythmia control is reached or prominent side effects occur, ↓ dose to 600-800 mg/d for one month and then to the maintenance dose, usually 400 mg/d; administer once daily (BID for severe GI intolerance). Use lowest effective dose.

**DOSAGE ADJUSTMENT** The following adverse effects may necessitate dose reduction or discontinuation of therapy: Amiodarone-induced interstitial/alveolar pneumonitis; elevation in hepatic enzymes > 3 x normal (2 x baseline if baseline liver enzymes elevated; hepatomegaly; hypothyroidism or hyperthyroidism; paroxysmal ventricular tachycardia (proarrhythmia); CHF

**DRUG INTERACTIONS** *Warfarin*: ↑ hypoprothrombinemic effect; *β-blockers*: may ↑ pharmacologic effects of *β*-blockers eliminated by hepatic metabolism; *Digoxin*: ↑ serum digoxin level; *Flecainide:* ↑ flecainide level; *Hydantoins*: ↑ hydantoin levels and ↓ amiodarone level; *Procainamide*: may ↑ procainamide level; *Quinidine:* may ↑ quinidine level; *Theophylline*: may ↑ theophylline level

**ADVERSE EFFECTS** Common with dose ≥ 400 mg/d (occur in 75% of patients and require discontinuation in 7-18% patients). Neurologic problems (20-40%); *GI complaints most common*; nausea/vomiting (10-33%), constipation, anorexia (4-9%); visual disturbances (4-9%); dermatologic reactions (15%); photosensitivity (10%), blue discoloration of skin; CHF (3%); bradycardia; abnormal liver function tests (4-9%); pulmonary inflammation or fibrosis (4-9%)

**MONITORING** Baseline work up should include, CXR, PFT's including diffusion capacity, thyroid function tests. Physical exam and CXR should be repeated q 3-6 months. Monitor LFT's regularly in patients receiving high maintenance doses. Monitor thyroid function tests q 3-6 months during therapy. Plasma concentrations (normal: 1-2.5 mcg/ml) may be helpful in evaluating non-responsiveness or unexpected severe toxicity. Monitor closely after dosage adjustments due to long half-life (9-44 days).

**CONTRAINDICATIONS** Severe sinus node dysfunction causing marked sinus bradycardia; second and third degree AV block; symptomatic bradyarrhythmias (except when used in conjunction with pacemaker).

## Amrinone lactate (Inocor, *Sanofi-Winthrop*)

**CLASS** Inotrope

**DOSE** **Short-term management CHF** Initial dose: 0.75 mg/kg IV bolus over 2-3 min, followed by continuous infusion of 5-10 mcg/kg/min. A second bolus (0.75 mg/kg) may be given 30 min after the initial bolus if needed. Maximum dose: 10 mg/kg/d

**DOSAGE ADJUSTMENT** Consider dose reduction if ↑ liver enzymes, or platelets ↓ to < 150,000/$mm^3$.

**ADVERSE EFFECTS** Arrhythmia (3%), ↓ BP, (1.3%), thrombocytopenia (2.4%).

**DISCONTINUATION** Marked ↑ in LFTs, severe dehydration, uncontrolled bleeding, arrhythmias, platelet count < 50,000/$mm^3$.

**CONTRAINDICATIONS** Caution in hypertrophic subaortic stenosis (may ↑ outflow obstruction).

**OTHER COMMENTS** In atrial fib/flutter, consider prior

## Amrinone lactate (cont.)

treatment with digitalis to prevent ↑ ventricular response rate from accelerated AV conduction. Correct hypokalemia before starting amrinone (↑ risk of arrhythmias).

## Anistreplase (APSAC) (Eminase, *Smith-Kline Beecham*)

**CLASS** Thrombolytic

**DOSE** **Acute MI:** 30 units; administered by direct venous injection or via IV line over 2-5 minutes.

**DRUG INTERACTIONS** *Heparin and/or warfarin:* ↑ risk of bleeding requires careful monitoring; *Antiplatelet agents*: no evidence of a synergistic or combined effect exists.

**ADVERSE EFFECTS** Bleeding overall (14.6%): non puncture site (2.8-10.6%); puncture site (4.6-5.7%); GI (2%), GU (2.4%), intracranial (0.57-1%); arrhythmia/conduction disorders associated with reperfusion (38%); hypotension (7.9%).

**CONTRAINDICATIONS** See Alteplace, p. 206.

**OTHER COMMENTS** Start treatment as soon as possible after onset of symptoms of acute MI (within 6-12 hrs). Readministration within 5 days to 6 months not recommended due to development of antistreptokinase antibodies.

## Aspirin

**DOSE** **Reduce risk of death and/or non-fatal myocardial infarction in patients with previous infarction or unstable angina:** 325 mg po QD; **Reduce risk of recurrent transient ischemic attacks or stroke in men who have had transient ischemia of the brain:** 325 mg QID.

**DRUG INTERACTIONS** *Warfarin:* may enhance the hypoprothrombinemic effect.

**ADVERSE EFFECTS** (non-enteric coated plain aspirin) Stomach pain (14.5%), heartburn (11.9%), nausea and/or vomiting (7.6%), gross gastrointestinal bleeding.

**DISCONTINUATION** Consider discontinuation 5-7 d before surgery to prevent or minimize excessive postoperative bleeding

**CONTRAINDICATIONS** Uricosuric therapy (probenecid); bleeding disorders.

**OTHER COMMENTS** Use with caution in patients with active GI lesions, history of recurrent GI lesions, impaired renal function, pre-existing hypoprothrombinemia, vitamin K deficiency, thrombocytopenia, thrombotic thrombocytopenic purpura or severe hepatic impairment.

## Atenolol (Tenormin, *ICI Pharma*)

**CLASS** $\beta$-blocker; $\beta$-1 selective

**DOSE** **Angina pectoris**: Initial dose: 50 mg po QD. If response is not achieved in 1 wk, ↑ to 100 mg/d. Some patients may require 200 mg/d; **Hypertension**: Initial dose: 50 mg/d, full effect seen within 1-2 wks. Can ↑ to 100 mg/d; dosage above this does not produce further benefit; **Acute MI**: 5 mg IV push over 5 min followed by another 5 mg IV push 10 minutes later; 10 min after the second IV dose, start 50 mg orally Q 12 hrs for 1 day and advance to 100 mg/d thereafter as tolerated.

**DOSAGE ADJUSTMENT** Renal impairment: CrCl 15-35 ml/min, maximum dosage 50 mg/d; if CrCl is < 15 ml/min, maximum dosage 50 mg every other day.

**DRUG INTERACTIONS** See Acebutolol, p. 205.

**ADVERSE EFFECTS** See Acebutolol, p. 205.

## Atenolol (cont.)

**DISCONTINUATION** See Acebutolol, p. 205.
**CONTRAINDICATIONS** See Acebutolol, p. 205.
**OTHER COMMENTS** For patients undergoing hemodialysis, give 50 mg after each dialysis.

## Atropine sulfate (Various manufacturers)

**CLASS** Anticholinergic
**DOSE** **Bradyarrhythmias:** Usual IV dose is 0.4-1 mg every 1-2 hrs as needed; larger doses up to 2.0 mg may be required.
**DRUG INTERACTIONS** *Atenolol:* may ↑ β-blocking effects; *Digoxin:* may ↑ digoxin effects.
**ADVERSE EFFECTS** *GI:* xerostomia, nausea/vomiting, paralytic ileus; *GU:* urinary hesitency/retention, impotence; *Ocular:* blurred vision, increased intraocular pressure, dilated pupils; *CV:* palpitations, bradycardia (after low-dose atropine), tachycardia (after higher doses); *CNS:* mental confusion or excitement (especially in the elderly), dizziness, insomnia, fever (especially in children), CNS stimulation with larger doses (restlessness, tremor).
**CONTRAINDICATIONS** (relative-i.e., may be required for symptomatic bradyarrhythmias or heart block even if one of the following conditions is present): Myocardial ischemia; obstructive GI disease, paralytic ileus, ulcerative colitis (especially with toxic megacolon), hepatic disease; obstructive uropathy, renal disease; myasthenia gravis; asthma; narrow-angle glaucoma.

## Benazepril (Lotensin, *Ciba*)

**CLASS** ACE Inhibitor
**DOSE** **Hypertension:** 10 mg po QD; Maintenance dose: 20-40 mg/d as single dose or 2 divided doses. **Administration**: Administer apart from antacids by 1-2 hrs.
**DOSAGE ADJUSTMENT** Renal impairment: CrCl < 30 ml/min initial dose 5 mg QD.
**DRUG INTERACTIONS** *Lithium*: ↑ serum lithium level; *Potassium, potassium sparing diuretics, heparin*: may ↑ serum potassium; *Diuretics, other antihypertensives, anaesthetics with BP lowering effects*: may cause excessive hypotension; *Antidiabetic meds*: may ↑ antidiabetic effect; *NSAID's*: may ↓ ACE inhibitor effect.
**ADVERSE EFFECTS** *CNS*: dizziness (3.3%), headache (5%), fatigue (2.6%); *GI*: nausea (1.4%); *CV*: hypotension (0.3%); *Hematologic*: neutropenia/agranulocytosis (rare); *Renal*: ↑ BUN & creatinine (more likely in CHF, renal artery stenosis, concurrent diuretic therapy); hyperkalemia (1%); *Other*: cough (1.9-3.4%).
**CONTRAINDICATIONS** Pregnancy or lactation; severe mitral or aortic stenosis; history of angioneurotic edema; significant renal artery stenosis (↑ risk of reducing renal perfusion to critical level). Life threatening anaphylactoid hypersensitivity reactions have been reported during dialysis with high-flux (e.g., polyacrylonitril) membranes and during LDL-apheresis with dextran sulfate.
**OTHER COMMENTS** Patients are more prone to hypotension when initiating therapy. Hypotension can be minimized by discontinuing diuretic 2-3 days prior to start. If diuretic cannot be discontinued, use an initial dose of 5 mg benazepril. Diuretic can be resumed if blood pressure is not controlled.

## Benzthiazide (Exna, *Robins*)

**CLASS** Diuretic

**DOSE Edema:** 50-200 mg po QD (administer BID if > 100 mg QD) Maintenance: 50-150 mg/d; **Hypertension**: 50-100 mg/d; give in 2 doses of 25 or 50 mg each (after breakfast and lunch). Maximum: 200 mg/d

**DRUG INTERACTIONS** *Calcium*: hypercalcemia; *Digitalis*: ↑ incidence of digitalis-induced arrhythmias; *Lithium*: ↑ serum lithium level; *Amphotericin B*: ↑ electrolyte depletion; *Bile acid sequestrants*: ↓ absorption of thiazide diuretics.

**ADVERSE EFFECTS** Hypotension, orthostatic hypotension, dizziness, vertigo, headache, insomnia, blurred vision, anorexia, nausea/vomiting, abdominal pain, diarrhea, constipation, jaundice, pancreatitis, impotence, renal dysfunction, interstitial nephritis, leukopenia, thrombocytopenia, agranulocytosis, aplastic anemia, hemolytic anemia, photosensitivity, rash, exfoliative dermatitis, Stevens-Johnson syndrome, hyperglycemia, hyperuricemia, respiratory distress.

**CONTRAINDICATIONS** Anuria.

## Bepridil (Vascor, *McNeil*)

**CLASS** Calcium channel blocker

**DOSE Chronic stable angina when other anti-anginal medications have failed:** Initially 200 mg po QD; adjust after 10 days depending on response. Usual dose: 300 mg/d. Maximum dose: 400 mg/d.

**DOSAGE ADJUSTMENT** May be necessary in renal or hepatic dysfunction, however no studies are available.

**DRUG INTERACTIONS** *β-blockers*: may ↑ depressant effect on contractility and AV conduction; *Antiarrhythmics, tricyclic antidepressants:* may further ↑ QT interval.

**ADVERSE EFFECTS** *CNS*: dizziness/lightheadedness (11.6-27%), nervousness (7.4-11.6%), headache (7-13.6%), asthenia (6.5-14%), tremor (9.3%); *GI*: nausea (7.26%), abdominal discomfort (7%), dry mouth (3.4%); *CV*: bradycardia (2%); tachycardia (2%), peripheral edema (2%), CHF (1%), Torsades de Pointes (↑ QT interval); *Other*: shortness of breath/dyspnea/wheezing (8.7%), agranulocytosis - (rare).

**MONITORING** Do not allow QT interval to exceed 0.52 sec.

**CONTRAINDICATIONS** History of serious ventricular arrhythmias due to proarrhythmic potential, sick sinus syndrome, second or third degree AV block (except with a functioning pacemaker), hypotension (< 90 systolic), decompensated LV dysfunction, congenital QT prolongation, patients taking other drugs that prolong QT interval.

**OTHER COMMENTS** The use of bepridil in patients within 3 months of acute MI cannot be recommended. Maintain normal potassium concentration during treatment. Use with caution in CHF patients.

## Betaxolol (Kerlone, *Searle*)

**CLASS** *β*-blocker; *β*-1 selective

**DOSE Hypertension:** 10 mg po QD; if desired response is not achieved within 14 days, increase the dose to 20 mg/d. Maximum dose: 40 mg/d.

**DOSAGE ADJUSTMENT** Initial dose in the elderly: 5 mg/d.

**DRUG INTERACTIONS, ADVERSE EFFECTS, DISCONTINUATION, CONTRAINDICATIONS** See Acebutolol p. 205.

## Bisoprolol (Zebeta, *Lederle*)

**CLASS** β-blocker; β-1 selective

**DOSE** **Hypertension**: 5 mg po QD; dosage may be ↑ to a maximum of 20 mg/d.

**DOSAGE ADJUSTMENT** Renal/hepatic impairment: CrCl < 40 ml/min or hepatic impairment (hepatitis/cirrhosis), initial dose 2.5 mg/d and use caution in dosage titration.

**DRUG INTERACTIONS** See Acebutolol, p. 205.

**ADVERSE EFFECTS** See Acebutolol, p. 205.

**DISCONTINUATION** See Acebutolol, p. 205.

**CONTRAINDICATIONS** See Acebutolol, p. 205.

## Bretylium Tosylate (Bretylol, *DuPont Critical Care*; also *Abbott, American Regent, Astra, Elkins-Sinn*)

**CLASS** Antiarrhythmic; Class IV

**DOSE** **Immediate life-threatening ventricular arrhythmias:** Initial dose 5 mg/kg by rapid IV injection (undiluted). If arrhythmia persists, ↑ dose to 10 mg/kg and repeat prn q 5-10 min up to a 30-35 mg/kg. For continued suppression administer the diluted solution by continuous IV infusion at 1-2 mg/min; alternative maintenance schedule is to infuse diluted solution at 5-10 mg/kg over a period > 8 minutes q 6 h; **Other ventricular arrhythmias**: *IV*: Initial dose 5-10 mg/kg of diluted drug by IV infusion over > 8 min; subsequent doses given at 1-2 hr intervals if arrhythmia persists. Maintenance dose: 5-10 mg/kg q 6 hrs or constant infusion of 1-2 mg/min; *IM*: Initial dose 5-10 mg/kg undiluted; may repeat at 1-2 hr intervals if arrhythmia persists. Maintainenance: same dose q 6-8 hrs. **Administration:** Keep patient supine during therapy or monitor for orthostatic hypotension. When administering IM do not give > 5 ml at any one site and alternate injection sites; there may be delay in onset of action of 20 minutes-2 hrs.

**DOSAGE ADJUSTMENT** Renal dysfunction: If CrCl 10-50 ml/min, ↓ dose by 50-75%.

**DRUG INTERACTIONS** Bretylium enhances pressor effects of catecholamines. Digoxin toxicity may be worsened by the initial release of norepinephrine.

**ADVERSE EFFECTS** *CV*: hypotension and postural hypotension (50%), bradycardia, ↑ frequency PVC's, transitory ↑ in BP, initial ↑ in arrhythmias (rare); *GI*: nausea/vomiting (3% incidence ↑ with rapid IV administration).

**OTHER COMMENTS** Avoid use in patients with fixed cardiac output (severe aortic stenosis or severe pulmonary hypertension). For a life-threatening arrhythmia in a digitalized patient, use bretylium only if digoxin toxicity is not the etiology and other agents are not ineffective.

## Bumetanide (Bumex, *Roche*)

**CLASS** Diuretic

**DOSE** **Edema**: *Oral*: 0.5-2 mg/d as a single dose; maximum daily dose 10 mg/d; *Parenteral*: 0.5-1 mg IV or IM; ↑ dose to achieve desired response at 2-3 hr intervals for a maximum daily dose of 10 mg. **Administration**: IV over a period of 1-2 minutes. Stable for > 24 hrs in D5W, normal saline and lactated ringers solutions.

**DRUG INTERACTIONS** *Anticoagulants*: ↑ effect of anticoagulants; *Lithium*: ↑ serum lithium level; *Cisplatin*: additive ototoxicity; *Probenecid*: ↓ action of loop diuretics; *Digoxin*: ↑ incidence of digitalis induced arrhythmias

## Bumetanide (cont.)

**ADVERSE EFFECTS** Asterixis, encephalopathy with preexisting liver disease, impaired hearing, vertigo, headache, upset stomach, dry mouth, nausea, vomiting, diarrhea, renal failure, muscle cramps, fatigue, hypotension, rash, thrombocytopenia.
**CONTRAINDICATIONS** Anuria, hepatic coma, severe electrolyte depletion.
**OTHER COMMENTS** Can be used in patients with furosemide allergy (cross-reactivity is rare). May cross-react in patients with hypersensitivity to sulfonamides.

## Captopril (Capoten, *Bristol-Myers Squibb*)

**CLASS** ACE Inhibitor
**DOSE** **Hypertension:** 25 mg po BID or TID; titrate every 1-2 wks by 25 mg increments BID-TID up to 100-150 mg BID-TID prn (maximum 450 mg/d). **Heart Failure**: Usual initial dose: 25 mg TID (6.25-12.5 mg TID for hyponatremic or hypovolemic patients). Titrate at 2 week intervals. Usual maintenance dose: 50-100 mg TID. Maximum dose: 450 mg/d. **Administration**: 1 hr before meals; food ↓'s bioavailability of captopril by 30-40%. Separate administration of captopril by 1-2 hrs from antacids.
**DOSAGE ADJUSTMENT** Decrease initial dose and use smaller increments for titration (1-2 week intervals) in patients with renal impairment.
**DRUG INTERACTIONS** See Benazepril, p. 209.
**ADVERSE EFFECTS** *CNS*: dizziness (0.5-2%), headache (0.5-2%), fatigue (0.5-2%); *GI*: nausea (0.5-2%), vomiting (0.5-2%), diarrhea (0.5-2%), dysgeusia (0.5-2%); *Hematologic*: neutropenia / agranulocytosis (rare); *Renal*: ↑ BUN and serum creatinine (more apt to occur in patients with CHF, renal artery stenosis, concurrent diuretic therapy); *Other*: cough.
**CONTRAINDICATIONS** See Benazepril, p. 209.
**OTHER COMMENTS** If possible, discontinue previous antihypertensive drug regimen 1 week before starting captopril to ↓ risk of hypotension. Diuretics should be discontinued 2-3 days prior to initiation of ACE inhibitor; if not possible, use lower initial dose of ACE inhibitor.

## Carteolol (Cartrol, *Abbott*)

**CLASS** $\beta$-blocker; non-selective with ISA
**DOSE** **Hypertension**: 2.5 mg po QD; gradually ↑ to 5-10 mg/d if adequate response is not achieved. Usual maintenance dose: 2.5-5 mg/d.
**DOSAGE ADJUSTMENT** Renal impairment: CrCl > 60 ml/min use dosage interval of 24 hrs, CrCl 20-60 ml/min use dosage interval of 48 hrs, CrCl < 20 ml/min, use dosage interval of 72 hrs.
**DRUG INTERACTIONS** See Acebutolol, p. 205.
**ADVERSE EFFECTS** See Acebutolol, p. 205.
**DISCONTINUATION** See Acebutolol, p. 205.
**CONTRAINDICATIONS** See Acebutolol, p. 205.

## Chlorothiazide (Diuril, *Merck*)

**CLASS** Thiazide diuretic
**DOSE** **Edema**: 0.5-1.0 g po/IV QD or BID: **Hypertension**: 0.5-1.0 g QD or BID. Maintenance: adjust according to blood pressure response. Maximum dose: 2 g/d in divided doses.

## Chlorothiazide (cont.)

**Administration**: IV: Reconstitute vials with 18 ml sterile water; add to sodium chloride or dextrose for IV infusion.

**DRUG INTERACTIONS** See Benzthiazide, p. 210.

**ADVERSE EFFECTS** See Benzthiazide, p. 210.

**CONTRAINDICATIONS** Anuria.

## Chlorthalidone (Hygroton, *Rhone-Poulenc Rorer*)

**CLASS** Diuretic

**DOSE Edema**: 50-100 mg po QD or 100 mg QOD; may ↑ to 150-200 mg QD or QOD; **Hypertension**: 25 mg QD; maintenance: 25-100 mg QD.

**DRUG INTERACTIONS** See Benzthiazide, p. 210.

**ADVERSE EFFECTS** See Benzthiazide, p. 210.

**CONTRAINDICATIONS** Anuria.

## Cholestyramine (Questran, Questran Light, *Bristol Labs;* Cholybar, *Parke-Davis*)

**CLASS** Bile acid sequestrant

**DOSE Type II A and II B hyperlipoproteinemia:** 12-24 gm po QD in 2-4 divided doses; **Administration:** Mix the powder with at least 2-6 oz. of water, juice, highly fluid soups, cereals, or pulpy fruits; cooling the preparation may increase palatability. Bars should be thoroughly chewed and plenty of fluid taken.

**DRUG INTERACTIONS** Can bind to many drugs in the GI tract and impair their absorption; therefore, administer other drugs 1 hr before or 4-6 hrs after cholestyramine. High dose, long term therapy may ↓ absorption of fat soluble vitamins (A,D,E,K,); actual vitamin deficiencies are rare.

**ADVERSE EFFECTS** *GI*: constipation (20%); abdominal distension, belching, flatulence, nausea, vomiting, diarrhea, heartburn, anorexia and steatorrhea are less common.

**CONTRAINDICATIONS** Complete biliary obstruction.

**OTHER COMMENTS** Therapy with an HMG - CoA reductase inhibitor or niacin provide the greatest additive effect on lowering LDL cholesterol.

## Clofibrate (Atromid-S, *Wyeth-Ayerst; Various*)

**CLASS** Fibric acid derivative

**DOSE Type III hyperlipoproteinemia:** 2 g po QD in divided doses.

**DRUG INTERACTIONS** *Warfarin, dicumarol:* ↑ hypoprothrombinemic effect.

**ADVERSE EFFECTS** *GI*: nausea (most common), vomiting, diarrhea, flatulence, bloating (less common), cholelithiasis, cholecystitis (twice rate of non users), myalgia, myopathy *CV*: cardiac arrhythmias *Other:* possible ↑ risk of malignancy.

**MONITORING** Periodic liver function tests and CBCs.

**DISCONTINUATION** After 3 months if response is inadequate; liver function tests steadily or excessively rise.

**CONTRAINDICATIONS** Significant hepatic or renal dysfunction, primary biliary cirrhosis, pregnancy and lactation.

## Clonidine (Catapres, Catapres - TTS, *Boehringer-Ingelheim*)

**CLASS** Central $\alpha$-adrenergic agonist

**DOSE Hypertension:** *Oral*: Initially 0.1 mg BID, ↑ by

## Clonidine (cont.)

increments of 0.1-0.2 mg/d until desired response (range: 0.2-0.8 mg/d, maximum dose: 2.4 mg/day). *Transdermal*: Initially 0.1 mg system every 7 days. If after 1-2 wks the desired reduction in blood pressure is not achieved increase dose by 0.1 mg. Dosage > two 0.3 mg systems usually does not improve efficacy.

**DOSAGE ADJUSTMENT** Elderly patients may benefit from lower initial dose; Renal impairment: CrCl < 10 ml/min, begin with 50-75% of usual initial dose.

**ADMINISTRATION** Discontinue therapy by reducing the dose gradually over 2-4 days to avoid a rapid rise in blood pressure ("rebound" hypertension).

**DRUG INTERACTIONS** *Tricyclic antidepressants*: may ↓ antihypertensive effects; *β-Blockers*: rebound hypertension with clonidine withdrawal may be enhanced (discontinue β-blockers several days before withdrawing clonidine).

**ADVERSE EFFECTS** *CNS*: insomnia, hallucinations, delirium, nervousness, agitation headache; *CV*: orthostatic hypotension (3%), congestive heart failure, tachycardia; *Dermatologic*: rash, angioneurotic edema; *GU*: impotence, ↓ sexual activity/loss of libido (3% with oral, rare with patch); *Other*: dry mouth (25-40%), drowsiness (12-35%), and dizziness.

**OTHER COMMENTS** Antihypertensive effect of transdermal system may not commence until 2-3 days after application.

## Colestipol (Colestid, *Upjohn*)

**CLASS** Bile acid sequestrant

**DOSE Type II A and II B hyperlipoproteinemia:** 5 gm po QD or BID; increase by 5 g/d at 1 or 2 month intervals. Range: 5-30 g/d in single or divided doses. **Administration**: Mix the powder with at least 2-6 oz. of water, juice, highly fluid soups, cereals or pulpy fruits; cooling the preparation may increase palatability.

**DRUG INTERACTIONS** See Cholestyramine, p. 213.

**ADVERSE EFFECTS** *GI*: Constipation (20%); abdominal distension, belching, flatulence, nausea, vomiting, diarrhea, heartburn, anorexia and steatorrhea are less common.

**CONTRAINDICATIONS** Complete biliary obstruction

**OTHER COMMENTS** See Cholestyramine, p. 213.

## Diazoxide (Hyperstat, *Schering*)

**CLASS** Direct acting vasodilator

**DOSE Hypertensive emergency:** 1-3 mg/kg (up to 150 mg) or 50-150 mg total q 5-15 min, subsequent doses at 4-24 hr intervals. **Administration**: Administer undiluted by rapid IV bolus (≤ 30 sec), directly into a peripheral vein; do not give IM, SC. Avoid extravasation.

**ADVERSE EFFECTS** *CNS*: dizziness/weakness (2%); *GI*: nausea/vomiting (4%); *CV*: hypotension (7%); *Other*: hyperglycemia, sodium and water retention.

**CONTRAINDICATIONS** Pregnancy; hypertension with aortic coarctation or A-V shunt; hypersensitivity to thiazides or sulfonamides.

**OTHER COMMENTS** Not to be given within 6 hrs of other antihypertensive agents. Ineffective in pheochromocytoma.

## Digitoxin (Crystodigin, *Lilly*)

**CLASS** Digitalis glycoside

**DOSE** **CHF, atrial fibrillation, atrial flutter, paroxysmal atrial tachycardia:** Loading dose *rapid*: 0.6 mg, followed by 0.4 mg, and 0.2 mg at intervals of 4-6 hrs; *slow*: 0.2 mg BID x 4 days. Maintenance dose: 0.05-0.3 mg QD.

**DRUG INTERACTIONS** *Quinidine*: ↓ digitoxin clearance; *Verapamil*: ↓ digitoxin clearance; *Cholestyramine, antacids, kaolin/pectin*: ↓ GI absorption; *Barbiturates, hydantoins (phenytoin), phenylbutazone, rifampin*: may ↑ digitoxin metabolism.

**ADVERSE EFFECTS** Signs and symptoms of toxicity: *CV*: ventricular premature contractions (most common), ventricular tachycardia, AV dissociation, accelerated junctional rhythm, atrial tachycardia, progressive pulse slowing and AV block; *GI*: anorexia, nausea, vomiting, diarrhea; *CNS*: visual disturbances, headache, weakness, dizziness, psychosis; *Other*: gynecomastia, eosinophilia, and thrombocytopenia are rare.

**CONTRAINDICATIONS** Ventricular fibrillation, ventricular tachycardia, digitalis toxicity; Beriberi heart disease; hypersensitive carotid sinus syndrome.

## Digoxin (Lanoxin, Lanoxicaps, *Burroughs Wellcome, Roxane, Elkins-Sinn, Wyeth-Ayerst*)

**CLASS** Digitalis glycoside

**DOSE** **Heart failure, atrial fibrillation, atrial flutter and paroxysmal atrial tachycardia:** Recommended doses are average values and may require modification; factors influencing dose include the disease being treated, lean body weight, renal function, concomitant disease states and drug therapy. Total body stores of 8-12 mcg/kg of lean body weight usually provide therapeutic effect in CHF and 10-15 mcg/kg for control of ventricular rate from rapid atrial arrhythmias: (For example 70 kg x 10 mcg/kg = 700 mcg loading dose). In renal insufficiency (CrCL < 10ml/min) give 6-10 mcg/kg as a loading dose. *For rapid loading give 50% of total dose initially and remainder at 4-8 hr intervals*. Assess clinical response prior to each dose. *For slow digitalization* an appropriate maintenance dose is given on a daily basis. Maintenance dose = (Total body stores) x (% daily loss) ÷ 100; % daily loss = 14 + CrCl/5. Usual maintenance range is 0.0625-0.325 mg/d.; **Administration:** Bioavailability of tablets is approximately 75-85%. When changing from oral to IV therapy, reduce digoxin dose by 20-25%; when changing from tablets or elixir to liquid filled capsules, reduce digoxin dose by 20%.

**DOSAGE ADJUSTMENT** Digoxin loading doses and maintenance doses require adjustment in renal insufficiency; the following conditions may also require a lower maintenance dose; hypokalemia, hypothyroidism, extensive myocardial damage, conduction disorders, and in geriatric patients. In heart failure accompanying acute glomerulonephritis, relatively low loading doses and maintenance doses are usually necessary.

**DRUG INTERACTIONS** *Potassium depleting corticosteroids and diuretics*: may contribute to digitalis toxicity; *Rapid administration of IV calcium*: may produce serious arrhythmias in digitalized patients; *Quinidine, flecainide, verapamil, amiodarone and propafenone*: may ↑ serum digoxin level; *Propantheline and diphenoxylate*: may ↑ digoxin absorption; *Antacids, kaolin-pectin, sulfasalazine, neomycin, cholestyramine, some anti-cancer drugs and metoclopramide:* may ↓ digoxin absorption; *Concomitant use of digoxin with sympathomimetics*: may ↑ risk cardiac arrhythmias;

## Digoxin (cont.)

*Succinylcholine*: may cause arrhythmias in digitalized patients; *β-Blockers and calcium channel blockers*: may have additive depressant effects on AV node conduction.

**ADVERSE EFFECTS** Signs and symptoms of toxicity: *CV*: ventricular premature contractions (most common), ventricular tachycardia, AV dissociation, accelerated junctional rhythm, atrial tachycardia, progressive pulse slowing and AV block. *GI*: anorexia, nausea, vomiting, diarrhea; *CNS*: visual disturbances, headache, weakness, dizziness, psychosis; *Other*: gynecomastia, eosinophilia, and thrombocytopenia (rare).

**MONITORING** Usual therapeutic range is 0.8-2 ng/ml; patients with atrial fibrillation or atrial flutter require and tolerate higher levels. Sampling of serum concentrations should be obtained, at least 6-8 hrs after last dose.

**CONTRAINDICATIONS** Ventricular fibrillation.

**OTHER COMMENTS** In Wolff-Parkinson-White syndrome with atrial fibrillation digoxin can ↑ transmission of impulse through accessory pathway. May worsen sinus bradycardia or sino-atrial block in patients with sinus node disease, and outflow obstruction in patients with idiopathic hypertrophic subaortic stenosis.

## Diltiazem (Cardizem, Cardizem CD, Cardizem SR, *Marion Merrell Dow*; Dilacor XR, *Rhone-Poulenc Rorer*)

**CLASS** Calcium channel blocker

**DOSE** **Vasospastic or chronic stable angina:** Initial dose 30 mg po QID; ↑ dose at 1-2 d intervals until control of angina. Usual dose: 180-360 mg/d in 3-4 divided doses. *Cardizem CD*: Initial dose: 120-180 mg/d; some patients may respond to higher doses up to 480 mg/d. **Hypertension**: *Cardizem SR*: Initial dose: 60-120 mg BID; may require 2 weeks before full effect is seen. Usual dose: 240-360 mg/d. *Cardizem CD*: Initial dose: 180-240 mg/d; maximum therapeutic effect achieved by 14 days chronic therapy; Usual dose: 240-360 mg/d. *Dilacor XR*: Initial dose: 180-240 mg/d; adjust as needed. Usual dose: 180-480 mg/d. **Atrial fibrillation, Atrial flutter, paroxysmal supraventricular tachycardia:** *Direct intravenous single injections*: 0.25 mg/kg actual body weight as a bolus given over 2 minutes (20 mg for the average patient); a second bolus (0.35 mg/kg over 2 minutes; 25 mg for the average patient can be given 15 minutes later if needed; subsequent doses need to be individualized). Patients with low body weight should be dosed on a mg/kg basis. Some patients may respond to 0.15 mg/kg. *Continuous IV infusion for continuous reduction of heart rate*: An infusion may be given immediately following bolus therapy as described above. Start initial infusion at 10 mg/hr and ↑ in 5 mg/hr increments up to 15 mg/hr as needed. Some patients may respond to an initial infusion rate of 5 mg/hr. Infusion duration >24 hrs and rate >15 mg/hr are not recommended.

**DOSAGE ADJUSTMENT** Titrate doses with caution in renal or hepatic impairment; use with caution in CHF patients.

**DRUG INTERACTIONS** *β-blockers*: may ↑ depressant effect on contractility and AV conduction; *Cimetidine and ranitidine*: may ↑ the bioavailability of diltiazem; *Digoxin*: may ↑ digoxin level; *Carbamazepine*: may ↑ carbamazepine level; *Cyclosporine*: may ↑ cyclosporine level.

**ADVERSE EFFECTS** *CNS*: dizziness/lightheadedness (1.5-7%), headache (2-12%), asthenia (2.8-5%); *GI*: nausea (1.6-1.9%), constipation (1.6%); *CV*: peripheral edema (2.4-9%), AV block (0.6-7.6%), bradycardia (1.5-6%), abnormal ECG

## Diltiazem (cont.)

(4.1%); *Other*: flushing (1.7-3%), dermatitis/rash (1-1.5%)
**CONTRAINDICATIONS** Sick sinus syndrome (unless functioning ventricular pacemaker is in place); second or third degree AV block; severe hypotension (systolic BP <90); acute MI with radiographically documented pulmonary congestion.

## Dipyridamole (Persantine, *Boehringer-Ingelheim*)

**CLASS** Antiplatelet
**DOSE** **Adjunct to coumarin anticoagulants in the prevention of postoperative thromboembolic complications of cardiac valve replacement**: 75-100 mg po BID.
**ADVERSE EFFECTS** Usually minimal and transient: dizziness, headache, abdominal distress, rash and diarrhea. Rare reports of angina.
**OTHER COMMENTS** Use with caution in patients with hypotension since it can cause peripheral vasodilation.

## Disopyramide (Norpace, Norpace CR, *Searle, Various Others*)

**CLASS** Antiarrhythmic; Class IA
**DOSE** **Treatment of documented life threatening ventricular arrhythmias (e.g. sustained ventricular tachycardia):** Recommended dose for most adults is 600 mg po QD (if < 50 kg, 400 mg/d) divided into 4 (immediate release capsules) or 2 (controlled release capsules) daily doses. For rapid control give initial loading dose of 300 mg immediate release capsules (200 mg if < 50 kg); may give 200 mg q6h prn thereafter. If no response by 48 hrs, either discontinue or carefully monitor subsequent doses of 250 or 300 mg q 6 h. **Administration**: Do not use extended release capsules when rapid control of ventricular arrhythmias is necessary. Normalize potassium prior to administration to minimize risk of proarrhythmia. The controlled release form is not recommended for patients with severe renal insufficiency (CrCl ≤ 40 ml/min).
**DOSAGE ADJUSTMENT** For adults < 50 kg or CrCl > 40 ml/min or hepatic insufficiency give 400 mg/d in divided doses (100 mg q 6 h for immediate release capsules, 200 mg q 12 h for controlled release capsules) Reduce dose in first degree heart block. For patients with severe renal insufficiency, 100 mg of immediate release with or without a load is given at ↑ dosing intervals depending on CrCl: 30-40 ml/min - q 8 hrs; 15-30 ml/min - q 12 hrs; < 15 ml/min - q 24 hrs: In patients with possible cardiac decompensation, an initial load should not be given and an initial dose of 100 q 6 h should not be exceeded.
**DRUG INTERACTIONS** *Procainamide, lidocaine*: widening of QRS complex may occur; *Erythromycin*: may ↑ disopyramide level; *Hydantoins, rifampin*: may ↓ disopyramide level; *Quinidine:* may result in ↑ disopyramide or ↓ quinidine level.
**ADVERSE EFFECTS** Most serious are CHF 1-3%, (potent negative inotrope) and hypotension; most common are anticholinergic; dry mouth (32%), urinary hesitancy (14%), constipation (11%), blurred vision, dry nose, eyes and throat (3-9%), urinary retention/frequency (3-9%), impotence (1-3%), dizziness, fatigue, headache (3-9%), bloating (3-9%) nervousness (1-3%).
**DISCONTINUATION** Discontinue with QRS prolongation > 25%. If hypotension occurs or CHF worsens, discontinue use and restart at lower dose. Second or third degree AV block or unifasicular, bifasicular or trifasicular block requires discontinuation unless ventricular rate controlled by pacemaker.

## Disopyramide (cont.)

**CONTRAINDICATIONS** Cardiogenic shock, pre-existing 2nd or 3rd degree AV block (if no pacemaker is present), congenital or acquired QT prolongation, sick sinus syndrome.

**OTHER COMMENTS** Use with caution in patients with sick sinus syndrome, Wolff-Parkinson-White or bundle branch block. Do not use in patients with urinary retention, glaucoma, myasthenia gravis, or uncompensated/marginally compensated CHF or hypotension unless caused by arrhythmia.

## Dobutamine (Dobutrex, *Lilly*)

**CLASS** Inotrope

**DOSE Inotropic support in cardiac decompensation:** Initial dose: 2.5-10 mcg/kg/min IV.

**DOSAGE ADJUSTMENT** ↑ dose in increments of 2.5 mcg/kg/min to desired response, up to a maximum rate of 40 mcg/kg/min; usual dose is 10 mcg/kg/min. Tolerance (↓ response with prolonged (> 24 hrs) continuous infusions) may occur and require ↑ dose. ↓ dose if preexisting hypertension.

**DRUG INTERACTIONS** *Bretylium*: potentiates pressor effect, possible arrhythmias; *Anesthetics (halothane, cyclopropane)*: possible serious arrhythmias - use with extreme caution; *Oxytocics*: possible severe persistent ↑BP, avoid; *Tricyclic antidepressants*: potentiates pressor effects.

**ADVERSE EFFECTS** ↑ HR, ↑ BP, PVCs (5%), phlebitis, anginal pain, nonspecific chest pain, palpitations, SOB (1-3%). Doses > 20 mcg/kg/min ↑ the risk for tachyarrhythmias.

**CONTRAINDICATIONS** Hypertrophic obstructive cardiomyopathy, severe aortic stenosis, sulfite allergy.

## Dopamine (Intropin, *DuPont;* Dopastat, *Warner-Chilcott, Abbott, others)*

**CLASS** Inotrope, Vasopressor

**DOSE Shock syndrome:** Initial dose: 2.5-10 mcg/kg/min IV; ↑ dose to desired response using 5-10 mcg/kg/min increments up to 20-50 mcg/kg/min (>50% respond to 20 mcg/kg/min). Usual maintenance dose 20-40 mcg/kg/min. **Renal vascular perfusion** Initial dose: 0.5-5 mcg/kg/min.

**DRUG INTERACTIONS** *Calcium channel and β-blockers*: block peripheral vasoconstriction (high doses) and cardiac effects, renal effects are not effected; *Anesthetics (halothane, cyclopropane)*: possible serious arrhythmias and ↓ BP - use with extreme caution; *MAO inhibitors (including furazolidone)*: pressor effect increased by 6-20 fold - administer phentolamine if given inadvertently; *Oxytocics*: possible severe persistent ↑BP, avoid; *Phenytoin*: possible seizures, severe ↓ BP and bradycardia; *Tricyclic antidepressants*: ↓ pressor effects.

**ADVERSE EFFECTS** Ectopy, nausea, vomiting, ↑ HR, anginal pain, palpitations, dyspnea, headache, vasoconstriction; high doses - ↓ urine output, dilated pupils, ventricular arrhythmia, gangrene.

**DISCONTINUATION** Excessive ↑ BP or HR, uncontrolled arrhythmias, ↓ urine output. Duration of action is very short; however, if discontinuation of infusion does not stabilize patient, phentolamine can be used to reverse exaggerated pressor effects. Taper gradually to avoid marked hypotension; additional IV fluids may be necessary.

**CONTRAINDICATIONS** Pheochromocytoma, uncorrected tachyarrhythmias, ventricular fibrillation, sulfite allergies - possible anaphylaxis.

## Doxazosin (Cardura, *Roerig*)

**CLASS** Peripheral alpha adrenergic blocker

**DOSE Hypertension:** Initial 1 mg po QD; postural effects are most likely to occur 2-6 hrs after a dose. Maintenance dose may be ↑ to 2 mg/d and up to 16 mg/d to achieve desired reduction in blood pressure; doses above 4 mg ↑ the likelihood of excessive postural effects.

**ADMINISTRATION** Marked postural hypotension and syncope may occur with first few doses. This phenomenon may be minimized by limiting the initial dose to 1 mg at bedtime

**ADVERSE EFFECTS** *CV*: palpitations (2%), postural hypotension/hypotension (0.3-1%); *CNS*: dizziness (19%), ↓ libido/sexual dysfunction (2%), asthenia (1-12%); *Other*: headache (14%), edema (4%).

## Enalapril Maleate (Vasotec, *Merck*)

**CLASS** ACE Inhibitor

**DOSE Hypertension:** Initial dose: 5 mg po QD. Maintenance dose: 10-40 mg/d as 1 or 2 doses/day. **CHF**: Initial dose: 2.5 mg/d or BID. Maintenance dose: 5-20 mg BID. Maximum daily dose: 40 mg; **Asymptomatic left ventricular dysfunction**: Initial: 2.5 mg QD; increase dose at 4d intervals to usual maintenance dose of 10 mg BID. Maximum dose 40 mg/d. **Administration**: Administer apart from antacids by 1-2 hrs.

**DOSAGE ADJUSTMENT** Renal impairment (creatinine > 1.6 mg/dl) or hyponatremia (NA+ < 130 mEq/L): Initial dose: 2.5 mg/d, ↑ dose as needed at 4 day or more intervals to maximum of 40 mg/d.

**DRUG INTERACTIONS** See Benazepril, p. 209.

**ADVERSE EFFECTS** *CNS*: dizziness; (4.3-7.9%), headache (1.8-5.2%), fatigue (1.8-3%); *GI*: nausea (1.3-1.4%), vomiting (1.3%), diarrhea (1.4-2.1%); *CV*: hypotension (6.7%); *Hematologic*: neutropenia / agranulocytosis (rare); *Renal*: ↑ BUN and serum creatinine (more apt to occur in patients with CHF, renal artery stenosis, concurrent diuretic therapy); *Other*: cough (1.3-2.2%).

**CONTRAINDICATIONS** See Benazepril, p. 209.

**OTHER COMMENTS** Patients are more prone to hypotension when initiating therapy. If possible, discontinue previous antihypertensive drug regimen 1 week before starting enalapril. Hypotension can be minimized by discontinuing diuretic or using a lower initial dose 2-3 days prior to start.

## Enalaprilat (Vasotec I.V., *Merck*)

**CLASS** ACE Inhibitor

**DOSE Hypertension:** 1.25 mg q 6 h IV over at least 5 minutes; doses up to 5 mg q 6 h for 36 hrs have been well tolerated. **Administration**: Administer IV over at least 5 minutes; may be administered undiluted, or diluted with up to 50 ml of a compatible diluent (D5W, NS, D5NS, D5LR).

**DOSAGE ADJUSTMENT** Renal impairment (creatinine > 3.0 mg/dL) or on a diuretic: Initial dose: 0.625 mg; if no response in 1 hour, repeat 0.625mg. Maintenance dose: 0.625-1.25 mg q6h.

**DRUG INTERACTIONS** See Benazepril, p. 209.

**ADVERSE EFFECTS** *CNS*: dizziness (4.3-7.9%), headache (1.8-5.2%), fatigue (1.8-3%); *GI*: nausea (1.3-1.4%), vomiting (1.3%), diarrhea (1.4-2.1%); *CV*: hypotension (6.7%); *Hematologic*: neutropenia/agranulocytosis (rare); *Renal*: ↑

## Enalaprilat (cont.)

BUN and serum creatinine (more apt to occur in patients with CHF, renal artery stenosis, concurrent diuretic therapy); *Other*: cough (1.3-2.2%).

**CONTRAINDICATIONS** See Benazepril, p. 209.

**OTHER COMMENTS** Can convert to oral therapy at a dose of 5mg/d (2.5mg/d in patients with creatinine clearance < 30 ml/min or other conditions in which a lower dose should be initiated; see enalapril).

## Enoxaparin Sodium (Lovenox, *Rhone-Poulenc Rorer*)

**CLASS** Anticoagulant (Low-molecular-weight heparin)

**DOSE** **Prevention of deep vein thrombosis following hip replacemnt surgery**: 30 mg BID by SC injection; initial dose given as soon as possible after surgery (not more than 24 hours postoperatively) and continued throughout post-operative course until DVT risk is diminished. Average duration: 7-10 d, up to 14 days has been well tolerated: **Administration**: Do not administer by IM injection. Use with caution in conditions associated with ↑ risk of hemorrhage; an unexplained ↓ in hematocrit or blood pressure should lead to a search for a bleeding site. Hemorrhagic complications may be reversed by slow IV injection of protamine.

**DOSAGE ADJUSTMENT** Use with caution in renal impairment and elderly (↑ risk of bleeding); no current recommendations for adjustment.

**DRUG INTERACTIONS** Use with care in presence of anticoagulants and platelet inhibitors.

**ADVERSE EFFECTS** Hemorrhage (5%), thrombocytopenia <100,000/mm$^3$ (2%); fever (4%), nausea (3%), hypochromic anemia (3%), edema (3%), peripheral edema (3%), confusion (2%), ecchymosis (2%), asymptomatic increases in transaminase levels (5%). Local irritation, pain, hematoma and erythema may follow SC injection.

**MONITORING** Periodic CBC, platelet count and stool occult blood tests are recommended during course of treatment.

**CONTRAINDICATIONS** Active major bleeding; thrombocytopenia associated with positive in-vitro test for anti-platelet antibody in the presence of enoxaparin; hypersensitivity to heparin or pork products.

## Ephedrine (Ephedrine, *Lilly, Abbott, LyphoMed, others*)

**CLASS** Vasopressor (*α*, *β*1, *β*2 agonist)

**DOSE** **Acute hypotensive states**: Initial dose: 25-50 mg IM or 10-25 mg slow IV push.

**DOSAGE ADJUSTMENT** Additional doses at 5-10 min intervals prn; not to exceed 150 mg/24 hrs.

**ADMINISTRATION** May be given slow IV push, IM or SC. IM administration: onset 10-20 min, duration 60 min.

**DRUG INTERACTIONS** *α and β-blockers:* block peripheral vasoconstriction (high doses) and cardiac effects; *Anesthetics (halothane, cyclopropane)*: possible serious arrhythmias and ↓ BP - use with extreme caution; *MAO inhibitors (including furazolidone)*: pressor effect increased by 6-20 fold; administer phentolamine if given inadvertently; *Oxytocics*: possible severe persistent ↑BP, avoid; *Tricyclic antidepressants*: ↓ or enhanced effects, ↑ cardiotoxicity use ↓ doses if pressor effects required; *Other sympathomimetics*: enhanced pressor effects, ↑ cardiotoxicity - use ↓ doses if required.

## Ephedrine (cont.)

**ADVERSE EFFECTS** Palpitations, tachycardia, arrhythmia, headache, insomnia, sweating, nervousness, vertigo, confusion, delirium, restlessness, anxiety, tremor, weakness, dizziness, hallucinations, nausea, vomiting, dysuria, urinary retention.
**DISCONTINUATION** Tolerance may develop; temporary discontinuation restores original response to the drug.
**CONTRAINDICATIONS** Narrow angle glaucoma, anesthetics (halothane, cyclopropane).
**OTHER COMMENTS** Use cautiously in patients with heart disease, correct intravascular volume depletion.

## Epinephrine (Adrenalin, *Parke-Davis & others*)

**CLASS** Vasopressor ($\alpha$, $\beta 1$, $\beta 2$ agonist)
**DOSE Ventricular fibrillation, pulseless ventricular tachycardia, pulseless electrical activity, asystole:** Initial dose: 1 mg IV push every 3-5 min. If inadequate response, consider intermediate dose: (2-5 mg IV push every 3-5 min); escalating dose (1 mg, 3 mg, 5 mg IV push 3 min apart), or high dose (0.1 mg/kg IV push every 3-5 min). **Bradycardia (not in cardiac arrest):** 2-10 mcg/min IV infusion. **Severe asthma, anaphylaxis:** Initial dose: 0.1-0.5 mg (0.1-0.5 ml of 1:1000) SC or IM; repeat dose prn at 20 min - 4 hr intervals. IV administration: Initial dose 0.1-0.25 mg (1.0-2.5 ml of 1:10,000) slow IV push over 5-10 min. every 5-15 min prn (or continuous infusion 1-4 mcg/min).
**DRUG INTERACTIONS** *α and ß-adrenergic blocking agents*: reverses the cardiac, bronchodilating and vasoconstrictor effects; *Anesthetics (halothane)*: PVC, ↑ HR, ventricular fibrillation. Use with extreme caution if at all; prophylactic administration of lidocaine or propranolol may be helpful. *Digitalis, tricyclic antidepressants, thyroid hormone*: potentiates arrhythmogenic effects of epinephrine; *Other sympathomimetics*: enhanced cardiac effects, ↑ cardiotoxicity; use ↓ doses if required.
**ADVERSE EFFECTS** Arrhythmias, ↑ BP, cerebral hemorrhage, hemiplegia, subarachnoid hemorrhage, anginal pain, palpitations, headache, tremor, weakness, dizziness, apprehensiveness, pallor, sweating, nausea, vomiting, metabolic acidosis, respiratory difficulty, tissue necrosis.
**CONTRAINDICATIONS** (Relative) narrow angle glaucoma, non anaphylactic shock, cerebral arteriosclerosis or organic brain damage, labor, cardiac dilatation, coronary insufficiency, circulatory collapse or ↓ BP due to phenothiazines (further lowers BP), anesthetics (chloroform, trichloroethylene, cyclopropane) - potentially fatal arrthymias.
**OTHER COMMENTS** Diabetics may require ↑ dosages of insulin or oral hypoglycemic agents since epinephrine ↑ blood glucose. Sulfite allergic patients may be treated with epinephrine injections despite its sulfite component since alternatives may not be as effective; D/C if paradoxical worsening of respiratory function occurs.

## Erythritol tetranitrate (Cardilate, *Burroughs-Wellcome*)

**CLASS** Nitrate
**DOSE Treatment & prevention of angina pectoris:** Initial dose: 5-10 mg SL or 10 mg po; titrate to lowest effective dose. Given before meals, and if necessary mid-morning, mid-afternoon and at bedtime. Maximum dose: 100 mg/d.
**ADMINISTRATION** Take ½ hr before or 1 hr after meals; do not crush or chew tablets.

## Erythritol tetranitrate (cont.)

**DRUG INTERACTIONS** *Drugs which effect vascular smooth muscle*: may see an ↑ or ↓ in effect of either drug *Dihydroergotamine*: ↑ bioavailability can ↑ BP and decrease antianginal effects.
**ADVERSE EFFECTS** Hypotension, flushing, headache.
**DISCONTINUATION** Excessive hypotension or tachycardia. Taper gradually to prevent withdrawal reactions (↑ angina).
**CONTRAINDICATIONS** Hypertrophic cardiomyopathy, severe anemia, cerebral hemorrhage/head trauma.
**OTHER COMMENTS** Dry mouth may ↓ absorption of sublingual tablets. Tolerance may develop; 10-12 hr nitrate-free interval may minimize this effect.

## Esmolol (Brevibloc, *Dupont, Merck*)

**CLASS** $\beta$-blocker; $\beta$-1 selective; Antiarrhythmic Class II
**DOSE** **Supraventricular tachycardia:** 50-200 mcg/kg/min IV (avg. dose 100 mcg/kg/min). Initial loading dose of 500 mcg/kg/min for 1 min followed by infusion of 50 mcg/kg/min for 4 min; if adequate effect not achieved, repeat loading dose and then infusion of 100 mcg/kg/min. Repeat loading dose and increasing infusion by 50 mcg increments (for 4 min). As desired HR or BP is approached, reduce incremental dose to 25 mcg/kg/min and omit loading infusion. Maintenance dosage > 200 mcg/kg/min does not significantly increase benefits.
**ADMINISTRATION:** Dilute to 250 mg/ml prior to infusion. After achieving desired HR transfer to alternative antiarrhythmic agent; ↓ dose of esmolol by half 30 min after the first dose of alternative agent. If satisfactory HR control is evident 1 hr after the second dose of alternative agent, discontinue esmolol.
**DRUG INTERACTIONS** See Acebutolol, p. 205.
**ADVERSE EFFECTS** *CV*: hypotension (most significant), bradycardia, heart failure, edema, pulmonary edema; *CNS*: dizziness, tiredness/fatigue, nervousness; *Endocrine*: hyperglycemia or hypoglycemia; *Respiratory*: bronchospasm; Raynaud's phenomenon.
**CONTRAINDICATIONS** See Acebutolol, p. 205.

## Ethacrynic Acid (Edecrin, *Merck*)

**CLASS** Loop diuretic
**DOSE** **Edema:** *Oral*: 50-200 mg po QD; adjust dose in 25-50 mg increments to produce gradual weight loss of 2.2-4.4 kg/d. *Parenteral*: 50 mg/d; may give second 50 mg dose if needed. **Administration**: IV slowly over several min. or by IV infusion.
**DRUG INTERACTIONS** *Aminoglycosides*: ↑ incidence of ototoxicity; *Anticoagulants*: ↑ effects of anticoagulants; *Lithium*: ↑ serum lithium level; *Cisplatin*: additive ototoxicity; *Probenecid*: ↓ action of loop diuretics; *Digoxin*: ↑ incidence of digitalis induced arrhythmias.
**ADVERSE EFFECTS** Anorexia, nausea, vomiting, diarrhea, acute pancreatitis, jaundice, GI bleeding, neutropenia, thrombocytopenia, fever, chills, hematuria, confusion, malaise, acute gout, abnormal LFT's, vertigo, headache, blurred vision, tinnitus, hyperuricemia, hyperglycemia.
**CONTRAINDICATIONS** Anuria, hepatic coma, severe electrolyte depletion.
**OTHER COMMENTS** Ethacrynic Acid has an additive effect when used with other diuretics. If using ethacrynic acid with other diuretics, start with an initial dose of 25 mg to avoid electrolyte depletion.

## Felodipine (Plendil, *Merck*)

**CLASS** Calcium channel blocker

**DOSE Hypertension:** 5 mg po QD; adjust based on response at intervals of not less than 2 weeks. Usual dose: 5-10mg/d. Maximum dose: 20mg/d.

**DOSAGE ADJUSTMENT** Adjust carefully in geriatric patients and those with impaired hepatic function; doses above 10mg in these patients should be avoided.

**DRUG INTERACTIONS** *β-blockers:* may ↑ depressant effect on contractility and AV conduction; *Digoxin*: may ↑ digoxin level; *Barbiturates*: may ↓ felodipine bioavailability; *Erythromycin*: may ↑ pharmacologic and toxic effects of felodipine; *Cimetidine, ranitidine*: may ↑ bioavailability of felodipine; *Hydantoins*: may ↓ felodipine levels; *Carbamazepine*: may ↓ felodipine levels.

**ADVERSE EFFECTS** *CNS*: dizziness/light-headedness (5.8%, headache (18.6%), asthenia (4.7%), paresthesia (2.5%); *GI*: nausea (1.9%), abdominal pain (1.8%); *CV*: peripheral edema (22.3%), chest pain (2.1%), palpitations (1.8%); *Other*: flushing (6.4%), muscle cramps (1.9%), upper respiratory infection (5.5%), cough (2.9%), dyspepsia (2.3%).

**OTHER COMMENTS** Use with caution in CHF patients.

## Flecainide (Tambocor, *3M*)

**CLASS** Antiarrhythmic; Class IC

**DOSE In patients without structural heart disease for (paroxysmal supraventricular tachycardia) and paroxysmal atrial fibrillation/flutter (PAF) associated with disabling symptoms:** Initial dose for PSVT and PAF is 50 mg po q 12 h; ↑ dose in increments of 50 mg BID every 4 days until efficacy achieved; for PAF may ↑ from 50 mg BID to 100 mg BID. Maximum dose for PSVT is 300 mg/d; **Prevention of documented life-threatening ventricular arrhythmias such as sustained ventricular tachycardia:** Initial dose 100 mg q 12 h; ↑ in increments of 50 mg BID every 4 days until efficacy achieved. Maximum dose 400 mg/d. **Administration**: For treatment of sustained ventricular tachycardia initiate therapy in the hospital.

**DOSAGE ADJUSTMENT** *Renal impairment*: CrCl ≤ 35 ml/min, initial dose 100 mg/d or 50 mg BID; less severe renal impairment initial dose is 100 mg q 12 h. ↑ dose cautiously at > 4 days in renal insufficiency and monitor plasma levels. *Hepatic impairment*: Do not use unless benefit outweighs risk; if used, cautious dose ↑ needed at > 4 d intervals.

**DRUG INTERACTIONS** *Amiodarone*: may ↑ flecainide level; *Cimetidine*: may ↑ flecainide bioavailability; *Disopyramide, verapamil*: ↑ negative inotropic effect, do not use unless benefits outweigh risks; *Smoking*: ↑ clearance of flecainide; *Digoxin*: may ↑ digoxin absorption and peak concentration; *Acidic urine*: ↑ elimination; *Alkaline urine*: ↓ elimination.

**ADVERSE EFFECTS** Dizziness (18.9%), dyspnea (10.3%), headache (9.6%), nausea (8.9%), fatigue (7.7%), palpitation (6.1%), chest pain (5.4%), asthenia (4.9%), tremor (4.7%), constipation (4.4%), edema (3.5%), abdominal pain (3.5%). Ventricular tachycardia reported in 0.4% of patients treated for PAF. When used to suppress PVC's post-MI (CAST study) excessive mortality or non fatal cardiac arrest was seen in flecainide treated patients compared to placebo (5.1% vs 2.3% respectively).

**MONITORING** Trough levels associated with therapeutic effect 0.2-1 mcg/ml; adverse effects ↑ with levels > 1 mcg/ml.

**DISCONTINUATION** If second or third degree AV block or bifassicular block (RBBB + left hemiblock) occurs, discontinue therapy unless a ventricular pacer is in place.

**CONTRAINDICATIONS** Pre-existing second or third degree AV block or bifasicular block unless a pacemaker is present to sustain cardiac rhythm if complete heart block occurs. Others include recent MI or cardiogenic shock.
**OTHER COMMENTS** Reserve use for patients in whom treatment benefits outweigh risk of proarrhythmic effect. Not recommended for use in patients with chronic atrial fibrilation or non life-threatening ventricular arrhythmias. Use only in extreme caution in sick sinus syndrome. May cause or worsen CHF, especially in patients with cardiomyopathy, pre-existing severe heart failure or low ejection fractions.

## Fosinopril (Monopril, *Mead-Johnson*)

**CLASS** ACE Inhibitor
**DOSE** **Hypertension:** 10 mg po QD. Maintenance dose: 20-40 mg QD; may ↑ to 80 mg/d. Divide dose to BID if inadequate response seen at end of dosing interval. **Administration**: Administer apart from antacids by 1-2 hrs.
**DRUG INTERACTIONS** See Benazepril, p. 209.
**ADVERSE EFFECTS** *CNS*: dizziness (1.6%), headache 3.2%), fatigue (1.5%); *GI*: nausea (1.2%), vomiting (1.2%), diarrhea (1.5%); *CV*: hypotension (1%); *Hematologic*: neutropenia / agranulocytosis (rare); *Renal*: ↑ BUN and serum creatinine (more apt to occur in patients with CHF, renal artery stenosis, concurrent diuretic therapy); *Other*: cough (2.2%).
**CONTRAINDICATIONS** See Benazepril, p. 209.
**OTHER COMMENTS** Patients are more prone to hypotension when initiating therapy. Hypotension can be minimized by discontinuing diuretic 2-3 days prior to start of ACE inhibitor. Diuretic can be resumed if blood pressure is not controlled. If diuretic cannot be discontinued use an initial dose of 10 mg fosinopril.

## Furosemide (Lasix, *Hoechst-Roussel*)

**CLASS** Loop diuretic
**DOSE** **Edema**: *Oral*: 20-80 mg/d; may titrate upward by 20 to 40 mg increments q 6-8h up to 600 mg/d in patients with severe edema; *IV push or IM* 20-40 mg/d may titrate upward by 20 mg increments q2h; **Hypertension**: 40 mg BID; adjust according to response. **Acute Pulmonary Edema**: 20-80 mg IV push over 1-2 minutes.
**DRUG INTERACTIONS** *Aminoglycosides*: ↑ incidence of ototoxicity; *Anticoagulants*: ↑ effects of anticoagulants; *Lithium*: ↑ serum lithium level; *Cisplatin*: additive ototoxicity; *Probenecid*: ↓ action of loop diuretics; *Digoxin*: ↑ incidence of digitalis induced arrhythmias.
**ADVERSE EFFECTS** Anorexia, nausea, vomiting, diarrhea, GI irritation, constipation, pancreatitis, jaundice, ischemic hepatitis, vertigo, headache, blurred vision, hearing loss, dizziness, restlessness, fever, photosensitivity, urticaria, pruritis, interstitial nephritis, rash, orthostatic hypotension, thrombophlebitis, glycosuria, muscle spasm, hyperuricemia, hyperglycemia, anemia, leukopenia, aplastic anemia, thrombocytopenia.
**CONTRAINDICATIONS** Anuria.

## Gemfibrozil (Lopid, *Parke-Davis*)

**CLASS** Fibric acid derivative

**DOSE** **Type IV or V hyperlipoproteinemia with hypertriglyceridemia, and for Type II B hyperlipoproteinemia:** (when HDL - cholesterol is also low and all other therapy has failed): 1200 mg po QD in 2 divided doses, 30 minutes before the a.m. and p.m. meals.

**DRUG INTERACTIONS** *Oral Anticoagulants*: ↑ pharmacologic effect of oral anticoagulants; *Lovastatin and other HMG CoA reductase inhibitors*: ↑ risk of rhabdomyolysis.

**ADVERSE EFFECTS** *GI*: dyspepsia (19.6%), abdominal pain (9.8%), diarrhea (7.2%) abnormal liver function tests and hematologic tests. Possible increased risk of myalgia and myopathy, cholelithiasis, cholecystitis and malignancy.

**DISCONTINUATION** Gallstones detected; myositis suspected; liver function test abnormalities persist.

**CONTRAINDICATIONS** Hepatic or severe renal dysfunction, primary biliary cirrhosis, pre-existing gallbladder disease, pregnancy and lactation.

## Guanabenz (Wytensin, *Wyeth-Ayerst*)

**CLASS** Central $\alpha$ adrenergic agonist

**DOSE** **Hypertension:** Initial dose: 4 mg BID; ↑ in increments of 4-8 mg/d every 1-2 wks. Maximum dose studied is 32 mg BID, but doses this high are rarely warranted.

**DOSAGE ADJUSTMENT** Monitor blood pressure carefully when administering to patients with hepatic or renal impairment

**ADVERSE EFFECTS** Drowsiness/sedation (39%), dry mouth (28-38%), dizziness (17%), weakness (10%), headache (5%), ↓ libido, impotence.

## Guanadrel (Hylorel, *Pennwalt*)

**CLASS** Peripheral antiadrenergic

**DOSE** **Hypertension:** Initial dose: 10 mg po QD or 5 mg BID if desired; Maintenance dose: 20-75 mg/d in BID dosages. Adjust the dosage weekly or monthly until blood pressure is controlled.

**DOSAGE ADJUSTMENT** Renal impairment: ↑ dosing interval based on CrCl: 10-50 ml/min (q 12-24 hrs); < 10 ml/min (q 24-48 hrs).

**DRUG INTERACTIONS** *Reserpine, alpha or β-blockers*: ↑ postural hypotension, bradycardia, depression; *MAO inhibitors*: ↓ antihypertensive effect; *Indirect acting sympathomimetics (e.g. ephedrine), tricyclic antidepressants, antipsychotics*: may ↓ antihypertensive effect; *Direct acting sympathomimetics (e.g. dobutamine)*: ↑ activity of sympathomimetic.

**ADVERSE EFFECTS** *CNS*: fatigue, headache, drowsiness, faintness; *GI*: ↑ bowel movements, gas pain, constipation, anorexia, nausea/vomiting; *GU*: nocturia, peripheral edema, ejaculation disturbances.

**CONTRAINDICATIONS** Known or suspected pheochromocytoma; within 1 week of MAO inhibitors; CHF.

## Guanethidine (Ismelin, *Ciba*)

**CLASS** Peripheral antiadrenergic

**DOSE** **Moderate and severe hypertension:** Initial dose: 10 mg po QD; ↑ dose every 5-7 days. Maintenance dose: 25-50 mg/d. In hospitalized patients, a 25-50 mg/d starting dose with increments of 25-50 mg/d may be used.

**DOSAGE ADJUSTMENT** Renal impairment: CrCl < 10 ml/min - dose every 24-36 hrs.

**ADMINISTRATION** During dosage adjustment, monitor for

## Guanethidine (cont.)

orthostatic hypotension.

**DRUG INTERACTIONS** *Reserpine*: ↑ postural hypotension, bradycardia, depression; *MAO inhibitors*: ↑ hypertensive effect; *Indirect acting sympathomimetics, tricyclic antidepressants, antipsychotics*: may ↓ antihypertensive effect; *Direct acting sympathomimetics*: ↑ activity sympathomimetics.

**ADVERSE EFFECTS** *CNS*: dizziness, weakness; *GI*: diarrhea; *CV*: bradycardia, syncope, orthostatic hypotension, fluid retention and edema; *Other*: inhibition of ejaculation

**CONTRAINDICATIONS** Pheochromocytoma, CHF not due to hypertension, use of MAO inhibitors.

## Guanfacine (Tenex, *Robins*)

**CLASS** Central α adrenergic agonist

**DOSE** **Hypertension:** Initial dose: 1 mg po QD given at bedtime to minimize daytime somnolence; if a satisfactory result is not reached in 3-4 weeks, ↑ dose to 2-3 mg/d. No evidence for ↑ efficacy with doses > 3 mg/d.

**DOSAGE ADJUSTMENT** Impaired renal function: use the low end of the dosing range.

**ADVERSE EFFECTS** Dry mouth (30%), somnolence (21%), fatigue (9%), dizziness (11%), constipation (10%), headache (4%), bradycardia, impotence, ↓ libido.

## Heparin

**CLASS** Anticoagulant

**DOSE** **Prophylaxis and treatment of venous thrombosis and its extension, pulmonary embolism, peripheral arterial embolism and atrial fibrillation with embolism:** *Full Dose Heparin Therapy*: For full dose continuous IV infusion therapy in a 68 kg adult, an initial loading dose is 5,000 units (IV bolus) followed by infusion of 20,000-40,000 units/d (800-1600 u/hr). For full dose intermittent IV therapy in 68 kg adult, initial dose is 10,000 units followed by 5,000-10,000 units q 4-6 hrs. For full dose subcutaneous therapy in a 68 kg adult, the usual initial dose is 5,000 units (IV bolus) + 10,000-20,000 units SC followed by SC injection of 8,000-10,000 units q 8 hrs or 15,000-20,000 q 12 hrs. Optimum duration determined by condition and severity; adjust according to clotting tests, (see monitoring); **Low dose prophylaxis for postoperative thromboembolism:** 5,000 units SC 2 hrs before surgery and q 8-12 hrs for 7 days or until full ambulation, whichever is longer. Reserve prophylaxis for patients > 40 years of age undergoing major surgery. **Surgery of heart and blood vessels**: Initial dose of not less than 150 units/kg to patients undergoing total body perfusion for open heart surgery - often 300 units/kg is used for procedures < 60 minutes and 400 units/kg is used for procedures > 60 minutes. **Disseminated Intravascular Coagulation:** 50-100 units/kg by IV infusion or IV injection q 4 hrs. **Administration**: To ensure continuous anticoagulation in patients in whom warfarin is being initiated, continue full heparin therapy for several days after therapeutic PT is obtained. Do not administer IM. Unexplained fall in HCT, BP or any other unexplained symptom should lead to consideration of hemorrhage; use with caution in diseases with increased risk of hemorrhage. When necessary, administer protamine to reverse heparin.

**DRUG INTERACTIONS** Drugs that interfere with platelet aggregation reactions may induce bleeding and should be used with caution; *Nitroglycerin*: may ↓ the pharmacologic effect of heparin although conflicting information exists.

**ADVERSE EFFECTS** Hemorrhage (≤10%),

## Heparin (cont.)

thrombocytopenia (≤30%), osteoporosis (after long term, high doses), cutaneous necrosis, suppression of aldosterone synthesis, rebound hyperlipidemia upon discontinuation, elevations in aminotransferases.

**MONITORING** Accepted therapeutic range for the PTT during full dose IV or SC heparin is 1.5-2.5 times the control value (in seconds), or an ACT value of 2-3 times control value (in seconds). Perform coagulation tests prior to initiation of therapy, q 4 hrs during early stages of treatment, and daily thereafter for continuous IV infusion therapy. For full dose therapy given by intermittent IV injection or deep SC injection, perform coagulation tests prior to initiation of therapy, prior to each dose during early therapy, and daily thereafter. Laboratory monitoring usually not performed for fixed, low dose SC heparin. Some clinicians recommend heparin dosage during cardiopulmonary bypass procedures to be adjusted to prolong the ACT to 480-600 seconds.

**CONTRAINDICATIONS** Severe thrombocytopenia; patients in whom blood coagulation tests cannot be performed at appropriate intervals (refers to full dose heparin therapy); uncontrollable bleeding state except when due to DIC.

**OTHER COMMENTS** Exclude patients from low dose heparin prophylaxis of postoperative thromboembolism if on oral anticoagulants or drugs that affect platelet function, or in bleeding disorders, brain or spinal cord injuries, spinal anesthesia, eye surgery or potentially sanguineous operations.

## Hydralazine (Apresoline, *Ciba & others*)

**CLASS** Direct acting vasodilator

**DOSE** **Essential hypertension:** Initial dose: 10 mg po QID first 2-4 days; titrate as needed to 25 mg QID; after 1 wk, 50 mg QID up to 400 mg/d. In some, BID dosing is adequate. **Severe hypertension, hypertensive emergency:** Initial: 10-50 mg IM, or 10-20 mg IV push. **Preeclampsia, eclampsia:** Initial: 5 mg IV, then 5-20 mg IV q 20-30 min. **CHF:** (afterload reduction): Initial oral dose: 50-75 mg in 3-4 divided doses. Maintenance dose: 200-600 mg/d. **Administration:** ↑ bioavailability with food.

**DOSAGE ADJUSTMENT** Lower doses in severe renal impairment. Dose not to exceed 200 mg/d in slow acetylators.

**DRUG INTERACTIONS** *Other parenteral antihypertensive agents*: profound ↓ BP *Sympathomimetics*: tachycardia, angina

**ADVERSE EFFECTS** *CNS*: headache; *CV*: palpitations, tachycardia, edema; *Other*: weight gain, SLE (> 200 mg/d).

**CONTRAINDICATIONS** Myocardial ischemia, mitral valvular rheumatic heart disease.

**OTHER COMMENTS** IV form unstable when in contact with metal, give immediately after drawing into syringe. Some tablets contain tartrazine and sulfites, which can cause allergic - type reactions.

## Hydrochlorothiazide (Hydrodiuril, *Merck, various others*)

**CLASS** Thiazide diuretic

**DOSE** **Edema:** 25-200 mg po QD. Maintenance dose: 25-100 mg QD or intermittently; may need up to 200 mg/d. **Hypertension:** 25-100 mg po QD.

**DRUG INTERACTIONS** See Benzthiazide, p. 210.

**ADVERSE EFFECTS** See Benzthiazide, p. 210.

**CONTRAINDICATIONS** Anuria.

## Hydroflumethiazide (Diucardin, *Wyeth-Ayerst;* Saluron, *Apothecon*)

**CLASS** Thiazide diuretic

**DOSE Edema: Initial:** 50 mg po QD or BID. Maintenance: 25-200 mg/d; administer in divided doses if dosage exceeds 100 mg/d. **Hypertension**: Initial: 50 mg po BID. Maintenance: 50-100 mg/d; do not exceed 200 mg/d

**DRUG INTERACTIONS** See Benzthiazide, p. 210.

**ADVERSE EFFECTS** See Benzthiazide, p. 210.

**CONTRAINDICATIONS** Anuria.

## Indapamide (Lozol, *Rhone-Poulenc Rorer*)

**CLASS** Diuretic

**DOSE Edema of CHF**: Initial: 2.5 mg po q a.m.; ↑ to 5 mg q a.m. if response not satisfactory after 1 wk. **Hypertension**: 1.25 mg po q a.m.; double dose at 4 wk intervals if satisfactory response not seen. Maximum dose: 5 mg QD.

**DRUG INTERACTIONS** *Allopurinol*: ↑ incidence of hypersensitivity reactions; *Anticoagulants*: ↓ effect of anticoagulant; *Calcium*: hypercalcemia; *Diazoxide*: may cause hyperglycemia; *Digitalis*: ↑ incidence of digitalis induced arrhythmias; *Lithium*: ↑ serum lithium level; *Corticosteroids, amphotericin B*: ↑ electrolyte depletion; *Bile acid sequestrants*: ↓ absorption of thiazide diuretics; *Nondepolarizing muscle relaxants*: ↑ blocking effects, prolonged respiratory depression.

**ADVERSE EFFECTS** Orthostatic hypotension (<5%); palpitations (<5%); dizziness (≥5%), vertigo (<5%), headache (≥5%), insomnia (<5%), fatigue (>5%), anxiety (>5%), nervousness (>5%), anorexia (<5%), GI effects (<5%), nausea/vomiting (<5%), abdominal pain (<5%), diarrhea/constipation (<5%), dry mouth (<5%), nocturia (<5%), impotence (<5%), rash (<5%), pruritis (<5%), hyperglycemia (<5%), hyperuricemia (<5%), muscle cramps (>5%). **CONTRAINDICATIONS** Anuria.

## Isoproterenol (Isuprel, *Sanofi-Winthrop, Abbott, Elkin-Sinn, IMS*)

**CLASS** Inotrope

**DOSE Acute unresponsive asthma attacks or bronchospasm during anesthesia:** Initial dose: 0.01-0.02mg IV push, repeat prn **Emergency cardiac arrhythmias:** Initial dose: 0.02-0.06 mg, repeat doses 0.01-0.02 mg prn; IV infusion initial rate: 5 mcg/min, adjusted to 2-20 mcg/min according to response. **Shock**: Initial infusion rate: 0.5-5 mcg (0.25-2.5 ml of 1:500,000 dilution) per min, adjusted to 2-20 mcg/min (advanced shock may require dose > 30 mcg/min). **Immediate temporary control of atropine resistant, hemodynamically significant bradycardia (with pulse) during ACLS:** Initial dose: 2-10 mcg/min IV infusion.

**DRUG INTERACTIONS** *Bretylium*: possible arrhythmias; *β-adrenergic blockers*: reverses the cardiac, bronchodilating and vasoconstriction effects; *Anesthetics (halothane, cyclopropane)*: ↑ arrhythmias, use with extreme caution; *Ergots*: enhances ↑ cardiac output, ↑ vasoconstriction, ↑ BP; *Other sympathomimetics*: enhanced effects, ↑ cardiotoxicity; *Tricyclic antidepressants*: possible ↑ BP.

**ADVERSE EFFECTS** Tachycardia, palpitations, ↑ or ↓ BP, ventricular arrhythmias (usually for doses that result in HR > 130 bpm), tachyarrhythmias, angina, Stokes-Adams seizures, flushing, sweating, tremors, nervousness, headache, dizziness, weakness, vomiting.

**CONTRAINDICATIONS** Tachycardia, tachyarrhythmias or

## Isoproterenol (cont.)

heart block caused by cardiac glycoside intoxication, ventricular arrhythmias, angina pectoris.
**OTHER COMMENTS** Contains sulfite, use cautiously in sulfite allergic patients if required. Correct intravascular volume depletion, hypoxia, acidosis, hypercapnia, ↓ or ↑ potassium before or concurrent with therapy.

## Isosorbide dinitrate sublingual & chewable **(Isordil, Sorbitrate, *Wyeth-Ayerst, ICI Pharma, others*)**

**CLASS** Nitrate
**DOSE** **Treatment & prevention of acute angina pectoris:** Initial dose: 2.5-5 mg SL, 5 mg chewable tablet.
**ADMINISTRATION** Place under the tongue or between cheek and gum while seated or reclined. Take at first sign of anginal attack; if no relief repeat q 5 min x 2. If pain persists, notify MD and report to ER. Do not crush or chew SL tabs. Do not crush chewable tabs. May be used prophylactically 5-10 min before activities that provoke an attack.
**DRUG INTERACTIONS, ADVERSE EFFECTS, DISCONTINUATION, CONTRAINDICATIONS** See Erythritol tetranitrate, p. 222.
**OTHER COMMENTS** Dry mouth may ↓ absorption of sublingual nitrates. Discard unused tablets 6 months after opening bottle. Keep original container closed tightly, protect from moisture.

## Isosorbide dinitrate sustained release **(Isordil Tembids, Sorbitrate SA, Dilatrate-SR, Iso-Bid, Isotrate Timecelles, *Various*)**

**CLASS** Nitrate
**DOSE** **Prevention of angina pectoris (not for acute attacks):** Initial dose: 40 mg po. Maintenance dose: 40-80 mg q 8-12 hrs.
**ADMINISTRATION** Tolerance to nitrates can be minimized by giving sustained release preparations QD or 8AM/2PM; anginal symptoms at night can be treated with a $\beta$-blocker or a calcium channel blocker. Must be swallowed whole.
**DRUG INTERACTIONS, ADVERSE EFFECTS, DISCONTINUATION,CONTRAINDICATIONS** See Erythritol tetranitrate, p. 222.
**OTHER COMMENTS** In general, avoid use of sustained release ISDN in acute MI (effects may be difficult to terminate).

## Isosorbide dinitrate tablet **(Isordil Titradose, Sorbitrate, *Wyeth, ICI Pharma, others*)**

**CLASS** Nitrate
**DOSE** **Prevention of angina pectoris (not for acute attacks):** Initial dose: 5-20 mg po. Maintenance dose: 10-40 mg q 6 hrs
**ADMINISTRATION** Tolerance to nitrates can be minimized by giving short-action preparations BID-TID (last dose not later than 7PM) instead of q 6 hrs; anginal symptoms at night can be treated with a $\beta$-blocker or a calcium channel blocker
**DRUG INTERACTIONS, ADVERSE EFFECTS, DISCONTINUATION, CONTRAINDICATIONS** See Erythritol tetranitrate, p. 222.

## Isosorbide mononitrate (IMDUR, *Key,* ISMO, *Wyeth Ayerst;* Monoket, *Schwarz-Pharma*)

**CLASS** Nitrate

**DOSE** **Prevention of angina pectoris (not for acute attacks):** IMDUR: 30 mg (1/2 of 60 mg tablet) or 60 mg po QD; may be ↑ to 120 mg/d after several days; rarely, 240 mg may be required. Others: Usual dose: 20 mg po BID.

**ADMINISTRATION** IMDUR: daily dose taken upon awakening in morning. Others: 1st dose on awakening, 2nd dose 7 hrs later.

**DRUG INTERACTIONS** *Drugs that affect vascular smooth muscle:* may see an ↑ or ↓ in effect of either drug.

**ADVERSE EFFECTS** Most common include headache, dizziness, flushing, other manifestations of hypotension. Methemoglobinemia is rare.

**CONTRAINDICATIONS** ↓ BP, hypertrophic cardiomyopathy (may ↑ angina), cerebral hemorrhage/head trauma (may ↑ intracranial pressure), severe anemia, nitrate allergy.

**OTHER COMMENTS** Avoid use in acute CHF and acute MI (↓ BP and ↑ HR effects difficult to terminate rapidly). A 10-12 hr. nitrate-free interval may minimize nitrate tolerance.

## Isradipine (DynaCirc, *Sandoz*)

**CLASS** Calcium channel blocker

**DOSE** **Hypertension:** Initial dose: 2.5 mg po BID; if satisfactory response does not occur after 2-4 weeks, the dose may be adjusted in 5 mg/d increments at 2-4 week intervals. Maximum dose: 20 mg/d; however, most patients show no additional response to doses above 10 mg/d and side effects are ↑.

**DRUG INTERACTIONS** *β-blockers*: may ↑ depressant effect on contractility and AV conduction.

**ADVERSE EFFECTS** *CNS*: dizziness (7.3%), headache (13.7%); *GI*: nausea (1.8%), abdominal discomfort (1.7%); *CV*: edema (7.2%), chest pain (2.4%), palpitations (4%), tachycardia (1.5%); *Other*: flushing (2.6%), fatigue (3.9%), rash (1.5%).

**OTHER COMMENTS** Use with caution in CHF patients. The bioavailability of isradipine is ↑ in the elderly, patients with hepatic impairment, and patients with mild renal impairment although no change in initial dose is needed.

## Labetalol (Normodyne, *Schering*) (Trandate, *Allen & Hanburys*)

**CLASS** *α* and *β*-blocker

**DOSE** **Hypertension**: *Oral*: 100 mg BID; titrate in increments of 100 mg BID q 2-3 days. Maintenance dose: 200-400 mg BID up to 1.2-2.4 g/d. *IV*: 20 mg slowly over 2 minutes; additional injections of 40-80 mg can be given at 10 min intervals until desired supine blood pressure is achieved or up to 300 mg administered.

**DOSAGE ADJUSTMENT** Use in impaired hepatic function with caution, drug metabolism may be diminished.

**DRUG INTERACTIONS** *Cimetidine:* ↑ bioavailability of oral labetalol; *Nitroglycerin*: labetolol blunts the reflex tachycardia that may be produced by nitroglycerin without preventing its hypotensive effect.

**ADVERSE EFFECTS** *CNS*: fatigue, headache, drowsiness; *GI*: diarrhea, reversible ↑ in transaminases, nausea, vomiting, dyspepsia; *Respiratory*: dyspnea, bronchospasm; *Musculoskeletal*: muscle cramps.

**CONTRAINDICATIONS** Not recommended for patients with mild arrhythmias, sinus bradycardia, greater than first degree heart block, CHF, cardiogenic shock, congenital or acquired long QT syndromes, bronchial asthma. Caution in patients with diabetes mellitus.

## Lidocaine **(Lidocaine HCl for IV injection: Astra, IMS, Fujisawa; Licocaine HCl for IV infusion: Abbott, Baxter, McGaw; Lidocaine for IM injection, LidoPen, STI)**

**CLASS** Antiarrythmic; Class IB

**DOSE** **Acute management of ventricular arrhythmias occurring during cardiac manipulation such as cardiac surgery or in relation to acute MI**: Single dose justified in following exceptional circumstances: **When ECG is not available to verify diagnosis but benefits outweigh risks; when facilities for IV administration are not available; patient in pre hospital phase of suspected acute MI when directed by qualified medical personnel viewing transmitted ECG.** *IM:* 300 mg in deltoid muscle, use only 10% solution. Lidopen Auto-Injector is for self administration in deltoid or anterolateral aspect of thigh. *IV:* Initial dose of 50-100 mg given at rate of 25-50 mg/min; if desired response not achieved, rebolus after 5 minutes. Do not give > 200-300 mg/hr. *Continuous IV infusion* for patients whose arrhythmias tend to recur and who cannot take oral antiarrhythmic therapy: 1-4 mg/min (20-50 mcg/kg/min); change to oral antiarrhythmic therapy as soon as possible. **Administration**: For IV use, administer lidocaine injection *without* preservatives.

**DOSAGE ADJUSTMENT** Reduce maintenance doses in heart failure, liver disease, receiving drugs known to ↓ clearance of lidocaine or ↓ liver blood flow, patients > 70 years of age, and digitalis toxicity accompanied by AV block. Widening of QRS complex and the appearance or aggravation of arrhythmias should be followed by dosage reduction and if needed discontinuation of drug.

**DRUG INTERACTIONS** *β-Blockers*: may ↑ lidocaine levels; *Cimetidine*: may ↓ lidocaine clearance; *Procainamide*: may have additive cardiodepressant action; *Tocainide*: may result in ↑ adverse effects; *Succinylcholine*: may prolong neuromuscular blockade.

**ADVERSE EFFECTS** *CNS*: lightheadedness, nervousness, drowsiness, confusion, mood changes, tremors, confulsions; *CV*: hypotension, bradycardia, CV collapse.

**MONITORING** Constant ECG monitoring is essential. Lidocaine plasma levels may correlate with CNS toxicity. Metabolites can contribute to toxicity.

**CONTRAINDICATIONS** Hypersensitivity to amide local anesthetics, Stokes-Adams attacks; Wolff-Parkinson-White syndrome, and severe degrees of sinoatrial, AV or intraventricular block in absence of an artificial pacemaker.

## Lisinopril **(Prinivil, *Merck*) (Zestril, *Stuart*)**

**CLASS** ACE Inhibitor

**DOSE** **Hypertension:** Initial dose: 10 mg po QD. Maintenance dose: 20-40 mg QD. **CHF**: Initial dose: 5 mg QD. Maintenance dose: 5-20 mg QD. **Administration**: Administer apart from antacids by 1-2 hrs.

**DOSAGE ADJUSTMENT** *CHF with hyponatremia*: Initial dose: 2.5 mg QD; *Renal impairment*: If creatinine > 3.0 mg/dl, initiate lisinopril at 1/2 recommended initial dose; if patient on dialysis, initiate lisinopril at 2.5 mg QD.

**DRUG INTERACTIONS** See Benazepril, p. 209.

**ADVERSE EFFECTS** *CNS*: dizziness (6.3%), headache (5.3%), fatigue (3.3%); *GI*: nausea (2.3%), vomiting (1.3%), diarrhea (3.2%); *CV*: hypotension (1.2-5%); *Hematologic*: neutropenia / agranulocytosis (rare); *Renal*: ↑ BUN and serum creatinine (more apt to occur in patients with CHF, renal artery stenosis, concurrent diuretic therapy); *Other*: cough (2.9-4.5%)

**CONTRAINDICATIONS** See Benazepril, p. 529.

## Lisinopril (cont.)

**OTHER COMMENTS** Patients are more prone to hypotension when initiating therapy. Hypotension can be minimized by discontinuing diuretic 2-3 days prior to start. Diuretic can be resumed if blood pressure is not controlled. If diuretic cannot be discontinued use an initial dose of 5 mg lisinopril.

## Lovastatin (Mevacor, *Merck*)

**CLASS** HMG CoA reductase Inhibitor

**DOSE Type II A and II B hyperlipoproteinemia:** Initial dose: 20 mg po QD with evening meal (40 mg/d if cholesterol > 300mg/dl); *Range*: 20-80 mg/d in single or divided doses. **Administration**: Take with meals (when lovastatin is given under fasting conditions, plasma concentrations ~ 2/3 of those achieved when administered after meals).

**DRUG INTERACTIONS** *Warfarin:* anticoagulant effect may be ↑; *Cyclosporine and other immunosuppressants*: ↑ risk of myopathy (30%) or rhabdomyolysis (avoid or adjust dose); *Erythromycin*: ↑ risk of myopathy or rhabdomyolysis (avoid); *Gemfibrozil:* ↑ risk of myopathy (5%) or rhabdomyolysis (avoid); *Niacin:* ↑ risk of myopathy (2%) or rhabdomyolysis (avoid).

**ADVERSE EFFECTS** *Skeletal muscle*: myalgia (1-3%) myopathy (0.5%), rhabdomyolysis (rare); *CNS*: headache (9%), dizziness, insomnia less frequent; *Hepatic*: serum transaminase levels > 3 x normal (2%); *Hypersensitivity*: varying severity, rare.

**MONITORING** Aminotransferase levels should be performed every 4-6 wks during first 3 months of therapy, every 6-8 wks during next 12 months, and at 6 month intervals thereafter; CPK levels in patients reporting muscle pain, tenderness, or weakness.

**DISCONTINUATION** Aminotransferase levels rise to 3 times normal and persist; markedly elevated CPK levels or if myopathy occurs. Consider discontinuation or temporary withdrawal in any patient with an acute, serious condition suggestive of a myopathy or with a risk factor predisposing to development of rhabdomyolysis including severe acute infection, hypotension, major surgery, uncontrolled seizures, and severe metabolic, endocrine or electrolyte disorders.

**CONTRAINDICATIONS** Active liver disease or unexplained persistent elevation of serum aminotransferases, pregnancy, lactation.

## Magnesium

**DOSE Mild Magnesium deficiency:** 1 g q 6 h x 4 doses (IM or IV). **Severe hypomagnesemia**: IM: up to 2 mEq/kg within 4 hrs; IV: 5 g/L in D5W or NS over 3 hrs. **Dietary Supplementation:** 27-54 mg po BID-TID or 100 mg po QID.

**ADVERSE EFFECTS** Usually a result of magnesium intoxication: flushing, sweating, hypotension, stupor, depressed reflexes, flaccid paralysis, hypothermia, cardiac & CNS depression.

**MONITORING** Serum magnesium levels, maintain urine output ≥ 100 ml q 4 hrs

**CONTRAINDICATIONS** Heart block, renal impairment, comatose patient (magnesium chloride).

**HOW SUPPLIED** Tablets: Magnesium Gluconate 550 mg (27 mg Mg); Magnesium Carbonate 250 mg; Injection: Magnesium Sulfate (1 mEq/ml, 4 mEq/ml, 0.8 mEq/ml); Magnesium Chloride (1.97 mEq/ml).

## Metaraminol (Aramine, *Merck*)

**CLASS** Vasopressor ($\alpha$, $\beta 1$ agonist)

**DOSE** **Hypotension:** Initial dose: 2-10 mg IM/SC, **Severe Shock:** Initial dose: 0.5-5 mg IV bolus; if needed, start continuous infusion at 5 mcg/kg/min (15-100 mg in 250-500 ml NS or 5% dextrose injection) to maintain desired BP. (150-500 mg in 250-500 ml has been used for higher doses.)

**DOSAGE ADJUSTMENT** Allow at least 10 min to elapse before additional doses are administered. Consider smaller doses in digitalized patients.

**DRUG INTERACTIONS** *Adrenergic blockers*: Phentolamine decreases but does not reverse or completely block the pressor effects; *β-adrenergic blockers*: propranolol blocks the cardiac stimulation and can be used to treat arrhythmias prophylactically; *Anesthetics (halothane, cyclopropane)*: potentially serious arrhythmias, avoid; *MAO inhibitors, ergots, tricyclic antidepressants, guanethidine*: possible hypertensive crisis; *Atropine*: blocks reflex bradycardia caused by metaraminol and enhances the pressor effects.

**ADVERSE EFFECTS** ↑ BP, palpitations, bradycardia, potentially fatal arrhythmias, ↓ renal perfusion, ↓ urine output, metabolic acidosis, ↓ cardiac output, apprehension, tremor, headache, precordial pain, respiratory distress, flushing, sweating, pallor, nausea, tissue sloughing, necrosis at injection site.

**DISCONTINUATION** D/C or ↓ rate if excessive ↑ or ↓ HR, uncontrolled ↑ BP, arrhythmias, excessive tremors, or nervousness, infiltration or thrombosis. Taper IV infusion gradually to avoid rapid ↓ HR. Hypotension may occur/recur when the drug is discontinued, especially after prolonged use; additional IV fluids may be necessary before D/C pressors.

**CONTRAINDICATIONS** Peripheral or mesenteric vascular thrombosis, profound hypoxia or hypercapnia, simultaneous use of cyclopropane, halothane.

**OTHER COMMENTS** Tachyphylaxis occurs with prolonged therapy; contains sulfite, use cautiously in sulfite-allergic patients if required; correct intravascular volume, hypoxia, hypercapnia, acidosis before or concurrent with therapy.

## Methoxamine (Vasoxyl, *Burroughs Wellcome*)

**CLASS** Vasopressor ($\alpha$ agonist)

**DOSE** **Hypotension during anesthesia:** Initial dose: 5-20 mg IM; 10-15 mg most common; in emergency: Initial dose: 3-5 mg IV; supplement with 10-15 mg IM; For prolonged effect, continuous IV infusion: Initial dose: 5 mcg/min. **Paroxysmal supraventricular tachycardia** Initial dose: 10 mg (range 5-15 mg) IV over 3-5 min, or 10-20 mg IM; allow at least 15 minutes to elapse before additional doses are administered.

**DRUG INTERACTIONS** *Alpha adrenergic blockers*: phentolamine does not completely block the pressor effects; *β-adrenergic blockers*: propranolol blocks the cardiac stimulation and can be used to treat arrhythmias prophylactically; *MAO inhibitors, ergots, tricyclic antidepressants, guanethidine*: possible hypertensive crisis; *Atropine*: blocks reflex bradycardia caused by metaraminol and enhances the pressor effects.

**ADVERSE EFFECTS** *CV*: ↑ BP, ventricular ectopy; *GI*: nausea, vomiting (often projectile), ↓ organ perfusion; *CNS*: headache, anxiety, nervousness.

**DISCONTINUATION** Systolic BP > 160 mmHg.

**CONTRAINDICATIONS** Severe hypertension.

## Methyclothiazide (Enduron, *Abbott*)

**CLASS** Thiazide diuretic

**DOSE** **Edema**: 2.5-10 mg po QD; **Hypertension**: 2.5-5 mg QD.

**DOSAGE ADJUSTMENT** If blood pressure control not satisfactory after 8-12 weeks with 5 mg/d, add another antihypertensive.

**DRUG INTERACTIONS** See Benzthiazide, p. 210.

**ADVERSE EFFECTS** See Benzthiazide, p. 210.

**CONTRAINDICATIONS** Anuria.

## Methyldopa (Aldomet, *Merck & various others*)

**CLASS** Central α adrenergic agonist

**DOSE** **Hypertension:** *Oral*: Initially 250 mg 2 to 3 times/d for first 48 hours; maintenance therapy is 500 mg to 3 g daily in 2-4 divided doses. *IV*: 250-500 mg q6h up to 1 g q6h

**DOSAGE ADJUSTMENT** Patients with impaired renal function may respond to smaller doses. Use lower doses in the elderly to reduce episodes of syncope.

**DRUG INTERACTIONS** *Lithium*: muscular weakness, lethargy & tremor *Propranolol*: paradoxical hypertension (rare).

**ADVERSE EFFECTS** *CNS*: sedation, headache, asthenia or weakness, dizziness, reversible mild psychosis; *CV*: bradycardia, aggravation of angina pectoris, orthostatic hypotension, edema, syncope; *GI*: nausea, vomiting, constipation, flatus, diarrhea, mild dry mouth, sore tongue; *Sensitivity/Hepatic*: abnormal liver function tests, jaundice, hepatitis; *Hypersensitivity*: fever, myocarditis, pericarditis, vasculitis, lupus-like syndrome; *Hematologic*: positive Coombs test (10-20%); *Other*: nasal stuffiness ↓ libido, impotence, gynecomastia.

**CONTRAINDICATIONS** Active hepatic disease, such as acute hepatitis or active cirrhosis.

## Metolazone (Zaroxolyn, Mykrox, *Fisons*)

**CLASS** Thiazide diuretic

**DOSE** *Zaroxolyn*: **Edema in renal disease or cardiac failure:** 5-20 mg po QD; **Mild to Moderate Hypertension:** 2.5-5 mg QD. *Mykrox*: **Mild to Moderate Hypertension:** 0.5 mg QD; may ↑ to 1.0 mg QD if response inadequate.

**DRUG INTERACTIONS** See Benzthiazide, p. 210.

**ADVERSE EFFECTS** See Benzthiazide, p. 210.

**CONTRAINDICATIONS** Anuria.

**OTHER COMMENTS** Metolazone preparations are not bioequivalent or therapeutically equivalent at the same doses. Mykrox is more rapidly and completely bioavailable. Do not interchange brands without dosage titration. Unlike other thiazides, useful when CrCl < 30 ml/min.

## Metoprolol (Lopressor, *Geigy*) (Toprol XL, *Astra*)

**CLASS** β-blocker; β-1 selective

**DOSE** **Hypertension:** 100 mg po QD in single or divided doses; ↑ to maintenance dose of up to 450 mg/d. **Angina:** 100mg/d in 2 divided doses up to a maximum dose of 400 mg/d; extended release tablets are used for once-a-day administration. **Acute MI**: administer 3 IV bolus injections of 5 mg each at approximately 2 minute intervals; 15 minutes later start oral dose of 50 mg every 6 hrs for 48 hrs followed by 100 mg twice daily. **Administration:** Food may enhance bioavailability; take at the same time each day.

## Metoprolol (cont.)

**DRUG INTERACTIONS** *Calcium channel blockers:* may potentiate β-blocker effects; $H_2$ *antagonists*: may ↑ bioavailability of metoprolol.

**ADVERSE EFFECTS** *CV*: bradycardia, heart failure, edema, pulmonary edema; *CNS*: dizziness, tiredness/fatigue, headache, peripheral neuropathy, nervousness; *GU*: sexual dysfunction, impotence, ↓ libido; *Endocrine*: hyperglycemia, hypoglycemia; arthralgia, arthritis, Raynaud's phenomenon.

**DISCONTINUATION** If sinus rate ↓ to 40 beats/min, particularly if associated with lowered cardiac output, give IV atropine. If heart block occurs, discontinue metaprolol, give atropine, and consider temporary pacemaker.

**CONTRAINDICATIONS** Acute MI in patients with a heart rate < 45 beats/min; > 1° AV block; systolic BP < 100 mmHg; moderate to severe CHF. Caution in bronchospastic disease, peripheral vascular disease, or diabetes mellitus.

## Mexiletine HCL (Mexitil, *Boehringer-Ingelheim*)

**CLASS** Antiarrhythmic; Class IB

**DOSE** **Documented life-threatening ventricular arrhythmias when rapid control is not essential**: 200 mg po q8h, adjust dose in 50-100 mg increments with minimum of 2-3 days between adjustments. If satisfactory response is not achieved with 300 mg q8h, ↑ to maximum of 1200 mg/d as tolerated. **For rapid control of ventricular arrhythmia**: Loading dose of 400 mg po followed by 200 mg q8h. **Administration**: Initiate therapy in the hospital; if adequate response is achieved on dose of ≤ 300 mg q8h, the same total daily dose may be given in divided doses every 12 hours. Take with food or antacids.

**DOSAGE ADJUSTMENT** Patients with severe liver disease or right sided CHF may require lower doses.

**DRUG INTERACTIONS** *Aluminum - magnesium hydroxide, atropine & narcotics:* may ↓ mexilitine absorption; *Metaclopramide*: may accelerate mexiletine absorption; *Hydantoins*: ↑ mexiletine clearance; *Rifampin*: may ↑ mexiletine clearance; *Urinary acidifiers*: may ↑ mexiletine clearance; *Urinary alkalinizers*: may ↓ mexiletine clearance; *Caffeine*: may ↓ clearance of caffeine by 50%; *Theophylline*: may ↑ theophylline levels.

**ADVERSE EFFECTS** *GI*: nausea/vomiting/heartburn (~40%), diarrhea (5.2%), constipation (4%), dry mouth (2.8%); *CNS:* dizziness/ lightheadedness (18.9-26.4%), tremor (13.2%), coordination difficulty (~10%), nervousness (5-11.3%), changes in sleep (7.5%), headache/blurred vision/visual disturbances (5.7-7.5%); *CV*: palpitations (4.3-7.5%), chest pain (2.6-7.5%), ↑ ventricular arrhythmias/PVC's (1-1.9%); *Other*: rash (3.8-4.2%), non-specific edema (3.8%), leukopenia/agranulocytosis (0.06%), thrombocytopenia (0.16%), LFT's 3 x nl (1-2%), dizziness/lightheadedness, tremor, coordination difficulty. GI distress can be minimized by ↓ dose, taking with food or antacid. Adverse reactions lead to 40% discontinuation in controlled trials.

**CONTRAINDICATIONS** Cardiogenic shock; pre-existing second or third degree AV block (if pacer not present).

**OTHER COMMENTS** Because of proarrhythmic effects, use of mexilitene in non life-threatening arrhythmias is not recommended. Use with caution in patients with hypotension, severe CHF, second or third degree AV block with operative ventricular pacemaker, sinus node dysfunction or intraventricular conduction abnormalities, patients with known seizure disorder.

## Milrinone acetate (Primacor, *Sanofi-Winthrop*)

**CLASS** Inotrope

**DOSE** **Short-term management CHF:** Initial dose: 50 mcg/kg IV slowly over 10 min: Maintenance dose as follows (in mcg/kg/min): minimum dose 0.375, standard 0.5, maximum dose 0.75.

**DOSAGE ADJUSTMENT** ↓ renal function may require ↓ dose, see manufacturer's dosage guidelines.

**ADMINISTRATION** Dilute with NS, one-half NS, or 5% dextrose injection to a final concentration of 100, 150, or 200 mcg/ml; regulate IV flow rate with a pump/controller. Incompatible with furosemide in same IV line.

**DRUG INTERACTIONS** Digitalis toxic effects may ↑ due to ↑ potassium loss.

**ADVERSE EFFECTS** Ventricular ectopy (8.5%), nonsustained ventricular tachycardia (2.8%), sustained ventricular tachycardia (1.0%), ventricular fibrillation (0.2%), supraventricular arrhythmias (3.8%), ↓ BP (2.9%), angina (1.2%), headache (2.9%), ↓ potassium (0.6%), tremor, thrombocytopenia (0.4%).

**CONTRAINDICATIONS** Severe aortic or pulmonary vascular disease, hypertrophic subaortic stenosis, post acute MI patients.

**OTHER COMMENTS** In atrial fib/flutter, consider prior treatment with digitalis to prevent ↑ ventricular response rate. Correct hypokalemia before starting milrinone. Correct ↓ intravascular volume to achieve optimal inotropic effects.

## Minoxidil (Loniten, *Upjohn*; Minodyl, *Quantum*)

**CLASS** Direct vasodilator

**DOSE** **Severe hypertension:** Initial dose 5 mg po QD; may be ↑ to 10, 20, 40 mg/d. Maximum dose: 100 mg/d. Hospitalization is recommended during initiation to assure ↓ BP is not more than intended. **Administration**: If supine diastolic BP ↓ < 30 mmHg, administer QD; if > 30 mmHg, administer BID.

**DOSAGE ADJUSTMENT** Smaller doses required in renal impairment or during dialysis; wait ≥ 3 days after dosage adjustments to see full response.

**DRUG INTERACTIONS** *Guanethidine:* profound ↓ BP; *β-blockers*: prevent ↑ HR; *Diuretics*: prevent sodium and water retention and possible CHF.

**ADVERSE EFFECTS** Temporary edema (7%), tachycardia (variable), pericardial effusion (3%), hypertrichosis (80%).

**CONTRAINDICATIONS** Pheochromocytoma, acute MI, dissecting aortic aneurysm.

## Moricizine (Ethmozine, *DuPont*)

**CLASS** Antiarrythmic; Class IC

**DOSE** **Life threatening ventricular arrhythmias, such as sustained ventricular tachycardia:** Usual dose is 600-900 mg po QD given in 3 equally divided doses. Adjust dose as tolerated in increments of 150 mg/d at 3 day intervals until desired effect. **Administration**: Initiate treatment in hospital. Some patients who are well controlled on q8h regimen may be given same total daily dose in a q12h regimen.

**DOSAGE ADJUSTMENT** With hepatic or renal impairment, start at ≤ 600 mg/d. Initiate with particular care in severe liver disease, if at all.

# Moricizine (cont.)

**DRUG INTERACTIONS** *Cimetidine*: may ↑ moricizine levels (begin moricizine at ≤ 600 mg/d); *Digoxin*: additive prolongation of PR interval, no significant ↑ in AV block or digoxin levels; *Propranolol*: small additive ↑ in PR interval; *Theophylline*: ↑ clearance and ↓ half-life.

**ADVERSE EFFECTS** Proarrhythmia is most serious (3.7%); *CV*: palpitations (5.8%), sustained ventricular tachycardia, chest pain, CHF, cardiac death (2-5%); *CNS*: dizziness (15.1%), headache (8%), fatigue (5.9%), hypesthesias, asthenia, nervousness, paresthesias, sleep disorder (2-5%); *Respiratory*: dyspnea (5.7%); *GI*: nausea (9.6%), abdominal pain, dyspepsia, vomiting, diarrhea (2-5%).

**DISCONTINUATION** Second or third degree AV block occurs unless a ventricular pacemaker is in place, proarrhythmias.

**CONTRAINDICATIONS** Pre-existing second or third degree heart block; (bifasicular block) unless a pacemaker is present; cardiogenic shock.

**OTHER COMMENTS** Because of proarrhythmic effects, reserve for patients in whom benefits outweigh risks. Use with extreme caution in patients with sick sinus syndrome; initiate therapy cautiously in patients with CHF (↑ risk of proarrhythmia).

# Nadolol (Corgard, *Bristol-Myers Squibb*)

**CLASS** β-blocker; non-selective

**DOSE** **Angina Pectoris:** Initial dose: 40 mg po QD; gradually ↑ in 40-80 mg increments at 3-7 day intervals until clinical response is obtained or there is pronounced slowing of heart rate. Maintenance dose: 40-80 mg/d up to 240 mg/d. **Hypertension**: Initial dose: 40 mg po qd; gradually ↑ dose by 40-80 mg increments as needed; maximum 240-320 mg/d.

**DOSAGE ADJUSTMENT** Renal impairment: adjust dosing interval based on CrCl: >50 ml/min (q 24 hrs); 31-50 ml/min (q 24-36 hrs); 10-30 ml/min (q 24-48 hrs); <10 ml/min (q 40-60 hrs).

**DRUG INTERACTIONS, ADVERSE EFFECTS, DISCONTINUATION, CONTRAINDICATIONS** See Acebutolol, p. 205.

# Niacin (Nicotinic Acid, *Various*)

**DOSE** **Type II, III, IV and V hyperlipoproteinemia with ↑ triglycerides:** Initial dose: Begin with 100 mg po TID to mute vasodilatory effects; ↑ weekly to 1-2 g TID over 5-6 wks. Maximum dose: 6-9 g/d. **Administration:** take with or following meals.

**DRUG INTERACTIONS** *Ganglionic blockers and other antihypertensives*: may potentiate the hypotensive effect; *Lovastatin and other HMG CoA reductase inhibitors*: ↑ risk of rhabdomyolysis (avoid).

**ADVERSE EFFECTS** Flushing of the face and upper body, headache, gastrointestinal upset, abnormal liver function tests, chronic liver damage, itching, tingling.

**MONITORING** Frequent liver function tests; blood glucose, particularly in patients with glucose intolerance.

**CONTRAINDICATIONS** Hepatic dysfunction, gout, active peptic ulcer, pregnancy and lactation, severe hypotension.

**OTHER COMMENTS** Flushing, headache, and tingling are transient and usually subside with continued therapy. If flushing is persistent, may give 325mg of aspirin 30 minutes before each dose of nicotinic acid.

## Nicardipine (Cardene, Cardene SR, *Syntex*)

**CLASS** Calcium channel blocker

**DOSE** **Chronic Stable Angina:** Initial dose: 20 mg po TID; allow 3 days before ↑ dose. Usual dose: 20-40 mg TID (sustained release capsules not recommended for angina); **Hypertension:** *Immediate release*: Initial dose: 20 mg po TID; usual dose: 20-40 mg TID; *Sustained release:* Initial dose: 30 mg po BID; usual dose: 30-60 mg BID. **Administration**: Therapy can be initiated with sustained release capsules by providing effective total daily dose of immediate release capsules as 2 divided doses.

**DOSAGE ADJUSTMENT** *Renal insufficiency*: 20 mg TID (immediate release capsules) or 30 mg BID (sustained released); *Hepatic insufficiency*: Initial dose is 20 mg BID (immediate release capsules); titrate and maintain BID schedule.

**DRUG INTERACTIONS** *β-blockers*: may ↑ depressant effect on contractility and AV conduction; *Cimetidine and ranitidine*: may ↑ the bioavailability of nicardipine; *Cyclosporine*: may ↑ cyclosporine levels with possible toxicity.

**ADVERSE EFFECTS** *CNS*: dizziness (4-6.9%), headache (6.4-8.2%), asthenia (4.2-5.8%), somnolence (1.1-1.4%), dry mouth (0.4-1.4%); *GI*: nausea (1.9-2.2%), abdominal discomfort (0.8-1.5%); *CV*: peripheral edema (7.1-8%), angina (5.6%), palpitations (3.3-4.1%), tachycardia (0.8-3.4%); *Other*: flushing (5.6-9.7%).

**MONITORING** Because of prominent BP lowering effect at peak blood levels, measure BP at peak effect (1-2 hrs after dosing) and just before next dose during initial titration.

**CONTRAINDICATIONS** Severe aortic stenosis.

**OTHER COMMENTS** Use with caution in CHF. ↑ in angina has been reported with initiation or at time of dosage ↑.

## Nifedipine (Procardia, Procardia XL, *Pfizer*; Adalat, *Miles & various others*)

**CLASS** Calcium channel blocker

**DOSE** **Vasopastic or Chronic Stable Angina:** *Capsules*: Initial dose: 10 mg po TID; Usual dose: 10-20 mg TID; daily dose > 120 mg/d rarely needed and > 180 mg not recommended. *Sustained release tablets*: Initial dose: 30-60 mg po qd; doses > 120 mg/d not recommended. **Hypertension**: Sustained release tablets as above.

**ADMINISTRATION** Sustained release tablets of nifedipine may be substituted for conventional capsules at the nearest equivalent total daily dose. Do not chew or divide extended release tablets.

**DRUG INTERACTIONS** *β-blockers*: may ↑ depressant effect on contractility and AV conduction; *Cimetidine*: may ↑ bioavailability of nifedipine; *Quinidine*: may ↓ quinidine level *Digoxin*: may ↑ digoxin level.

**ADVERSE EFFECTS** *CNS*: dizziness (4.1-27%), headache (10-23%), nervousness/mood change (7%); *GI*: nausea or heartburn (3.3-11%); *CV*: peripheral edema (7-30%), palpitation (7%), CHF (2-6.7%), acute MI (4-6.7%); *Other*: flushing (3-25%), weakness (12%), muscle cramps (8%), dyspnea, cough, wheezing (6-8%); nasal congestion/sore throat (6%).

**OTHER COMMENTS** Use with caution in CHF patients.

## Nimodipine (Nimotop, *Miles*)

**CLASS** Calcium channel blocker

**DOSE** **Subarachnoid Hemorrhage:** Initiate within 96 hrs of event; 60 mg po q 4 hr x 21 days. **Administration**: If the patient

## Nimodipine (cont.)

cannot swallow, capsule may be punctured at both ends with an 18-gauge needle and contents emptied into an NG tube.
**DOSAGE ADJUSTMENT** Hepatic failure can ↓ nimodipine clearance; therefore, ↓ dose to 30 mg q 4 hrs.
**DRUG INTERACTIONS** *Hypotensive agents*: ↑ hypotension; *Phenytoin*: ↑ risk of phenytoin toxicity.
**ADVERSE EFFECTS** *CV*: hypotension (5%; most common), edema; *CNS*: headache.

## Nitroglycerin injection **(Tridil, Nitro-Bid IV, Nitroglycerin in 5% Dextrose, *DuPont, Marion Merrell Dow, Abbott, Baxter, others*)**

**CLASS** Nitrate
**DOSE** **BP control in perioperative hypertension, CHF associated with acute MI, or angina pectoris unresponsive to recommended doses of nitrates, β-blockers:** Initial dose: 5 mcg/min via IV infusion pump (non-PVC tubing); 25 mcg/min (PVC tubing).
**DOSAGE ADJUSTMENT** Titrate dose with 5 mcg/min increments q 3-5 min; if no response use increments of 10-20 mcg/min until desired BP attained; up to 100 mcg/min may be required. Patients with normal-low LV filling pressures are extremely sensitive to drug and may respond fully to 5 mcg/min. Higher doses required when PVC IV tubing is used (NTG absorbs to several plastics). Tolerance will develop to continuous infusion.
**DRUG INTERACTIONS** *Drugs which effect vascular smooth muscle*: May see an ↑ or ↓ in effect of either drug; *Dihydroergotamine*: ↑ bioavailability can ↑ BP and decrease antianginal effect; *Heparin*: may ↓ anticoagulation effect.
**ADVERSE EFFECTS** Hypotension, flushing, headache, alcohol intoxication with prolonged high dose infusions.
**DISCONTINUATION** Excessive hypotension or tachycardia. Taper gradually to prevent withdrawal reactions (↑ angina episodes).
**CONTRAINDICATIONS** Hypertrophic cardiomyopathy, severe anemia, cerebral hemorrhage/head trauma.

## Nitroglycerin ointment **(Nitrol, Nitro-Bid, *Adria, Marion Merrell Dow*)**

**CLASS** Nitrate
**DOSE** **Treatment & prevention angina pectoris, ↓ cardiac workload in CHF (unlabeled)**: Initial dose: ½ inch (12.5 mm) q8h applied to skin; ↑ dose by ½ inch with each application prn.
**ADMINISTRATION** Spread thin layer on skin using applicator or dose measuring papers; do not use fingers or rub or massage. Apply over 2¼ x 3½ inch area of chest or back. 1 inch (25mm) ointment = 15 mg NTG. A 10-12 hr nitrate free interval has been recommended to minimize tolerance.
**DRUG INTERACTIONS** See Erythritol tetranitrate, p. 222.
**ADVERSE EFFECTS** *CV*: hypotension, flushing, headache; *Dermatologic*: allergic reactions, erythematous, vesicular, pruritic lesions, anaphylactoid reactions (oral mucosal and conjuctival edema).
**DISCONTINUATION** See Erythritol tetranitrate, p. 222.
**CONTRAINDICATIONS** See Erythritol tetranitrate, p. 222.
**OTHER COMMENTS** Keep tube tightly capped; In general, use of long acting nitrates in acute MI should be avoided.

## Nitroglycerin sustained release

(*Various*)

**CLASS** Nitrate

**DOSE** **Treatment & prevention angina pectoris:** Initial dose: 2.5-9.0 mg po TID dose may be ↑ by 2.5 or 2.6 mg (tablets) increments 2-4 times a day over days to weeks.

**ADMINISTRATION** Tolerance to sustained release preparations can be minimized by giving QD or 8AM/2PM; anginal symptoms at night can be treated with a *β*-blocker or a calcium channel blocker. Must be swallowed whole; not chewed, crushed or used sublingually.

**DRUG INTERACTIONS, ADVERSE EFFECTS, DISCONTINUATION, CONTRAINDICATIONS** See Erythritol tetranitrate, p. 222.

**OTHER COMMENTS** In general, avoid use of sustained release NTG preparations in acute MI.

## Nitroglycerin sublingual (Nitrostat, *Parke-Davis*)

**CLASS** Nitrate

**DOSE** **Treatment & prevention acute angina pectoris:** Initial dose: 0.15-0.6 mg SL. **Administration:** Place under tongue or between cheek and gum while seated or reclined. Take at first sign of anginal attack; if no relief, repeat q 5 min x 2; if pain persists notify MD and report to ER. Do not crush SL tablets. May be used prophylactically 5-10 min before activities that provoke an attack.

**DRUG INTERACTIONS, ADVERSE EFFECTS, DISCONTINUATION, CONTRAINDICATIONS** See Erythritol Tetranitrate, p. 222.

**OTHER COMMENTS** Dry mouth may ↓ absorption of sublingual nitrates. Discard unused tablets 6 months after opening bottle. Keep original container closed tightly and protected from moisture.

## Nitroglycerin transdermal systems (patch) (Deponit, Minitran, Nitrodisc, Nitro-Dur, Transderm-Nitro, *Various*)

**CLASS** Nitrate

**DOSE** **Treatment & prevention angina pectoris (not for acute attacks):** Initial dose: 0.2-0.4 mg/hr. Doses up to 0.8 mg/hr may be needed. **Administration:** Apply patch to dry skin, free of hair, excessive moisture; avoid below knee or elbow, cuts and irritated areas. May take up to 1-2 hrs. for onset of action. Effects persist after patch is removed for up to 24 hrs. Drug absorption ↑ with exercise and high temperature (sauna). A 10-12 hr nitrate free interval has been recommended to minimize tolerance.

**DRUG INTERACTIONS, ADVERSE EFFECTS, DISCONTINUATION, CONTRAINDICATIONS** See Erythritol tetranitrate, p. 222.

**OTHER COMMENTS** Used patches contain residual NTG; avoid exposure to children, pets when discarding. Avoid placing cardioverter/defibrillator on NTG patch; may cause arcing, burns to patient. Products differ in ease of application/removal, adhesiveness, comfort, size, release rate, total NTG content.

**HOW SUPPLIED** Patches available in NTG release rate of 0.1, 0.2, 0.3, 0.4, 0.6, 0.8 mg/hr.

## Nitroprusside (Nipride, *Roche*, Nitropress, *Abbott*)

**CLASS** Direct vasodilator

**DOSE** **Hypertensive crisis; controlled hypotension during surgery; (unlabeled); refractory CHF, acute MI:** Initial dosage for all indications: 0.3 mcg/kg/min IV; gradual upward titration every few minutes until desired effect is achieved or 10 mcg/kg/min is reached. Doses > 2 mcg/kg/min cause accumulation of cyanide. **Administration**: 50 mg vial must be diluted only with dextrose in water (2-3 ml) and further diluted in 250-1000 ml D5W. Infusions must be wrapped to protect from light; do not administer discolored solutions. Must use an electronic infusion device.

**DOSAGE ADJUSTMENT** Reduced doses required with severe liver impairment and renal dysfunction. Dose increase not recommended when tachyphylaxis to ↓ BP effects are attributable to concomitant cyanide toxicity.

**ADVERSE EFFECTS** Rapid ↓ BP, brady/tachycardia, ECG changes, lactic acidosis, ↓ platelet aggregation, cyanide toxicity, methemoglobinemia, thiocyanate toxicity.

**DISCONTINUATION** Signs and symptoms of cyanide/thiocyanate toxicity (bright red venous blood, lactic acidosis, air hunger, confusion), ataxia, seizures, stroke.

**CONTRAINDICATIONS** Compensatory hypertension (aortic coarctation), AV shunting, to ↓ BP during surgery in patients with known inadequate cerebral circulation or moribund patients requiring emergency surgery.

**OTHER COMMENTS** Elderly patients are more sensitive to the drug. Cyanide toxicity is treated with 3% sodium nitrate, 4-6 mg/kg (0.2 ml/kg) over 2-4 min immediately followed by an infusion of sodium thiosulfate (10 or 25%) 150-250 mg/kg; regimen may be repeated at half original doses after 2 hrs.

## Norepinephrine (Levophed, *Sanofi-Winthrop*)

**CLASS** Vasopressor

**DOSE** Dosage in terms of norepinephrine (2 mg norepinephrine bitartrate = 1 mg norepinephrine) **Hypotension:** Initial dose: 8-12 mcg/min IV; titrate to desired BP. Usual maintenance dose: 2-4 mcg/min.

**DRUG INTERACTIONS** *α-adrenergic blocker*: phentolamine blocks some peripheral vasoconstriction; use to prevent tissue sloughing; pressor effects are unaltered; *β-blockers*: propranolol blocks cardiostimulating effects and can be used to treat cardiac arrhythmias associated with norepinephrine; ↑ BP effects may be potentiated; *Anesthetics (cyclopropane, halothane), digitalis, other sympathomimetics*: enhanced effects, ↑ cardiac arrhythmias; *MAO inhibitors, tricyclic antidepressants, some antihistamines, ergots, methyldopa*: severe prolonged ↑ BP; *Furosemide, other diuretics*: ↓ arterial responsiveness; *Atropine*: blocks reflex tachycardia and enhances pressor response.

**ADVERSE EFFECTS** ↑ BP, arrhythmias, ↓ HR (reversed by atropine), ↓ cardiac output, ↓ blood flow (kidney, others), ↓ urine output, acidosis, headache, restlessness, anxiety, nervousness, weakness, dizziness, precordial pain, tremor, respiratory distress, pallor, blanching of skin, pilomotor response, paresthesias, necrosis/tissue sloughing if extravasation occurs and after SC administration.

**MONITORING** BP (every 2 min until desired BP achieved, then every 5 min during infusion), EKG, filling pressures, cardiac output, circulation to extremities. Maintain SBP at 80-100 mmHg if previously normotensive, or 30-40 mmHg below usual BP if hypertensive. If large doses are required, occult blood loss should be suspected.

**DISCONTINUATION** Excessive ↑ BP, ↓ or ↑ HR,

## Norepinephrine (cont.)

uncontrolled arrhythmias. Gradual tapering, especially after prolonged use, may prevent recurrence of hypotension when discontinued. Reinstitute if Systolic BP falls to 70-80 mmHg. Fluid administration may be necessary when tapering the drug.

**CONTRAINDICATIONS** (Relative): Shock caused by MI, severe CHF (norepinephrine increases arterial resistance and cardiac workload) severe CAD or CV disease, hypertension, ventricular tachycardia, acute pancreatitis or hepatitis, peripheral or mesenteric vascular thrombosis simultaneous use of halothane or cyclopropane.

**OTHER COMMENTS** If norepinephrine extravasates into SC tissues; treat with 5-10 mg phentolamine diluted in 10-15 ml NS; infiltrate liberally to affected area. Addition of 5-10mg phentolamine per liter of infusion may prevent tissue sloughing without altering pressor effects.

## Penbutolol (Levatol, *Reed & Carnrick*)

**CLASS** $\beta$-blocker; non-selective with ISA

**DOSE** **Hypertension**: Initial dose: 20 mg po qd, (full effect is seen by the end of two wks); titrate as needed to maximum dose of 80 mg/d. **Administration:** Should be taken on an empty stomach - absorption is slowed by the presence of food.

**DRUG INTERACTIONS, ADVERSE EFFECTS, DISCONTINUATION, CONTRAINDICATIONS** See Acebutolol, p. 205.

## Pentaerythritol tetranitrate (Peritrate, *Parke-Davis*, Duotrate, *Jones Medical*)

**CLASS** Nitrate

**DOSE** **Treatment & prevention angina pectoris:** Initial dose: 10-20 mg po TID-QID; can titrate to 40 mg 4 times daily. Take ½ hr before or 1 hr after meals and at bedtime. *Sustained release*: 1 tab/capsule q12h. **Administration:** Take on empty stomach; do not crush, chew, or take sublingually.

**DRUG INTERACTIONS, ADVERSE EFFECTS, DISCONTINUATION, CONTRAINDICATIONS** See Erythritol tetranitiate, p. 222.

**OTHER COMMENTS** Tolerance may develop; 10-12 hr nitrate-free interval may minimize this effect.

## Phenylephrine (Neo-Synephrine, *Sanofi-Winthrop, Others*)

**CLASS** Vasopressor ($\alpha$ agonist)

**DOSE** **Moderate hypotension**: Initial dose: IM or SC: 2-5 mg (range 1-10 mg); slow IV push: 0.2 mg (range: 0.2-0.5 mg). Adjust dose to desired BP response, giving additional doses IM or SC q 1-2 hrs prn, or via IV route q 10-15 min. **Severe hypotension/ shock**: Initial IV infusion rate: 0.1-0.18 mg/min; as BP stabilizes adjust rate to 0.04-0.06 mg/min. **Paroxysmal supraventricular tachycardia**: Initial dose not to exceed 0.5 mg via direct IV injection over 20-30 sec. Adjust dose in increments of 0.1-0.2 mg such that SBP does not exceed 160 mmHg. **Hypotension during spinal anesthesia** *(prophylaxis)*: 2-3 mg IM; *(emergencies)*: 0.2-0.5 mg IV injection.

**DRUG INTERACTIONS** *α-adrenergic blockers*: phentolamine

## Phenylephrine (cont.)

reverses its effects, phenothiazines may ↓ its effects and shorten its duration of action; *β-blockers*: block cardiostimulating effects and can be used to treat cardiac arrhythmias associated with phenylephrine; *Oxytocics*: may cause persistent hypertension and possible rupture of cerebral vessels (post-partum); *Other sympathomimetics*: enhanced effects, ↑ cardiac arrhythmias; *MAO inhibitors, ergots, tricyclic antidepressants*: potentiate ↑ BP; use with extreme caution if at all; *Furosemide, other diuretics*: ↓ arterial responsiveness.

**ADVERSE EFFECTS** ↑ BP, arrhythmias (much less than norepinephrine or metaraminol), ↓ HR (reversed by atropine), ↓ cardiac output, ↓ blood flow (kidney, others), ↓ urine output, acidosis, headache, restlessness, anxiety, nervousness, weakness, dizziness, precordial pain, tremor, respiratory distress, pallor, blanching of skin, pilomotor response, paresthesias, necrosis/tissue sloughing if extravasation occurs and after SC administration.

**CONTRAINDICATIONS** (Relative): Shock caused by MI, severe CHF (phenylephrine ↑ arterial resistance and cardiac workload), severe CAD or CV disease, hypertension, ventricular tachycardia, acute pancreatitis or hepatitis, peripheral or mesenteric vascular thrombosis.

**OTHER COMMENTS** May be useful in treating hypotension associated with halothane, cyclopropane, and others where cardiac stimulation is undesirable (e.g. hypertrophic obstructive cardiomyopathy). Contains sulfite, use cautiously in sulfite-allergic patients; correct intravascular volume, Correct hypoxia, hypercapnia, acidosis before or concurrent with therapy.

## Pindolol (Visken, *Sandoz*)

**CLASS** β-blocker; non-selective with ISA

**DOSE** **Hypertension**: Initial dose: 5 mg po BID; if a satisfactory ↓ in BP does not occur within 3-4 wks, adjust dose by 10 mg/d at 3-4 wk intervals (maximum: 60 mg/d).

**DOSAGE ADJUSTMENT** Adjust dose in patients with poor liver function which may cause plasma levels to increase.

**DRUG INTERACTIONS, ADVERSE EFFECTS DISCONTINUATION, CONTRAINDICATIONS** See Acebutolol, p. 205.

## Polythiazide (Renese, *Pfizer*)

**CLASS** Thiazide diuretic

**DOSE** **Edema**: 1-4 mg po QD. **Hypertension**: 2-4 mg/d.

**DRUG INTERACTIONS, ADVERSE EFFECTS** See Benzthiazide, p. 210.

**CONTRAINDICATIONS** Anuria.

## Potassium Chloride (Kaon-Cl, *Adria;* Slow-K, *Summit*; Kay Ciel, *Forest;* K-Dur, *Key*; Klotrix, *Bristol*; K-Tab, *Abbott*); (Potassium Bicarbonate, Klorvess, *Sandoz*; K-Lyte, *Bristol*)

**DOSE** **Prevention of hypokalemia**: 16-24 mEq/d; **Potassium depletion**: 40-100 mEq/d; **Administration**: Mix or dissolve soluble powders and effervescent tablets in 3-8 ounces of cold water, juice or other suitable beverage and drink slowly. Injectable KCl may not be administered undiluted - must be diluted in a suitable volume and administered by slow IV infusion (generally not > 20 mEq/hr).

## Potassium Chloride (cont.)

**DRUG INTERACTIONS** *ACE Inhibitors:* ↑ serum potassium; *Potassium sparing diuretic*: ↑ serum potassium; *Digitalis*: use caution if discontinuing potassium supplementation (hypokalemia may cause digitalis toxicity).

**ADVERSE EFFECTS** *GI*: nausea, vomiting, diarrhea, flatulence, GI obstruction, GI bleeding, ulceration or perforation; *Other*: hyperkalemia.

**CONTRAINDICATIONS** Severe renal impairment with oliguira or azotemia, untreated Addison's disease, hyperkalemia, concomitant use of potassium-sparing diuretics.

**OTHER COMMENTS** mEq/g of various potassium salts: potassium gluconate 4.3, citrate 9.8, bicarbonate 10.0, acetate 10.2, chloride 13.4.

## Pravastatin (Pravachol, *Bristol-Myers Squibb*)

**CLASS** HMG CoA reductase inhibitor

**DOSE** **Type II A and II B hyperlipoproteinemia:** Initial dose: 10-20 mg po QD at bedtime. Range: 10-40 mg once daily at bedtime. Adjust dose at 4 week intervals based on response.

**Administration:** May give without regard to meals.

**DRUG INTERACTIONS** *Warfarin*: anticoagulant effect may be ↑; *Cyclosporine and other immunosuppressants*: ↑ risk of myopathy (30%) or rhabdomyolysis (avoid or adjust dose); *Erythromycin*: ↑ risk of myopathy or rhabdomyolysis (avoid); *Gemfibrozil:* ↑ risk of myopathy (5%) or rhabdomyolysis (avoid); *Niacin:* ↑ risk of myopathy (2%) or rhabdomyolysis (avoid).

**ADVERSE EFFECTS** *Skeletal muscle*: myalgia (1-3%), myopathy (0.5%), rhabdomyolysis (rare); *CNS*: headache (9%), dizziness, insomnia less frequent; *Hepatic*: serum transaminase levels > 3 times normal (2%); *Hypersensitivity*: rare.

**MONITORING, DISCONTINUATION** See Lovastatin, p. 232. **CONTRAINDICATIONS** Active liver disease or unexplained persistent elevation of serum aminotransferases. pregnancy, lactation.

## Prazosin (Minipress, *Pfizer*)

**CLASS** Peripheral α blocker

**DOSE** **Hypertension:** Initial dose: 1 mg po BID-TID. Maintenance dose: 6-15 mg/d in divided doses. Doses > 20 mg/d usually do not ↑ efficacy.

**ADMINISTRATION** Take the first dose at bedtime due to high incidence of first dose effect (marked hypotension and syncope). When adding a diuretic or other antihypertensive agent, reduce dosage to 1-2 mg TID then retitrate.

**ADVERSE EFFECTS** *CV*: palpitations (5.3%), postural hypotension/hypotension; *CNS*: dizziness (10.3%), ↓ libido/sexual dysfunction, asthenia (~7%); *Other*: headache (7.8%), edema.

## Probucol (Lorelco, *Marion Merrell Dow*)

**DOSE** **Type II A and II B hyperlipoproteinemia:** 500 mg po BID (with morning and evening meals).

**DRUG INTERACTIONS** *Drugs that ↑ the QT interval, affect atrial rate, or cause AV block* (avoid).

**ADVERSE EFFECTS** *Cardiac*: prolongation of the QT interval, ventricular arrhythmias, syncope; *GI*: diarrhea or loose stools (10%).

**DISCONTINUATION** Marked prolongation of the QT interval, persistent abnormal lab findings, satisfactory

## Probucol (cont.)

cholesterol reduction not achieved within 3 months of therapy. **CONTRAINDICATIONS** Evidence of recent or progressive myocardial damage, serious ventricular arrhythmias, unexplained syncope or syncope of cardiovascular origin, abnormally long QT interval.

## Procainamide HCl (Pronestyl, Pronestyl Filmlok; *Apothecon;* Procan SR, *Parke-Davis*)

**CLASS** Antiarrhythmic; Class IA

**DOSE** **Ventricular tachycardia or other life-threatening ventricular arrhythmias:** Usual initial dose of conventional tablets or capsules: up to 50 mg/kg/d in divided doses q 3 hrs. Maintenance therapy: ¼ of the total required daily dose q 6 hrs; with extended release tablets usual dose 50 mg/kg in divided dose q6h. **Conversion of atrial fib and paroxysmal atrial tachycardia:** Initial dose: 1.25 gm of conventional tablets or capsules. If no change in the ECG, administer 750 mg 1 hr later; additional doses of 0.5-1 gm of conventional tablets or capsules have been administered q 2 h until normal sinus rhythm or toxic effects. Maintenance therapy: conventional tablets or capsules 0.5-1g q4-6h; extended release tablets ¼ of total daily dose q6h with usual dose of 1g q6h. **Administration:** *Oral therapy* should replace IM or IV therapy as soon as possible. For initial oral therapy, conventional tablets or capsules should be used; extended release tablets should only be used for maintenance dosage and should not be crushed or chewed; *Parenteral*: **Treatment of arrhythmias that occur during surgery and anesthesia** 100-500 mg administered parenterally (preferably IM). **Arrhythmias:** *Initial control*: IV doses of 50-100 mg may be given q 5 min until the arrhythmia is controlled, adverese effects occur, or 500 mg has been given; **consider** waiting 10 min or longer for distribution before additional doses are given. Alternatively, a loading dose IV infusion of 500-600 mg may be given at a constant rate over a 25-30 minute period (rate not to exceed 25-50 mg/min). 600 mg is usually sufficient, maximum is 1g to achieve control. *Maintenance*: continuous IV infusion of 1-6 mg/min (0.02-0.08 mg/kg/min).

**DOSAGE ADJUSTMENT** Reduce dose in renal insufficiency, congestive heart failure, and critically ill patients. ↓ dose if QRS widening of > 50% or marked prolongation of QT interval.

**DRUG INTERACTIONS** *Propranolol:* may ↑ procainamide serum levels; *Cimetidine and ranitidine*: appear to ↑ the bioavailability of both procainamide and NAPA; *Quinidine, trimethoprim*: may ↑ the plasma levels of both procainamide and NAPA, *lidocaine, phenytoin, propranolol, quinidine*: cardiac effects may be additive or antagonistic, and toxic effects may be additive; *Amiodarone:* may ↑ plasma procainamide and NAPA concentration up to 55% and 33%, respectively.

**ADVERSE EFFECTS** Hypotension and serious disturbances of cardiac rhythm such as ventricular asystole or fibrillation are more common after IV administration; *Skin*: Angioneurotic edema, urticaria, pruritus, flushing, maculopapular rash. A lupus-like syndrome is fairly common after prolonged administration and in slow acetylators. Positive ANA found in at least 50% of patients receiving long term therapy (usually within 2-18 months); *Hematologic*: neutropenia, thrombocytopenia, hemolytic anemia (rare), agranulocytosis; *CNS*: dizziness, giddiness, weakness, mental depression, psychosis with hallucinations; *GI*: anorexia, nausea, vomiting, abdominal pain, bitter taste, diarrhea (3-4%).

**MONITORING** Desired plasma concentrations are 4-8 mcg/ml; toxicity is associated with levels > 12 mcg/ml. NAPA also has significant antiarrhythmic activity and has a slower renal clearance than procainamide; NAPA's antiarrhythmic level

## Procainamide HCl (cont.)

is between 10-30 mcg/ml, toxic level is > 30 mcg/ml.
**CONTRAINDICATIONS** Complete heart block, idiosyncratic hypersensitivity, Lupus Erythematosus, Torsades de Pointes.

## Propafenone HCl (Rythmol, *Knoll*)

**CLASS** Antiarrhythmic; Class IC
**DOSE** **Life-threatening ventricular arrhythmias, (e.g. sustained ventricular tachycardia):** Titrate to response and tolerance: Initial dose: 150 mg po q8h; ↑ q 3-4 days up to 225-300 mg q8h.
**DOSAGE ADJUSTMENT** *Impaired hepatic function*: ↓ dose by 70-80%. *Impaired renal function*: administer with caution; consider ↓ dose if QRS widens, and for 2-3° AV block.
**DRUG INTERACTIONS** *Local anesthetics*: may ↑ risk of CNS side effects; *Cimetidine*: may ↑ propafenone level and effect; *Quinidine*: may ↑ level and effect of propafenone; *Rifampin*: may ↑ the clearance of propafenone resulting in ↓ level and effect; *Warfarin*: may ↑ warfarin level and PT; *β-blockers metabolized by the liver*: β-blocker effects may be ↑; *Cyclosporine:* whole blood cyclosporin trough level; may ↑ and renal function may ↓; *Digoxin*: may ↑ digoxin level/effect.
**ADVERSE EFFECTS** Dizziness (12.5%), nausea/vomiting (10.7%), unusual taste (8.8%), constipation (7.2%), fatigue (6%), dyspnea (5.3%), proarrhythmia (4.7%), angina (4.6%), headache (4.5%), blurred vision (3.8%), CHF (3.7%), palpitation (3.4%), ventricular tachycardia (3.4%), dyspepsia (3.4%), First degree AV block (2.5%), ↑ QRS duration (1.9%), PVC's (1.5%); Less frequent: *CNS*: abnormal dreams, apnea, coma, confusion, memory loss, seizures and tinnitus; *CV*: Atrial flutter, AV dissociation, cardiac arrest, sick sinus syndrome; *Hematologic*: agranulocytosis, anemia, bruising, granulocytopenia, ↑ bleeding time, leukopenia, thrombocytopenia, positive ANA titers.
**CONTRAINDICATIONS** Uncontrolled CHF; cardiogenic shock; SA, AV and intraventricular disorders in the absence of an artificial pacemaker; bradycardia; marked hypotension; bronchospastic disorder; manifest electrolyte imbalance.

## Propranolol (Inderal, *Wyeth-Ayerst*)

**CLASS** β-blocker; non-selective
**DOSE** **Arrhythmias**: 10-30 mg po TID-QID; **Hypertension:** 40 mg po BID or 80 mg/d (SR). Usual dose: 120-240 mg/d (BID-TID) or 120-160 mg/d (SR). Maximum dose: 640 mg/d. **Angina:** 80-320 mg/d (BID, TID, QID) or 80 mg/d (SR); 160 mg/d SR. **MI:** 180-240 mg/d (given TID-QID). **Hypertrophic subaortic stenosis:** 20-40 mg TID-QID or 80-160 mg/d (SR). **Pheochromocytoma:** 60 mg/d x 3 d pre-operatively. **Migraine:** 80-240 mg/d in divided doses. **Essential tremor:** 40 mg BID up to 320mg/d. **Administration:** reserve IV use for life threatening arrhythmias: 1-3 mg under careful monitoring; do not exceed 1 mg/min; for pheochromocyoma, administer concomitantly with an alpha-adrenergic blocking agent.
**DRUG INTERACTIONS, ADVERSE EFFECTS, DISCONTINUATION, CONTRAINDICATIONS** See Acebutolol, p. 205.
**OTHER COMMENTS** β-adrenergic blockade may blunt premonitory signs and symptoms (e.g. tachycardia, BP changes) of acute hypoglycemia.

## Protamine Sulfate (Protamine Sulfate, *Lilly, Fujisawa, Elkins-Sinn*)

**CLASS** Heparin antagonist

**DOSE** **Treatment of heparin overdose:** Dose is determined by dose of heparin administered, its route of administration and time elapsed since given. If < 15-30 minutes have elapsed since heparin was administered by IV injection, most clinicians recommend 1-1.5 mg protamine be given for every 100 units of heparin administered; if 30-60 minutes have elapsed since IV injection of heparin, 0.5-0.75 mg protamine should be given for every 100 units; if $\geq$ 2 hrs have elapsed since IV injection, 0.25-0.375 mg of protamine should be given for every 100 units of heparin. If heparin was given by IV infusion, some clinicians recommend a dose of 25-50 mg of protamine be given after stopping the infusion. **Administration**: Protamine sulfate injection should be given by very slow intravenous injection over a 10 minute period in doses not to exceed 50 mg. Use with caution in patients with fish allergy. Previous exposure to protamine may predispose susceptible individuals to hypersensitivity reactions; antiprotamine antibodies are present in serum of infertile or vasectomized men (may predispose to hypersensitivity reactions).

**ADVERSE EFFECTS** Rapid IV injection has caused hypotension and anaphylactoid reactions: bradycardia, hypersensitivity reactions, pulmonary edema, circulatory collapse. Heparin rebound with bleeding has been reported several hrs after adequate neutralization by protamine.

**MONITORING** Monitor PTT or ACT to determine the effect of protamine in neutralizing heparin. Coagulation tests usually performed 5-15 minutes after administration of protamine; another set 2-8 hrs later may detect heparin rebound.

**CONTRAINDICATIONS** Known intolerance to protamine.

## Quinapril (Accupril, *Parke-Davis*)

**CLASS** ACE Inhibitor

**DOSE** **Hypertension:** Initial dose: 10 mg po QD. Usual dosage: 20, 40 or 80 mg/d in single dose or 2 divided doses; adjust dose at intervals of at least 2 weeks. **Administration:** Administer apart from antacids by 1-2 hrs.

**DOSAGE ADJUSTMENT** Renal impairment: Initial dose: 5 mg qd (CrCl 30-60 ml/min), 2.5 mg qd (CrCl 10-30 ml/min).

**DRUG INTERACTIONS** See Benazepril, p. 209.

**ADVERSE EFFECTS** *CNS*: Dizziness (3.9%), headache (5.6%), fatigue (2.6%); *GI*: nausea (1.4%), vomiting (1.4%); *Hematologic*: neutropenia / agranulocytosis (rare); *Renal*: ↑ BUN and serum creatinine (more apt to occur in patients with CHF, renal artery stenosis, concurrent diuretic therapy); *Other*: cough (2%).

**CONTRAINDICATIONS** See Benazepril, p. 209.

**OTHER COMMENTS** Patients are more prone to hypotension when initiating therapy, which can be minimized by discontinuing diuretic 2-3 days prior to start. Diuretic can be resumed if blood pressure is not controlled. If diuretic cannot be discontinued use an initial dose of 5 mg quinapril.

## Quinethazone (Hydromox, *Lederle*)

**CLASS** Thiazide diuretic

**DOSE** **Edema:** 50-100 mg po QD (occasionally 50 mg BID, 150-200 mg/d infrequently necessary).

**DRUG INTERACTIONS** See Benzthiazide, p. 210.

**ADVERSE EFFECTS** See Benzthiazide, p. 210.

**CONTRAINDICATIONS** Anuria.

## Quinidine Sulfate

**(Quinidex, *Robins*) Quinidine Gluconate (Quiniglute, *Berlex*) Quinidine Polygalacturonate (Cardioquin, *Purdue Frederick*)**

**CLASS** Antiarrhythmic; Class IA

**DOSE** **Premature atrial and ventricular contractions:** 200-300 mg po 3 or 4 times daily. **Paroxysmal supraventricular tachycardias:** 400-600 mg po q 2-3 hrs until the paroxysm is terminated. **Atrial Flutter**: administer after digitalization. **Conversion of atrial fibrillation**: 200 mg po q 2-3 hrs for 5-8 doses with daily increases until sinus rhythm is restored or toxic effects occur; do not exceed a total daily dose of 3-4 g. Prior to quinidine administration, control the ventricular rate and CHF (if present) with digoxin. Maintenance therapy: 200-300 mg po 3-4 times daily; sustained release forms 300-600 mg q 8-12 hrs. **Acute tachycardia:** *IM:* 600 mg of quinidine gluconate IM; subsequently, 400 mg quinidine gluconate can be repeated as often as q 2 hrs prn. *IV*: 800 mg of quinidine gluconate (diluted with 40 ml of Dextrose 5%) infused at an initial rate of 16 mg/min in adults; usual dose is 300 mg, although 500-750 mg may be required. Note: quinidine sulfate is 83% quinidine; quinidine gluconate is 62% quinidine; quinidine polygalacturonate is 80% quinidine; *the oral dosages listed above are based on the quinidine content, not the salt.*
**Administration:** IM administation may be used if the patients condition is not critical; IV administration reserved for poorly-tolerated ventricular tachycardia; extended release tablets are primarily used for maintenance therapy. Adverse GI effects can be minimized by taking with food or antacid. To determine possible idiosyncrasy to quinidine, a test dose of 200 mg of quinidine sulfate orally or 200 mg of quinidine gluconate IM should be administered before full therapy is started.

**DOSAGE ADJUSTMENT** Use with caution in patients with renal or hepatic insufficiency.

**DRUG INTERACTIONS** *Amiodarone*: may ↑ quinidine level; *Certain antacids*: may ↑ quinidine level; *Barbiturates*: may ↓ quinidine level; *Cholinergic drugs*: may antagonize quinidine vagolytic effect; *Anticholinergics*: additive vagolytic effects; *Cimetidine, verapamil*: may ↑ quinidine level and effects; *Nifedipine, sucralfate*: may ↓ quinidine level and effects; *Hydantoins*: may ↓ therapeutic effect of quinidine; *Rifampin*: ↑ metabolism of quinidine; *Anticoagulants*: may ↑ anticoagulant effect; *Digoxin*: ↑ digoxin level; *Disopyramide*: ↑ disopyramide level and ↓ quinidine level; *Procainamide, propafenone*; may ↑ levels of each; *Tricyclic antidepressants, β-blockers (metoprolol, propranolol), neuromuscular blockers*: may ↑ quinidine effect.

**ADVERSE EFFECTS** More frequent: bitter taste, diarrhea, flushing of skin with itching, loss of appetite, nausea, vomiting, stomach pain or cramping. Less frequent: allergic reaction, cinchonism, hypotension, anemia, thrombocytopenia, confusion, depression, widening of QRS complex.

**MONITORING** Quinidine levels (maintain between 2-6 mcg/ml), periodic blood counts, LFT's, BUN, creatinine.

**DISCONTINUATION** 25% or greater increase in duration of QRS complex, disappearance of P waves. Discontinue use if signs of blood dyscrasia, hepatic or renal disorder occur.

**CONTRAINDICATIONS** Complete AV block, condution defects with a marked grade of QRS widening, history of drug-induced Torsade de Pointes, long QT syndrome; thrombocytopenic purpura associated with quinidine, digitalis intoxication, myasthenia gravis, escape rhythms.

## Ramipril (Altace, *Hoechst-Roussel*)

**CLASS** ACE Inhibitor

**DOSE Hypertension:** Initial dose: 2.5 mg po QD. Maintenance dose: 2.5-20 mg/d as single dose or in two equally divided doses. **Heart failure post-MI:** Initial dose: 2.5 mg po BID, increasing to 5 mg BID after 2 days as tolerated. **Administration**: Administer apart from antacids by 1-2 hrs.

**DOSAGE ADJUSTMENT** Renal impairment: Initiate therapy at 1.25 mg QD for CrCl < 40 ml/min (creatinine > 2.5 mg/dl); titrate dosage upward based on blood pressure response to a maximum of 5 mg/d. Liver disease: Maximum dose 2.5 mg QD.

**DRUG INTERACTIONS** See Benazepril, p. 209.

**ADVERSE EFFECTS** *CNS*: dizziness (2.2%), headache (5.4%), fatigue (2%); *GI*: nausea (1.1%), vomiting (1.1%), jaundice; *CV*: hypotension (0.5%); *Hematologic*: neutropenia / agranulocytosis (rare); *Renal*: ↑ BUN/creatinine (more likely in CHF, renal artery stenosis, concurrent diuretic therapy); *Others*: cough (3%), skin rashes, angioneurotic edema (rare).

**CONTRAINDICATIONS** See Benazepril, p. 209.

**OTHER COMMENTS** Patients are more prone to hypotension when initiating therapy; hypotension can be minimized by discontinuing diuretic 2-3 days prior to start. Diuretic can be resumed if blood pressure is not controlled. If diuretic cannot be discontinued, use an initial dose of 1.25 mg ramipril.

## Reserpine (Serpasil, *Ciba*; Serpalan, *Lannett*)

**CLASS** Peripheral antiadrenergic

**DOSE Hypertension:** Initial dose: 0.5 mg/d for 1-2 wks; then reduce to a maintenance dose of 0.1-0.25 mg/d. **Administration**: Take with food or milk.

**DOSAGE ADJUSTMENT** Lower dosages may be necessary in the elderly and patients with renal insufficiency.

**DRUG INTERACTIONS** *MAO inhibitors*: ↑ risk of hypertensive reaction; *Sympathomimetics Direct Acting (e.g. dobutamine)*: ↑ sympathomimetic effect; *Indirect Acting e.g. ephedrine)*: ↓ sympathomimetic effect; *Digitalis*: proarrhythmia; *Tricyclic antidepressants*: hypotension, flushing manic reactions.

**ADVERSE EFFECTS** *GI*: ↑ intestinal motility, nausea and vomiting, anorexia, diarrhea, dry mouth; *CV*: angina-like symptoms, arrhythmias, bradycardia, syncope; *CNS*: drowsiness, depression, dizziness, headache, extrapyramidal symptoms; *GU*: impotence, gynecomastia, ↓ libido.

**CONTRAINDICATIONS** Mental depression, peptic ulcer, ulcertative colitis, electroconvulsive therapy.

## Simvastatin (Zocor, *Merck*)

**CLASS** HMG CoA reductase inhibitor

**DOSE Type II A and II B hyperlipoproteinemia:** Initial dose: 5-10 mg po QD in the evening (5 mg/d for patients with LDL ≤ 190 mg/dl). Maintenance dose: 5-40 mg/d as a single dose in the evening; adjust dose at 4 wk intervals based on response.

**DRUG INTERACTIONS** *Warfarin*: anticoagulant effect may be ↑; *Cyclosporine and other immunosuppressants*: ↑ risk of myopathy (30%) or rhabdomyolysis (avoid or adjust dose); *Erythromycin*: ↑ risk of myopathy or rhabdomyolysis (avoid); *Gemfibrozil*: ↑ risk of myopathy (5%) or rhabdomyolysis (avoid); *Niacin*: ↑ risk of myopathy (2%) or rhabdomyolysis (avoid)

**ADVERSE EFFECTS** *Skeletal muscle*: myalgia, myopathy, rhabdomyolysis; *CNS*: headache, dizziness, insomnia less

## Simvastatin (cont.)

frequent; *Hepatic*: serum transaminase levels > 3 times normal (1.0%); *Hypersensitivity*: varying severity (rare).
**MONITORING, DISCONTINUATION** See Lovastatin, p. 232. **CONTRAINDICATIONS** Active liver disease or unexplained persistent elevation of serum aminotransferases, pregnancy, lactation.

## Sodium Nitroprusside

**See Nitroprusside, p. 241.**

## Sotalol (Betapace, *Berlex*)

**CLASS** Antiarrhythmic - Class III; β-blocker (non-selective)
**DOSE** **Ventricular arrhythmias**: 80 mg po BID; ↑ to 240-320 mg/d given in 2-3 divided doses if necessary. Some patients with refractory ventricular arrhythmias may require doses up to 640 mg/d. Adjust dosage gradually, allowing 2-3 days between dosing increments in order to achieve steady state.
**Administration**: Take on empty stomach (food may ↓ absorption); do not use in patients with hypokalemia or hypomagnesemia (can exaggerate the degree of QT prolongation and ↑ the risk of Torsade de Pointes).
**DOSAGE ADJUSTMENT** Modify dosing interval based on renal function: CrCl > 60 ml/min (q 12 hrs), CrCl 30-60 ml/min (q 24 hrs), CrCl 10-30 ml/min (q 36-48 hrs), CrCl < 10 ml/min; individualize dose: Dosage escalations in renal impairment should be after 5-6 doses at the appropriate intervals.
**DRUG INTERACTIONS** See Acebutolol, p. 205.
**ADVERSE EFFECTS** See Acebutolol, p. 205.
**DISCONTINUATION** QT interval > 550 msec
**CONTRAINDICATIONS** See Acebutolol, p. 205.
**OTHER COMMENTS** As the clinical status of the patient allows, discontinue previous antiarrhythmic therapy for 2-3 plasma half-lives before starting sotolol. After discontinuation of amiodarone, do not initiate sotalol until the QT interval is normalized. Proarrhythmic events can occur at initiation of therapy and with each upward dosage adjustment.

## Spironolactone (Aldactone, *Searle*)

**CLASS** Potassium sparing diuretic
**DOSE** **Primary hyperaldosteronism**: 100-400 mg po QD. **Edema**: 100 mg/d; may ↑ dose after 5 days if adequate response not achieved (range: 25-200 mg/d). **Essential hypertension**: 50-100 mg/d in single or divided doses; titrate dosage at 2 week intervals to maximize response. **Hypokalemia**: 25-100 mg/d to treat diuretic-induced hypokalemia.
**Administration**: Administration of spironolactone with food ↑ absorption of spironolactone.
**DRUG INTERACTIONS** *Anticoagulants*: ↓ hypoprothrombinemic effect; *Potassium preparation*: hyperkalemia; *ACE Inhibitors*: ↑ serum potassium; *Digoxin*: may ↑ or ↓ half-life of digoxin.
**ADVERSE EFFECTS** Abdominal cramping, diarrhea, gastric bleeding, ulceration, gastritis, vomiting, drowsiness, lethargy, headache, ataxia, gynecomastia, irregular menses/amenorrhea, postmenopausal bleeding, urticaria, drug fever, agranulocytosis.
**CONTRAINDICATIONS** Anuria, renal insufficiency, hyperkalemia, concomitant use of amiloride or triamterene.

## Streptokinase (Kabikinase, Streptase, *Smith-Kline-French, Hoechst-Roussel*)

**CLASS** Thrombolytic

**DOSE** **Acute evolving transmural MI**: IV infusion: 1.5 million units over 60 minutes; or Intracoronary (IC) infusion 20,000 units bolus dose followed by 2,000 units IV/min x 60 min for total dose 140,000 units. **PE, DVT, arterial thrombosis, embolism**: Loading dose 250,000 units IV over 30 min, followed by 100,000 units/hr IV for 24-72 hr (arterial thrombosis/embolis), 72 hr (DVT), 24 hr (PE; if concurrent DVT is suspected, then 72 hr).

**DRUG INTERACTIONS** *Heparin:* usually stopped before initiating SK (both may ↑ bleeding, careful monitoring is advised); *Antiplatlet agents (aspirin, dipyridamole, indomethacin, phenylbutazone, sulfinpyrazone) and warfarin (Coumadin)*: May ↑ bleeding if given before, during or after SK.

**ADVERSE EFFECTS** See p. 50. Others include noncardiogenic pulmonary edema after large MI and intracoronary administration, polyneuropathy, Guillain-Barre.

**CONTRAINDICATIONS:** See Alteplace, p. 206.

**OTHER COMMENTS** May be ineffective if given between 5 days - 6 mo of previous SK administration, or recent streptococcal infection.

## Terazosin (Hytrin, *Abbott, Burroughs-Wellcome*)

**CLASS** Peripheral $\alpha$ adrenergic blocker

**DOSE** **Hypertension:** Initial dose: 1 mg po at bedtime; slowly ↑ to a maintenance dose of 1-5 mg/d. May see benefit at doses as high as 20 mg/d.

**ADMINISTRATION** Can cause marked hypotension and syncope with first few doses; this effect can be minimized by limiting the initial dose to 1 mg at bedtime. If terazosin is discontinued for several days or longer, reinstitute therapy using the initial dosing regimen.

**ADVERSE EFFECTS** *CV*: palpitations (4.3%), postural hypotension/hypotension (1.3%); *CNS*: dizziness (19.3%), ↓ libido/sexual dysfunction, asthenia (11.3%); *Other*: headache (16.2%), edema (<1%).

## Ticlopidine (Ticlid, *Syntex*)

**CLASS** Antiplatelet

**DOSE** **Reduce risk of thrombotic stroke in patients who have experienced stroke precursors and in patients who have had a completed thrombotic stroke**: 250 mg po BID with food.

**DOSAGE ADJUSTMENT** ↓ or discontinuation may be necessary in patients if hemorrhagic or hematopoietic problems are encountered.

**DRUG INTERACTIONS** *Aspirin*: concomitant use with ticlopidine is not recommended; *Digoxin*: ↓ digoxin levels by 15%; *Theophylline*: ↑ theophylline half life and ↓ clearance; *Cimetidine*: ↓ clearance of single dose of ticlopidine by 50%; *Antacids*: ↓ ticlopidine levels by 18%.

**ADVERSE EFFECTS** Diarrhea (12.5%), nausea and dyspepsia (7%), rash (5%), GI pain (4%), neutropenia (2%), purpura (2%), vomiting (1%), flatulence (2%), ↑ LFTs (1%).

**DISCONTINUATION** If clinical evaluation and repeat laboratory testing confirm neutropenia (<1200/mm$^3$).

**CONTRAINDICATIONS** Hematopoietic disorders such as neutropenia and thrombocytopenia; hemostatic disorder or active pathological bleeding; severe liver impairment.

## Timolol (Blocadren, *Merck*)

**CLASS** β-blocker; non-selective

**DOSE** **Hypertension:** Initial dose: 10 mg po BID used alone or added to diuretic. Maintenance dose: 20-40 mg/d. **Acute MI**: 10 mg BID.

**DRUG INTERACTIONS, ADVERSE EFFECTS DISCONTINUATION, CONTRAINDICATIONS** See Acebutolol, p. 205.

## Tocainide HCl (Tonocard, *Merck*)

**CLASS** Antiarrhythmic; Class IB

**DOSE** **Life-threatening ventricular arrhythmias:** Initial dose: 400 mg po q8h. Maintenance dose: 1200-1800 mg/d divided into 3 doses; doses > 2400 mg/d are infrequent. Patients who tolerate the TID regimen may be tried on a BID regimen with careful monitoring. **Administration**: patients who do not tolerate the drug may benefit from administration with meals.

**DOSAGE ADJUSTMENT** Patients with renal or hepatic impairment may be adequately treated with < 1.2 g daily.

**DRUG INTERACTIONS** *Metoprolol*: may have additive effects inotropicity; *Lidocaine*: may ↑ incidence of adverse reactions, including seizures.

**ADVERSE EFFECTS** *Most serious*: agranulocytosis, bone marrow depression, leukopenia, neutropenia, aplastic anemia, thrombocytopenia, pulmonary fibrosis, *Most frequent*: dizziness/vertigo (15.3%), nausea (14.5%), paresthesia (9.2%), tremor (8.4%), skin lesion/rash (8.4%), vomiting (4.6%), headache (4.6%), diarrhea/loose stools (3.8%), altered mood/awareness (3.4%); *Less frequent*: *CNS*: Coma, seizures, agitation, confusion disorientation, depression, anxiety; *Dermatologic*: Stevens-Johnson syndrome, exfoliative dermatitis, urticaria, pruritis.

**DISCONTINUATION** Development of a hematologic or pulmonary disorder (e.g. pulmonary fibrosis).

**CONTRAINDICATIONS** Hypersensitivity to amide - type local anesthetics; patients with second or third degree AV block in the absence of an artificial ventricular pacemaker.

## Triamterene (Dyrenium, *Smith Kline Beecham*)

**CLASS** Potassium sparing diuretic

**DOSE** **Edema**: 100 mg po BID; do not exceed 300 mg/d. **Administration**: Administer after meals to prevent nausea.

**DRUG INTERACTIONS** *Amantadine*: may cause ↑ amantadine plasma levels and toxicity; *Potassium preparation*: hyperkalemia; *ACE Inhibitors*: ↑ serum potassium; *Cimetidine*: ↑ bioavailability and ↓ renal clearance of triamterene; *Indomethacin*: may cause acute renal failure.

**ADVERSE EFFECTS** *GI*: diarrhea, nausea, vomiting, jaundice, ↑ LFTs; *Renal*: azotemia, ↑ BUN/creatinine, interstitial nephritis; *Hematologic*: thrombocytopenia, megaloblastic anemia; *CNS*: weakness, fatigue, dizziness, headache; *Other*: hyperuricemia, hyperkalemia, dry mouth, anaphylaxis, photosensitivity, rash.

**CONTRAINDICATIONS** Concomitant administration of spironolactone or amiloride, anuria, servere hepatic disease, hyperkalemia, severe or progressive kidney disease.

## Trichlormethiazide (Methahydrin, *Marion Merrell Dow*) (Naqua, *Schering*)

**CLASS** Thiazide diuretic

**DOSE** **Edema**: 2-4 mg po QD; **Hypertension**: 2-4 mg QD; when initiating therapy, patients may be given doses twice daily.

**DRUG INTERACTIONS, ADVERSE EFFECTS** See Benzthiazide, p. 210. **CONTRAINDICATIONS** Anuria.

## Trimethaphan camsylate (Arfonad, *Roche*)

**CLASS** Direct vasodilator

**DOSE** **Controlled hypotension during surgery:** Initial: 3-4 mg/min; usual range 0.3-6 mg/min IV. **Hypertensive emergency, severe hypertension, pulmonary edema with pulmonary hypertension associated with systemic hypertension**: Initial: 0.5-1 mg/min. **Dissecting aortic aneurysm (unlabeled)**: Initial: 1-4 mg/min.

**DOSAGE ADJUSTMENT** Marked variation in response occurs. Aggressive dosing may result in respiratory arrest; use with great caution in elderly and debilitated patients.

**DRUG INTERACTIONS** *Anesthetic agents (especially spinal):* may exaggerate ↓ BP; *Neuromuscular blocking agents, nondepolarizing agents, succinylcholine:* effects are potentiated.

**ADVERSE EFFECTS** Use with caution in allergic patients (releases histamine); dilates pupils (does not indicate anoxia or depth of anesthesia), respiratory arrest with higher doses.

**CONTRAINDICATIONS** Uncorrected anemia, hypovolemia, shock, asphyxia, uncorrected respiratory insufficiency, unavailability of fluids or inability to replace blood, pregnancy (serious consequences to fetus); ineffective in preeclampsia.

## Urokinase (Abbokinase, Abbokinase Open Cath, *Abbott*)

**CLASS** Thrombolytic

**DOSE** **Coronary artery thrombosis/Acute MI**: *Intracoronary:* 6000 IU/min for up to 2 hrs; average dose = 500,000 IU; *Intravenous*: 2-3 million units over 45 to 60 minutes; ½ the dose give rapidly over 5 minutes followed with the remainder by continuous infusion; **IV catheter clearance**: 5000 IU, repeat x 1 for resistant cases; inject slowly and gently an amount (5,000 IU/ml) of UK (Open Cath) equal to volume of catheter with a 1 ml TB syringe, replace TB syringe with 5 ml syringe, wait 5 min, aspirate, repeat q 5 min; if still not open within 30 min, cap catheter, allow UK to remain in catheter for 30-60 min, then reattempt to aspirate; a 2nd dose may be necessary; when patency is restored aspirate 4-5 ml blood to remove all drug and clot, irrigate catheter with NS using a 10 ml syringe; **PE**: 4400 IU/kg IV over 10 minutes, then 4400 IU/kg/hr IV for 12 hrs.

**DRUG INTERACTIONS** *Heparin:* if given before, during and after UK, careful monitoring is advised since both may cause bleeding; *Antiplatelet agents (aspirin, dipyridamole, indomethacin, phenylbutazone, sulfinpyrazone) and warfarin (Coumadin)*: may ↑ bleeding if given before, during, or after UK.

**ADVERSE EFFECTS** See p. 50.

**DISCONTINUATION** Thrombin time should be < 2 x normal control before UK is initiated and before heparin is initiated following UK (≈ 3-4 hrs after UK is stopped), anaphylactic reaction, uncontrolled bleeding.

**CONTRAINDICATIONS** See Alteplace, p. 206.

**OTHER COMMENTS** Start treatment as soon as possible after onset of symptoms of acute MI, and within 7 d after PE.

## Verapamil (Calan, Calan SR, *Searle*), (Isoptin, Isoptin SR, *Knoll*), (Verelan, *Lederle*)

**CLASS** Calcium channel blocker; antiarrhythmic - Class IV

**DOSE** **Chronic stable, unstable, vasospastic angina:** 80-120 mg po TID; adjust dose daily (unstable) or weekly based on clinical response. **Hypertension:** 80 mg TID; sustained release 240 mg Q AM. Consider 40 mg TID or 120 mg/d of sustained release product in patients with decreased hepatic function, elderly or small stature. Hypotensive effect seen during first week; titrate upward as needed; Maximum dose: 360 mg/d of regular release tablets, 480 mg/d of sustained release products. **Arrhythmias**: *Oral dosing:* Digitalized patient with chronic atrial fibrillation: 240-320 mg/d in 3 or 4 divided doses; PSVT prophylaxis in non-digitalized patients: 240-480 mg/d in 3 or 4 divided doses; do not exceed 480 mg/d; **Arrhythmias** - *Parenteral dosing:* SVT: Initial: 5-10 mg (0.075-0.15 mg/kg), over 2 minutes; repeat 10 mg IV (0.15 mg/kg) 30 minutes after initial dose if response is not adequate.

**ADMINISTRATION** When switching from immediate release tablets to sustained release, total daily dose remains the same.

**DRUG INTERACTIONS** *β-blockers*: may ↑ depressant effect on contractility and AV conduction; *Digoxin*: may ↑ serum digoxin level; *Lithium*: may ↓ serum lithium level; *Theophylline*: may ↑ theophylline level; *Cyclosporine*: may ↑ cyclosporine level; *Carbamazepine*: may ↑ carbamazepine level.

**ADVERSE EFFECTS** *CNS*: dizziness/ lightheadedness (3.5%); headache (2.2%); *GI*: constipation (7.3%); nausea (2.7%), *CV*: hypotension (2.5%), peripheral edema (2.1%); bradycardia (1.4%); AV block (1%); pulmonary edema (1.8%); *Other*: shortness of breath/dyspnea/wheezing (1.4%).

**CONTRAINDICATIONS** Sick sinus syndrome or second or third degree AV block except with a functioning pacemaker, ventricular tachycardia, hypotension (< 90 mmHg systolic), severe left ventricular dysfunction, cardiogenic shock and severe CHF unless secondary to supraventricular tachycardia amenable to verapamil therapy, atrial flutter or fibrillation with an accessory bypass tract (may ↑ ventricular response). Do not give IV verapamil within a few hours of IV β-blockers.

**OTHER COMMENTS** Avoid concomitant use of verapamil with quinidine in patients with hypertrophic cardiomyopathy (IHSS). The incidence of CHF, arrhythmia and severe hypotension may be ↑ when verapamil is administered concurrently with β-blockers. Disopyramide should not be administered concomitantly with verapamil. IV verapamil may cause fatal hypotension if given during ventricular tachycardia.

## Warfarin (Coumadin, *DuPont*) Warfarin (Sofarin, *Lemmon*) Warfarin (Panwarfin, *Abbott*)

**CLASS** Anticoagulant

**DOSE** **Prophylaxis and treatment of venous thrombosis and its extension; Prophylaxis and treatment of atrial fibrillation with embolization; Prophylaxis and teatment of pulmonary embolism; Adjunct in prophylaxis of systemic embolism after acute MI:** 10 mg po QD for 2-4 days. Adjust daily according to PT or INR determinations. Maintenance regimen: 2-10 mg/d based on INR or PT. **Administration**: Brand interchange is not recommended. When transferring from heparin, use concurrent therapy until a therapeutic PT or INR is reached; optimum duration of overlap has not been defined. Numerous factors including travel, changes in diet, environment, physical state and medication may influence response. Use with caution in elderly, debilitated or when given in any physical condition where added risk of

## Warfarin (cont.)

hemorrhage is present.

**DOSAGE ADJUSTMENT** Use with caution in renal and hepatic impairment; elderly may require lower doses.

**DRUG INTERACTIONS** Check tertiary sources for complete list of drug interaction as list is exhaustive; must consider prescription and over-the-counter medications.

**ADVERSE EFFECTS** Hemorrhage, necrosis of skin and other tissues (purple toe syndrome), alopecia, urticaria, dermatitis, fever, nausea, diarrhea, systemic cholesterol, microembolization.

**MONITORING** Adjust dose based on daily PT or INR; the following indications have a desired therapeutic range of PT ratio of 1.3-1.5 times control (INR of 2-3); prophylaxis and treatment of venous thrombosis, atrial fibrillation to prevent systemic embolism, acute myocardial infarction, treatment of PE. Once stable, monitor PT or INR q 4-6 wks.

**CONTRAINDICATIONS** When risks of hemorrhage may be greater than benefits of anticoagulation, pregnancy, hemorrhagic tendencies or blood dyscrasias, recent or contemplated CNS or eye surgery, traumatic surgery resulting in large open surfaces, bleeding tendencies associated with active ulceration or overt bleeding of GI, GU or respiratory tracts. Others include cerebrovascular hemorrhage, aneurysms (cerebral, dissecting aorta); pericarditis and pericardial effusions, bacterial endocarditis; threatened abortion, eclampsia and preeclampsia; inadequate laboratory facilities or unsupervised senility, alcoholism, psychosis or lack of patient cooperation; spinal puncture and other diagnostic or therapeutic procedures with potential for uncontrollable bleeding. Miscellaneous: major regional or lumbar block anesthesia, malignant hypertension, continuous tube drainage of small intestine. May be contraindicated patients with diverticulitis, vasculitis, severe renal or hepatic impairment, polyarthritis, visceral carcinoma, bleeding granuloma, severe diabetes mellitus, severe allergic and anaphylactic disorders, Vitamin C or Vitamin K deficiency.

**OTHER COMMENTS** Use with caution in disturbances of intestinal flora, surgery or trauma, known or suspected protein C deficiency and severe to moderate hypertension.

## INTRAVENOUS CARDIAC DRUGS

| Drug | Dosage |
|---|---|
| Adenosine | **Supraventricular tachycardia:** 6 mg bolus over 1-2 sec; follow with 12 mg in 1-2 min. x 2 prn. |
| Amrinone | **CHF:** Initial dose: 0.75 mg/kg bolus over 2-3 min. followed by 5-10 mcg/kg/min. A second bolus (0.75 mg/kg) may be given 30 min after the initial bolus if needed. Maximum dose: 10 mg/kg/d |
| Bumetanide | **Edema:** 0.5-1 mg over 1-2 min; increase dose at 2-3 hr intervals to maximum daily dose of 10 mg. |
| Diazoxide | **Hypertensive emergency:** 1-3 mg/kg (up to 150 mg) as undiluted rapid bolus directly into a peripheral vein. |
| Dobutamine | **Inotropic support:** Initial dose: 2.5-20 mcg/kg/min. Maximum rate: 40 mcg/kg/min. |
| Dopamine | **Shock:** Initial dose: 2.5-10 mcg/kg/min; maximum: 20-50 mcg/kg/min. **Renal perfusion**: 0.5-5 mcg/kg/min. |
| Enalaprilat | **Hypertension:** 1.25-5 mg q 6 hr IV over at least 5 min. Creatinine > 3.0 mg/dL or on diuretics: Initial dose 0.625 mg (may repeat in 1 hr). Maintenance dose: 0.625-1.25 mg q 6 hrs. |
| Ephedrine | **Hypotension:** 10-25 mg slow IV push. Additional doses q 5-10 min. prn; do not exceed 150 mg/24 hrs. |
| Epinephrine | **Bradycardia (not in cardiac arrest):** 2-10 mcg/min. |
| Esmolol | Loading dose: 500 mcg/kg/min x 1 min followed by 50 mcg/kg/min x 4 min; repeat loading dose and ↑ infusion by 50 mcg/kg/min q 4 min prn. Maintenance: 50-200 mcg/kg/min. |
| Furosemide | **Acute pulmonary edema:** 20-80 mg IV push over 1-2 min. High doses (> 200 mg) occasionally required. |
| Hydralazine | **Severe hypertension:** 10-20 mg IV push. **Preeclampsia:** Initial: 5 mg IV, then 5-20 mg IV q 20-30 min. |
| Isoproterenol | **Atropine-resistant bradycardia:** 1-10 mcg/min. |
| Labetalol | **Hypertension:** 20 mg over 2 min. followed by injections of 40-80 mg at 10 min. intervals prn. |
| Lidocaine | Initial dose: 50-100 mg over 2-4 min; may rebolus after 5 min. Maintenance: 1-4 mg/min (20-50 mcg/kg/min). |

## INTRAVENOUS CARDIAC DRUGS

| Drug | Dosage |
|---|---|
| Metaraminol | **Shock:** Initial dose: 0.5-5 mg bolus; if needed, continuous infusion starting at 5 mcg/kg/min. |
| Methyldopa | **Hypertension:** 250-1000 mg q 6 hrs. |
| Metoprolol | **Acute MI:** 5 mg bolus x 3 (each 2 min apart); 15 min after last bolus, start 50 mg po q 6 hr x 48 hrs. followed by 100 mg po BID. |
| Milrinone | **CHF:** 50 mcg/kg over 10 min; maintenance dose: 0.375-0.75 mcg/kg/min. |
| Nitroglycerin | **Perioperative hypertension, CHF with acute MI, unstable angina:** Initial dose: 5 mcg/min (non-PVC tubing); 5-20 mcg/min increments q 3-5 min. Doses exceeding 100 mcg/min may be required. |
| Nitroprusside | **Hypertensive crisis, refractory CHF:** 0.3-10 mcg/kg/min. Doses > 2 mcg/kg/min may accumulate cyanide. |
| Norepinephrine | **Hypotension:** Initial dose: 8-12 mcg/min; titrate to desired BP. Usual maintenance: 2-4 mcg/min. |
| Phenylephrine | **Severe hypotension:** 0.1-0.18 mg/min; as BP stabilizes, adjust rate to 0.04-0.06 mg/min. |
| Procainamide | Loading dose: 500-1000 mg over 25-30 min (rate not to exceed 25-50 mg/min). Maintenance: 1-6 mg/min. |
| Propranolol | 1-3 mg under careful monitoring; rate not to exceed 1 mg/min. |
| Trimethaphan | **Hypertensive emergency:** 0.5-1 mg/min. May result in respiratory arrest. |
| Verapamil | **Supraventricular tachycardia**: Initial dose: 5-10 mg (0.075-0.15 mg/kg) over 2 min; repeat 10 mg (0.15 mg/kg) 30 min. later if response inadequate. |
| Others | Alteplace tPA (p. 205), Anistreplase (APSAC, p. 208), Bretylium (p. 211), Digoxin (p. 215), Diltiazem (p. 216), Heparin (p. 226), Methoxamine (p. 233), Protamine (p. 247), Quinidine (p. 248), Streptokinase (p. 251), Urokinase (p. 253). |

# INDEX

# Additional Information also includes:

- ***Essentials of ECG Interpretation:*** Arrhythmias and Conduction Disturbances, "Wide-Complex" Tachycardia, Acute MI, Pacemakers, and the Effects of Drugs, Electrolytes and Medical Disorders. More than 90 ECG strips in all.

- ***Recent Clinical Trials:***

| Trial | Design | Results |
|---|---|---|
| Gusto (N Engl J Med) 1993; 329:673) | 41,021 patients randomized to one of four regimens: (1) accelerated tPA... | Accelerated tPA + IV heparin with slight reduction in 30-day mortality compared to streptokinase (6.3% vs. 7.3%),... |

***More Than 100 Trials Reviewed***

- ***Management of the Cardiac Surgical Patient:***
    - **Pre-op Preparation**
    - **Post-op Complications**

---

**• SAME STYLE**
**• LARGER PRINT**
**• 650 PAGES - 51/2" x 7"**
**• FITS LABCOAT POCKET**

---

*SEE INSIDE BACK COVER FOR ORDERING INFORMATION*

## FAX / MAIL ORDER FORM

*(see reverse side for fax number / mailing address)*

| TION | DESCRIPTION | # | UNIT COST (U.S. dollars) | TOTAL |
|---|---|---|---|---|
| 1 | Essentials of Cardiovascular Medicine (ECM) | | **29.95** | |
| 2 | ECM: Shirt-Pocket (Abridged) Edition | | **12.95** | |
| 3 | Book Set (Options 1 + 2) | | **37.90** (save $5) | |
| pping & Handling (see below)<br>es Tax: Michigan residents add 6% | | | | |
| **TAL AMOUNT DUE (U.S. FUNDS)** | | | | |

**PING & HANDLING** (all costs are in U.S. dollars; option numbers refer to those d above): **USA:** Option #1 or #3: $4 first book or book set; each additional copy $2; on #2: $2 per book. **Canada/Mexico:** Option #1 or #3: $6 per book or book set; on #2: $2 per book. **All Other:** Option #1: $16 per book; Option #2: $5 per book; on #3: $19 per book set. Prices subject to change.

_ VISA ___ MasterCard ___ Check Enclosed *(U.S. dollars from U.S. bank only)*

rd #:

piration date: Purchase Order #:

ease print
me: ______________________________

dress: ______________________________
clude
one #)

______________________________

______________________________

**MAIL TO:** **PHYSICIANS' PRESS**
555 South Woodward Ave., Suite 908
Birmingham, Michigan 48009 USA

**FAX TO:** **(810) 642-4949**

For discount pricing (more than 20 copies), comments or suggestions, please write. Also check with your local bookstore for availability.

# FAX / MAIL ORDER FORM

***(see reverse side for fax number / mailing address)***

| OPTION | DESCRIPTION | # | UNIT COST (U.S. dollars) | TOTAL |
|---|---|---|---|---|
| 1 | Essentials of Cardiovascular Medicine (ECM) | | **29.95** | |
| 2 | ECM: Shirt-Pocket (Abridged) Edition | | **12.95** | |
| 3 | Book Set (Options 1 + 2) | | **37.90** (save $5) | |
| Shipping & Handling (see below)<br>Sales Tax: Michigan residents add 6% | | | | |
| **TOTAL AMOUNT DUE (U.S. FUNDS)** | | | | |

**IPPING & HANDLING** (all costs are in U.S. dollars; option numbers refer to those ited above): **USA:** Option #1 or #3: $4 first book or book set; each additional copy $2; tion #2: $2 per book. **Canada/Mexico:** Option #1 or #3: $6 per book or book set; tion #2: $2 per book. **All Other:** Option #1: $16 per book; Option #2: $5 per book; tion #3: $19 per book set. Prices subject to change.

__ VISA ___ MasterCard ___ Check Enclosed *(U.S. dollars from U.S. bank only)*

ard #:

xpiration date: Purchase Order #:

lease print
ame: ________________________________

ddress: ________________________________
nclude
none #)

________________________________

________________________________

**MAIL TO:** **PHYSICIANS' PRESS**
555 South Woodward Ave., Suite 908
Birmingham, Michigan 48009 USA

**FAX TO:** **(810) 642-4949**

For discount pricing (more than 20 copies), comments or suggestions, please write. Also check with your local bookstore for availability.

# FAX / MAIL ORDER FORM

*(see reverse side for fax number / mailing address)*

| PTION | DESCRIPTION | # | UNIT COST (U.S. dollars) | TOTAL |
|---|---|---|---|---|
| 1 | Essentials of Cardiovascular Medicine (ECM) | | **29.95** | |
| 2 | ECM: Shirt-Pocket (Abridged) Edition | | **12.95** | |
| 3 | Book Set (Options 1 + 2) | | **37.90** (save $5) | |
| ipping & Handling (see below)<br>les Tax: Michigan residents add 6% | | | | |
| **TAL AMOUNT DUE (U.S. FUNDS)** | | | | |

**PPING & HANDLING** (all costs are in U.S. dollars; option numbers refer to those ed above): **USA:** Option #1 or #3: $4 first book or book set; each additional copy $2; on #2: $2 per book. **Canada/Mexico:** Option #1 or #3: $6 per book or book set; on #2: $2 per book. **All Other:** Option #1: $16 per book; Option #2: $5 per book; on #3: $19 per book set. Prices subject to change.

_ VISA ___ MasterCard ___ Check Enclosed *(U.S. dollars from U.S. bank only)*

ard #:

xpiration date: Purchase Order #:

ease print
ame: ____________________

ddress: ____________________
clude
one #)

____________________

____________________

**MAIL TO:** **PHYSICIANS' PRESS**
555 South Woodward Ave., Suite 908
Birmingham, Michigan 48009 USA

**FAX TO:** **(810) 642-4949**

For discount pricing (more than 20 copies), comments or suggestions, please write. Also check with your local bookstore for availability.

## FAX / MAIL ORDER FORM

*(see reverse side for fax number / mailing address)*

| ͻPTION | DESCRIPTION | # | UNIT COST (U.S. dollars) | TOTAL |
|---|---|---|---|---|
| 1 | Essentials of Cardiovascular Medicine (ECM) | | **29.95** | |
| 2 | ECM: Shirt-Pocket (Abridged) Edition | | **12.95** | |
| 3 | Book Set (Options 1 + 2) | | **37.90** (save $5) | |
| hipping & Handling (see below)<br>ales Tax: Michigan residents add 6% | | | | |
| **ͻTAL AMOUNT DUE (U.S. FUNDS)** | | | | |

**IPPING & HANDLING** (all costs are in U.S. dollars; option numbers refer to those ted above): **USA:** Option #1 or #3: $4 first book or book set; each additional copy $2; ion #2: $2 per book. **Canada/Mexico:** Option #1 or #3: $6 per book or book set; tion #2: $2 per book. **All Other:** Option #1: $16 per book; Option #2: $5 per book; tion #3: $19 per book set. Prices subject to change.

__ VISA ___ MasterCard ___ Check Enclosed *(U.S. dollars from U.S. bank only)*

ard #:

xpiration date: Purchase Order #:

ease print ame: ______________________________

ddress: ______________________________
nclude
one #)

______________________________

______________________________

**MAIL TO:** **PHYSICIANS' PRESS**
555 South Woodward Ave., Suite 908
Birmingham, Michigan 48009 USA

**FAX TO:** **(810) 642-4949**

For discount pricing (more than 20 copies), comments or suggestions, please write. Also check with your local bookstore for availability.